I0759910

DIANE WOLFF

Cooking for Dysphagia

and Other Swallowing Disorders

101 *Delicious Recipes and Techniques for Safe, Easy Eating*

MAYO CLINIC PRESS

With contributions by Karen Sheffler and Theresa Richard.

Please note: Photos throughout this book show garnishes that may or may not be suitable for specific levels of dysphagia. The use of garnishes should be carefully considered for safety. Please visit *https://www.iddsi.org* for more information.

Proceeds from the sale of every book benefit important medical research and education at Mayo Clinic.

To stay informed about Mayo Clinic Press, please subscribe to our free e-newsletter at *MCPress.MayoClinic.org* or follow us on social media. For bulk sales contact Mayo Clinic at *SpecialSalesMayoBooks@mayo.edu.*

MAYO CLINIC PRESS
200 First St. SW
Rochester, MN 55905
MCPress.MayoClinic.org

ISBN: 979-8-88770-391-6 Hardcover
ISBN: 979-8-88770-392-3 eBook

Library of Congress Control Number: 2024057118
Library of Congress Cataloging-in-Publication Data is available upon request.

Printed in China

First printing: 2025

In memory of my mother,
the late great Cathie G.

The biggest complaint I hear from all of them is about boring tasteless food.

HEIDI PINES
Former director Long Term Care, Aetna, after visiting a range of healthcare facilities, from low cost to high cost

If you make it yourself, you know what's in it. It's cheaper, tastes better, and it's healthier.

CHEF WOLFGANG PUCK
on the best reason for cooking at home

Good cooking is no mystery. You don't need years of culinary training, or rare and costly foodstuffs or an encyclopedic knowledge of world cuisines. You need only your own senses. You need good ingredients, too.

ALICE WATERS
Chez Panisse proprietor and founding mother of the California food revolution, in *The Art of Simple Food*

The healing power of food created with love must not be underestimated.

DENISE PICKETT-BERNARD, PHD, RDN, LDN
Integrative and Functional Nutrition Academy, noted chef and nutritionist

Contents

7 **Foreword: The Importance of Nutrition**
Dr. Walter Willett

Part I

9 **Introduction**

12 **What Is a Swallowing Disorder? Coping with Change**
Theresa Richard

- 17 *Common Myths*
- 19 *FAQs When Facing a Diagnosis*

24 **You Have Dysphagia: What's Next?**
Karen Sheffler

- 39 *IDDSI*

Part II

55 **The Puree Kitchen System**

56 **Setting Up the Puree Kitchen**

60 **Batch Cooking Method**

63 **The Pantry and Freezer**

Part III

69 **Before You Start**

- 74 *How to Make a Beautiful Plate Using Piping Techniques*
  Andrew Cullum

76 **Recipes**

- 79 *Soups*
- 89 *Salads*
- 99 *Poultry*
- 110 *Vegetable-Based*
- 120 *Seafood*
- 132 *Meat*
- 154 *Pasta*
- 170 *Vegetable Side Dishes*
- 194 *Whole Grains*
- 203 *Legumes and Pulses*
- 208 *Breakfasts*
- 215 *Smoothies*
- 221 *Desserts*

235 **Acknowledgments**

237 **Resources**

241 **Sources**

245 **About the Author and Contributors**

246 **Index**

250 **Recipes and Ingredients Index**

Foreword

The Importance of Nutrition

DR. WALTER WILLETT
Frederick John Stare Professor of Epidemiology and Nutrition at the Harvard T.H. Chan School of Public Health

The first question an individual must ask in setting up a dysphagia kitchen is this: What are you going to eat?

The answer is simple: lean protein, a variety of fruit and vegetables, good carbohydrates, good fats, low-sodium foods, and low-sugar foods. Missing from this list are junk food and highly processed foods.

The good news is that the choices for healthy eating are under the control of those who have dysphagia, their families, and their caregivers. Nutrition is the most overlooked element of maintaining general good health, a good immune system, and quality of life.

My research on choosing foods with the best types of carbohydrates, fats, and proteins, and on the relative importance of various food groups and supplements, informs *Cooking for Dysphagia and Other Swallowing Disorders.* Diane has built on this research to help anyone facing a diagnosis of dysphagia ensure that they or their loved one is able to maintain and enjoy a healthy eating plan.

Diane has laid out in an easy-to-use fashion how to plan for the transition to a pureed diet, with excellent recipes and helpful techniques that make it easy to get food on the table. She incorporates expert advice from dysphagia experts to help with this transition as well.

Cooking for Dysphagia and Other Swallowing Disorders is an important and useful book for all who are dealing with this condition, and one I highly recommend.

Part I

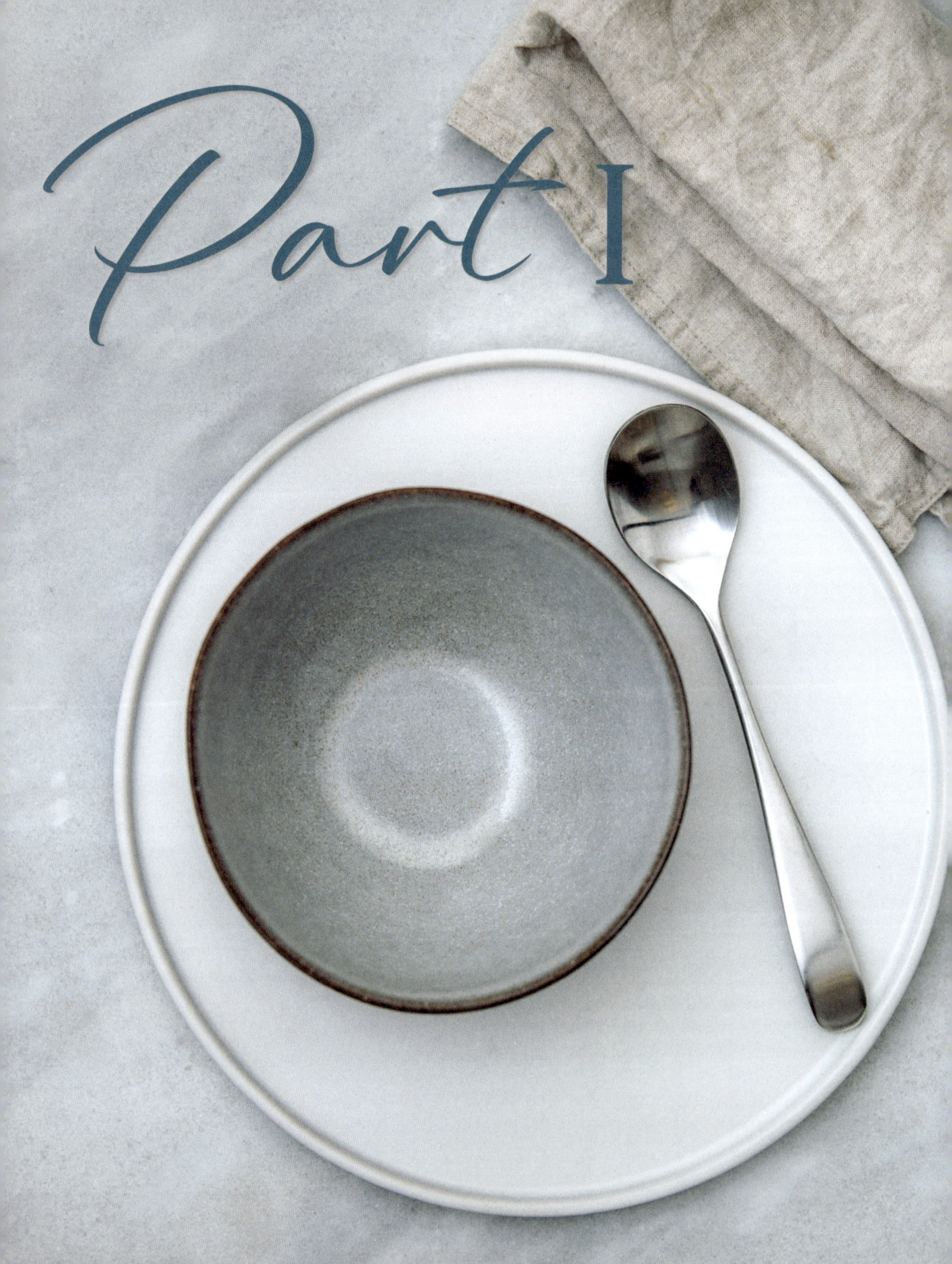

Introduction

I had been cooking for my mom for two years when she was diagnosed with dysphagia, a swallowing disorder, along with the onset of dementia. *Boom!* Once the diagnosis was made, every meal from that point forward had to be pureed, and every beverage, including liquid medicines, needed to be of the prescribed consistency. I had to put food on the table that night. What was I to do? My mother had to eat, or she would lose weight, lose immune function, and decline in health.

The transition to a dysphagia kitchen is a huge adjustment for you or your loved one and the whole family. My sister, a registered nurse, recommended baby food, but baby food is not nutritious enough for an adult. I checked the pharmacy where I bought thickener. The food that was available commercially was canned or vacuum-packed and not appetizing. The labels indicated the meals were not created with nutrition in mind. I am an experienced researcher. I kicked into high gear and began reporting my story. I read everything that was available. I ordered books. I read articles online. I spoke to healthcare professionals. I shopped like a maniac. I could not find a book of practical advice, so you hold in your hands the book I wish I'd had when my mom was diagnosed.

Dysphagia impacts people of all age groups. It develops as a consequence of numerous medical conditions, including neurological conditions related to age, cancer treatment, accidents, and war injuries. It is widespread—fifteen million Americans have a swallowing disorder—and life-threatening. The condition affects a million new people a year, according to the Centers for Disease Control and Prevention. Feeding is basic to life, and a person has to eat or they will die. Additionally, if a person with swallowing difficulties coughs and aspirates their food (that is, if food enters the airway or lungs), they can get bacterial pneumonia, which is life-threatening, difficult to cure, and requires hospitalization.

The diagnosis of dysphagia is an emotional time for both the patient and their family. It involves not only a change in diet but also a change in how food is prepared, stored, and served. You will need to rethink your kitchen setup to include appliances like a food processor. I have given much thought to how to make the process of transitioning to the requirements of this type of cooking and meal-making easy.

From the moment you or your loved one receives a diagnosis of dysphagia, you, your family, and any other caregivers have to rethink the home healthcare situation, as feeding yourself or your loved one becomes all about purees. While this might sound quite simple, it is not. I come from a family of great cooks and have traveled all over the world looking for great food and great stories. So when my mother received the diagnosis of swallowing difficulties, I researched all the available cookbooks, experimented with different brands of commercially available products, and tried out a variety of kitchen tools. I also consulted with many healthcare professionals in different medical fields and found resources for ordering such useful products as thickened water and thickened ice cream. All of this research took time, organization, and testing. Now I have gathered all of this experience and information into this easy-to-use practical guide and recipe book.

The recipes included are both nutritious and delicious. They make use of fresh ingredients and foods like lean proteins, fruits, vegetables, and whole grains. I like to use organic foods when possible, whole foods (meaning foods that have been processed as little as possible), and foods without chemical additives and preservatives. I recommend using the best-quality ingredients you can. Additionally, in putting together these recipes I used the guidelines recommended by the International Dysphagia Diet Standardisation Initiative (IDDSI) and the Healthy Eating Plate of the Harvard T.H. Chan School of Public Health.

Many healthcare professionals have told me that nutrition for the elderly and dysphagia patients is a completely overlooked area. The Covid-19 pandemic focused the nation's attention on senior health because nutrition plays a key role in boosting the immune system, and this in turn helps prevent illness and reduce the need for hospitalization. I realized early on that if my mother was to have a healthy diet, it was up to me. That is how this guidebook came about, and I truly hope it will be of use to all people affected—patients, healthcare professionals, caregivers, and family members who are facing similar challenges.

But this book is more than a collection of recipes and food tips. It is meant to offer a one-stop resource for dysphagia patients and their caregivers. Theresa Richard, a speech-language pathologist, provides an excellent overview of what dysphagia is and how it is diagnosed. She addresses common myths and answers FAQs. Karen Sheffler, also a speech-language pathologist (SLP), and an IDDSI expert, provides essential information about the levels of IDDSI, the testing of food for compliance with IDDSI, and a description of good practices for home healthcare.

Additionally, I take you step-by-step through my system for the setup and organization of a dysphagia kitchen, with planning tips on how to cook on a schedule, how many portions to cook at one time, ideas for batch cooking, how to store food safely, and how to label the stored food so that a great meal is always on hand. I cover the best cooking techniques for food that will be pureed, and how to puree it for the perfect texture for ease of swallowing. I talk about equipment to make pureeing easier, what to have on hand in the freezer and the pantry, and more. These recipes may be enjoyed by family and friends as well as by the patient and caregiver, as I have been reminded by a noted SLP of the importance of social interaction, a component of happiness, during meals. Isolation does not contribute to quality of life.

Ina Garten, author of the Barefoot Contessa cookbooks, says that a cook needs to master ten dishes. So, if you are the person with dysphagia, make a list of your ten favorite dishes. If you are the caregiver, speak to the person with the swallowing disorder to discover their ten dishes. Most have variations. Once you have a list of favorites and variations, this means an end to boredom.

And note that the meal is not only what's on the plate, it's also the atmosphere, the smells and look of the food. Enjoy yourself. Involve the person with the swallowing disorder. Pick flowers and make bouquets. Play music. Have a dance in the kitchen.

Remember these mantras:

Food is medicine, food is love.

Life is too short to eat boring, tasteless food.

Even though the form of the food changes, food can still have the delish factor.

It is better to have a tweaked version of the dish than not to have the dish at all!

Swirl Away!

What Is a Swallowing Disorder?

Coping with Change

THERESA RICHARD, M.A., CCC-SLP, BCS-S,
Founder/CEO of the MedSLP Collective and MedSLP Education, Host of the "Swallow Your Pride" podcast

Swallowing is a task that is completed several hundred times per day, even up to seven hundred times per day, yet it's not often thought of. A swallow is a very complex and coordinated process that involves precise timing and movement of various muscles and structures in the mouth, throat, and esophagus. Its main function is to safely and efficiently transport food and liquid from the mouth to the stomach for the purposes of nutrition and quality of life.

A swallow can be broken down into three phases, but it's important to note that the process of swallowing should be considered a continuum, as each phase can impact the others.

1. **Mouth/oral phase.** This phase is voluntary and involves chewing food and mixing it with saliva to form a cohesive bolus (ball of food). The tongue then propels the bolus toward the back of the mouth and into the throat (pharynx).

2. **Throat/pharyngeal phase.** This phase is triggered without having to think about it when the bolus reaches the back of the tongue and touches the soft palate, the walls of the throat, and the area around the tonsils. A complex sequence of events then occurs in rapid succession: breathing temporarily stops, the muscles and cartilages of the vocal cords close tightly to further protect the airway, and the muscles of the pharynx contract in a wave-like motion (peristalsis) to squeeze the bolus downward and into the esophagus.

3. **Food tube/esophageal phase.** This phase is also involuntary and begins when the bolus enters the esophagus (a muscular tube connecting the throat to the stomach). The esophageal muscles propel the bolus downward toward the stomach.

This entire process occurs in a matter of seconds and requires precise coordination of more than thirty pairs of muscles and multiple cranial nerves that control these muscles. Any disruption in the timing, strength, or coordination of these muscles can result in dysphagia. It's important to note that individuals' anatomies can differ drastically, and although something may seem "disordered" to a professional, it can still be considered "functional" for a person if it is not bothersome to their quality of life.

A swallow is considered "safe" if food and liquid are transferred from the mouth to the stomach without allowing any material to enter the airway or lungs (aspiration). A completely safe swallow every time is not a realistic expectation, as even healthy individuals occasionally aspirate small amounts of food or liquid without any negative consequences. However, frequent or significant aspiration can lead to serious complications such as pneumonia, malnutrition, and dehydration.

Coughing during or after swallowing is a common sign that the body is trying to protect the airway from aspiration. When sensory receptors in the larynx (or voice box) detect foreign material, they trigger a cough reflex to forcefully expel the material out of the airway. In this sense, a cough can be seen as a positive indication that the body's protective mechanisms are functioning properly.

However, if coughing during or after swallowing occurs frequently, it may be a sign of an underlying swallowing problem that needs further evaluation. In addition to coughing, these signs and symptoms may include choking during or after meals, a wet or gurgly voice during or after eating or drinking, feeling like food or liquid is "going down the wrong pipe," a sensation of food getting stuck in the throat, pain during swallowing, or recurrent pneumonia. If any of these symptoms are present, it is important to seek an evaluation by a speech-language pathologist (SLP) who specializes in swallowing disorders.

Sometimes the SLP may determine that your cough is simply your body protecting itself. However, a cough can be downright annoying and bothersome, and it can impact your quality of life if it happens frequently. In this case, it is still important to speak to an SLP about possible cough management solutions.

It is important to note that not all individuals with dysphagia will cough when aspirating. In some cases, the sensory receptors in the larynx/voice box may be impaired, leading to "silent aspiration," in which material enters the lungs without triggering a cough reflex. This is particularly concerning because the aspiration can go undetected and lead to serious complications over time. An instrumental swallowing evaluation can identify silent aspiration and guide appropriate management strategies. If your SLP concludes that your swallowing problems are potentially serious, they will ask you to undergo a more formal evaluation and dysphagia assessment.

Dysphagia Assessment

Dysphagia is usually assessed using a combination of clinical and instrumental evaluations. The specific tests used will depend on your symptoms, medical history, and overall health status.

The first step in assessing dysphagia is typically a clinical swallowing evaluation (CSE), which is performed by an SLP. The CSE will include a thorough review of your medical history, current symptoms, and medications that may impact swallowing. An oral peripheral exam or cranial nerve exam may be performed to assess the strength and coordination of the muscles of the mouth, tongue, and cheeks, and to evaluate the function of the nerves that control swallowing. An SLP may also observe you swallowing different textures of food and liquid to assess swallowing efficiency and determine which textures are safe for you. SLPs may also administer swallowing-related quality-of-life questionnaires or patient-reported outcome measures (PROMs) to gain insight on the impact of the dysphagia from your perspective.

Based on the findings of the CSE, the SLP may recommend further instrumental testing (using specialized technology and equipment) to assess the safety and efficiency of the swallow and directly visualize the swallowing process. A videofluoroscopic swallow study (VFSS), also known as a modified barium swallow study (MBSS), involves having you swallow various textures of food and liquid mixed with barium while a series of X-ray images is taken (barium is a radiopaque contrast agent that shows up on X-rays). The SLP and radiologist analyze the images to assess the timing and coordination of swallowing, identify any structural abnormalities, and determine if aspiration is occurring. The study provides a comprehensive view of all phases of swallowing (oral, pharyngeal, and esophageal) and can help guide treatment recommendations.

Another common instrumental test used to assess swallowing function is the fiberoptic endoscopic evaluation of swallowing (FEES). It involves a thin, flexible endoscope being passed through the nose and into the throat to directly visualize the pharynx and larynx during swallowing. FEES allows for assessment of the throat phase of swallowing, including laryngeal closure, muscle coordination, and presence of residue (food stuck in the mouth, throat, and/or esophagus) or aspiration.

It is important to advocate for a thorough and comprehensive evaluation to accurately diagnose and assess the nature and severity of dysphagia. If you have concerns about the tests being recommended or the results of the evaluation, don't hesitate to ask questions and seek a second opinion if needed. The results of these various tests are then used to diagnose the specific type and severity of dysphagia and guide personalized treatment recommendations (more on this in the next chapter). The SLP will work closely with you, your family, and other members of your healthcare team to develop a comprehensive management plan that addresses the physical, nutritional, and psychosocial aspects of dysphagia. Regular follow-up assessments are important to monitor progress and adjust the treatment plan as needed to ensure optimal outcomes.

The Emotional Impact of Dysphagia

The emotional impact of a dysphagia diagnosis can be profound. A diagnosis of dysphagia can have far-reaching effects on your physical health, emotional well-being, and social functioning. It can also significantly impact the lives of caregivers and family members, who may need to take on additional responsibilities and adapt to new routines.

Fear and anxiety around mealtimes due to the risk of choking or aspiration are common. Difficulty participating in social activities that involve eating and drinking, such as family meals, dining out, or attending parties and events, can be challenging. Relationships may become strained if family and friends do not understand the challenges and limitations imposed by dysphagia. You may feel embarrassed or self-conscious about eating and drinking in front of others, leading to social isolation and withdrawal.

Stigma and misunderstanding from others who may not be familiar with dysphagia and its effects can further compound these social difficulties. The loss of enjoyment and pleasure associated with eating and drinking, which can be a significant source of quality of life for many individuals, can be particularly difficult to cope with. Frustration, anger, or depression related to the loss of independence and control over a basic life function may also occur.

Caregivers may experience stress and burden as they take on additional responsibilities and devote more time to meal planning, preparation, assistance with feeding, and monitoring. The emotional stress and burden related to managing a loved one's nutrition, hydration, and safety needs can be significant. Balancing caregiving responsibilities with work, family, and personal obligations can be challenging. There is also a potential for caregiver burnout and physical strain, particularly if the loved one requires significant assistance with positioning and feeding.

If you are experiencing social and emotional difficulties with a diagnosis of dysphagia, it is very important for

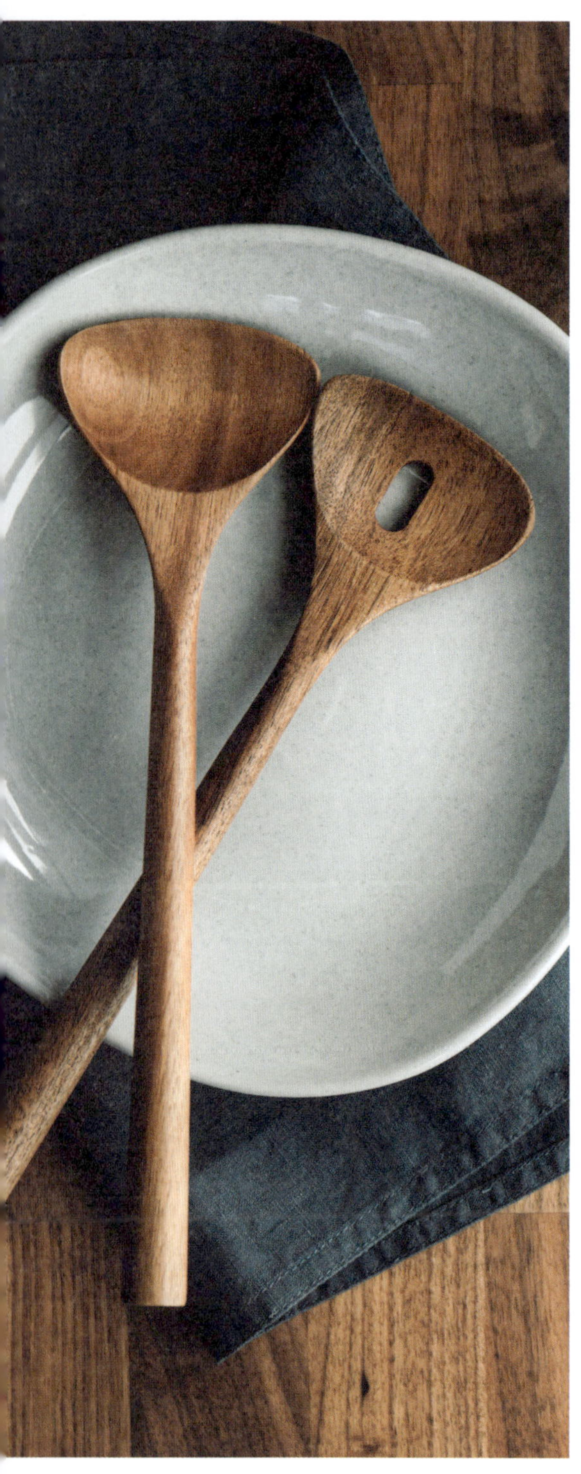

you to discuss your feelings with your SLP. The SLP can recommend psychologists or social workers who can assist you with taking a holistic approach to dysphagia management that addresses not only the physical aspects of swallowing but also the emotional, social, and financial impacts on you and your family.

This approach may involve:

- Providing education and counseling to help you and your caregivers understand the diagnosis and adapt to new routines and strategies for managing dysphagia.
- Offering support groups or peer mentoring programs to connect you and your caregivers with others who have similar experiences and challenges.
- Assisting with navigating insurance coverage and identifying community resources and support services to help alleviate financial burdens.

By taking a comprehensive, person-centered approach to dysphagia management, which prioritizes the individual's comfort and safety, healthcare professionals can help you and your family adapt to the challenges of living with dysphagia and maintain the highest possible quality of life.

Common Myths

There are several common myths and misconceptions about dysphagia that can lead to misunderstandings about the condition and its management. Here are some of the top myths and the facts to counter them:

MYTH 1

Thickened liquids are always safer for individuals with dysphagia.

FACT: While thickened liquids can be beneficial for some individuals with dysphagia, they are not always the safest or most appropriate choice. The decision to use thickened liquids should be based on a thorough swallowing evaluation and the specific needs and goals of the individual.

In some cases, thickened liquids may actually increase the risk of aspiration or other complications. Additionally, some individuals may find thickened liquids unpalatable or may have difficulty meeting their hydration needs with thickened liquids alone.

In other cases, individuals may prefer to continue using thickener. This shared decision-making should be made with the SLP.

MYTH 2

The chin tuck technique should be used by everyone with dysphagia.

FACT: The chin tuck is a commonly used postural technique that involves tucking the chin down toward the chest while swallowing. It can be helpful for some individuals with dysphagia by protecting the airway and reducing the risk of aspiration. The effectiveness of the chin tuck depends on the specific nature and severity of the individual's swallowing impairment. In some cases, the chin tuck may actually make swallowing more difficult or less efficient. Through an instrumental evaluation, the SLP will identify if the chin tuck is likely to be effective for you.

MYTH 3

There is nothing that can be done to improve swallowing function in individuals with dysphagia.

FACT: While dysphagia can be a challenging and persistent condition, there are many strategies and interventions that can help improve swallowing function and quality of life.

The specific approach will depend on the underlying cause and severity of the dysphagia, as well as the individual's goals and preferences. Some common interventions include:

- Swallowing exercises and therapy techniques to strengthen the muscles of the mouth and throat and improve coordination and timing of swallowing.
- Postural adjustments to protect the airway and facilitate safe swallowing.
- Diet modifications to alter the texture, consistency, or volume of foods and liquids to make them easier and safer to swallow.
- Neuromuscular electrical stimulation (NMES) to stimulate the muscles of the throat and improve swallowing function.
- Biofeedback techniques to help individuals visualize and control their swallowing movements.
- Surgical interventions to correct anatomical abnormalities or improve swallowing function in specific cases.

MYTH 4

Feeding tubes are always a last resort and indicate a poor prognosis.

FACT: Feeding tubes can be a valuable tool for managing dysphagia and ensuring adequate nutrition and hydration in some individuals. The decision to use a feeding tube should be based on a careful assessment of the individual's nutritional status, swallowing abilities, overall health, and goals of care.

In some cases, a feeding tube may be used as a temporary measure to support nutrition and hydration while the individual participates in swallowing therapy and works toward resuming oral eating. In other cases, a feeding tube may be a long-term solution for individuals who are unable to meet their nutritional needs safely or efficiently through oral intake alone.

It is important to recognize that the use of a feeding tube does not necessarily indicate a poor prognosis or quality of life. Many individuals with feeding tubes are able to maintain active and fulfilling lives with proper support and management. The key is to approach the decision to use a feeding tube as part of a comprehensive, person-centered care plan that prioritizes, as noted above, the individual's comfort, safety, and quality of life.

FAQs When Facing a Diagnosis

When facing a diagnosis of dysphagia, you and your family may have many questions and concerns. Here are some of the most frequently asked questions and some guidance on how to advocate for person-centered care.

1 What caused my dysphagia and is it treatable?

Dysphagia can result from a variety of conditions, including neurological disorders, muscular disorders, structural abnormalities, and other medical conditions. The specific cause of dysphagia will determine the most appropriate treatment approach. Some causes of dysphagia may be reversible with treatment, while others may require ongoing management to minimize complications and maintain quality of life. It is important to work with a healthcare team to identify the underlying cause of your dysphagia and develop an individualized treatment plan.

2 Will I need to change my diet, and how will I meet my nutritional needs?

If you have dysphagia, you may need to modify your diet to ensure safe and efficient swallowing and to maintain adequate nutrition and hydration. The specific diet modifications recommended will depend on your swallowing abilities and risks, as determined by the swallowing evaluation. Some common diet modifications include:

- Altering the texture of foods to make them easier to chew and swallow (e.g., pureeing, chopping, or softening foods).
- Thickening liquids to slow their flow and reduce the risk of aspiration.
- Limiting or avoiding foods that are difficult to chew or swallow (e.g., hard, crunchy, or stringy foods).
- Using special techniques or strategies to facilitate safe swallowing (e.g., chin tuck, multiple swallows, alternating bites of food with sips of liquid).

It is important to work with an SLP and a registered dietitian to develop an individualized meal plan that meets your nutritional needs while minimizing the risk of complications. If you have concerns about the taste, texture, or variety of the recommended diet, let your healthcare team know so that they can help you find solutions that work for you.

3 What are the risks and complications of dysphagia?

Dysphagia can lead to a variety of complications if not properly managed, including:

- **Aspiration pneumonia.** A lung infection that occurs when food, liquid, or saliva enters the lungs.
- **Malnutrition.** Insufficient intake of nutrients due to difficulty swallowing or avoidance of certain foods.
- **Dehydration.** Insufficient intake of fluids due to difficulty swallowing or avoidance of liquids.
- **Choking.** A blockage of the airway by food or other objects.
- **Social isolation.** Avoidance of social situations involving eating or drinking due to embarrassment or fear of choking.

It is important to work with your healthcare team to minimize the risks and complications of dysphagia through proper evaluation, treatment, and management.

If you experience any signs or symptoms of complications, such as coughing or choking during meals, unexplained weight loss, or recurrent respiratory infections, let your healthcare team know right away.

4 How can I continue to enjoy meals and social situations with dysphagia?

Eating and drinking are important social and cultural activities that can be challenging for individuals with dysphagia. However, there are many strategies and adaptations that can help you continue to enjoy meals and participate in social situations:

- **Plan ahead.** Call ahead to restaurants to inquire about their menu options and their ability to accommodate special diets or requests.
- **Bring your own food.** If you are going to a social event where the food options may be limited or unsuitable for your needs, consider bringing your own food or snacks that you know you can eat safely.
- **Use adaptive equipment.** Special utensils, cups, and plates can make it easier to eat and drink independently and safely.
- **Take your time.** Don't feel rushed to finish your meal or keep up with others. Take your time and focus on eating and drinking safely and comfortably.
- **Communicate your needs.** Let your dining companions know about your dysphagia and any special accommodations you may need. Most people will be understanding and willing to help.

- **Focus on the social aspect.** Remember that meals are about more than just the food. Enjoy the conversation, company, and atmosphere, even if you are not able to eat or drink as much as you would like.

5 How can I advocate for myself and ensure I receive person-centered care?

Advocating for yourself and ensuring that you receive person-centered care is essential for individuals with dysphagia. Here are some tips for being an effective self-advocate:

- **Educate yourself.** Learn as much as you can about your dysphagia, its causes, and its management. This will help you ask informed questions and participate actively in your care.
- **Communicate your needs and preferences.** Let your healthcare team know what is important to you, what you are willing and not willing to do, and what you hope to achieve through treatment.
- **Ask questions.** If you don't understand something or have concerns about your care, speak up and ask for clarification or additional information.
- **Bring a support person.** Consider bringing a trusted family member or friend to your appointments to help you take notes, ask questions, and advocate for your needs.
- **Know your rights.** Familiarize yourself with your rights as a patient, including the right to informed consent, the right to refuse treatment, and the right to a second opinion.
- **Be persistent.** If you feel that your needs are not being met or that your concerns are not being addressed, don't hesitate to speak up and advocate for yourself.
- **Seek support.** Connect with other individuals and families affected by dysphagia through support groups, online forums, or advocacy organizations. These connections can provide valuable information, support, and resources.

Remember, you are the expert on your own experiences, needs, and preferences. Your healthcare team should work collaboratively with you to develop a care plan that is tailored to your individual goals and priorities.

6 How can I ensure I receive appropriate care in a healthcare facility?

If you have dysphagia and are in a healthcare facility, such as a hospital or nursing home, it is important to advocate for appropriate care and management. Here are some tips:

- **Inform the staff.** Make sure that all members of the healthcare team, including doctors, nurses, and therapists, are aware of the dysphagia diagnosis and any special needs or accommodations required.
- **Provide documentation.** Bring copies of any relevant medical records, test results, or treatment plans to the facility and make sure they are included in your chart.
- **Request a swallowing evaluation.** If a swallowing evaluation has not been done recently or if there have been changes in your swallowing function, request a new evaluation by an SLP.
- **Review the care plan.** Ask to see your care plan and make sure that it includes appropriate interventions and accommodations for dysphagia, such as diet modifications, feeding assistance, and oral care.
- **Monitor for complications.** Be vigilant for signs of complications, such as coughing or choking during meals, weight loss, or signs of aspiration pneumonia (fever, chills, night sweats), and report them to the healthcare team immediately.
- **Advocate for person-centered care.** Remind the healthcare team of your personal preferences, goals, and values, and make sure that the care plan is aligned with these priorities.
- **Escalate concerns.** If you feel that your needs are not being met or that their care is not appropriate, don't hesitate to escalate your concerns to a supervisor, patient advocate, or ombudsman.

Remember, healthcare facilities have a responsibility to provide safe, appropriate, and person-centered care to all individuals, including those with dysphagia. By advocating for yourself and working collaboratively with the healthcare team, you can help ensure that you receive the care and support you need.

7 Where can I find more information and support?

There are many resources available for individuals and families affected by dysphagia. Some good places to start include the American Speech-Language-Hearing Association (ASHA), the National Foundation of Swallowing Disorders (NFOSD), the Dysphagia Research Society (DRS), and local hospitals, rehabilitation centers, or universities. There are also many online communities and forums where individuals with dysphagia and their caregivers can connect with others, share experiences and advice, and find support. See the list of resources at the end of this book.

Remember, you are not alone on this journey. There is a wealth of information, support, and resources available to help you navigate the challenges of living with dysphagia.

8 What should I do if I suspect someone I know has dysphagia?

If you suspect that someone you know may have dysphagia, it is important to encourage them to seek evaluation and treatment from a qualified healthcare professional. Here are some steps you can take:

- **Share your concerns.** Talk to the person about what you have observed and why you are concerned. Be gentle, nonjudgmental, and supportive.
- **Encourage them to see a doctor.** Suggest that they make an appointment with their primary care physician to discuss their symptoms and get a referral to an SLP or other specialist if needed.
- **Offer to help.** Offer to accompany them to their appointment, take notes, or help them prepare questions to ask their doctor.
- **Provide information.** Share reliable information about dysphagia and its management with the person and their family, but avoid giving medical advice or making diagnoses.
- **Be supportive.** Let the person know that you are there to support them and that there are resources and treatments available to help them manage their dysphagia.

Dysphagia is a serious condition that can have significant impacts on a person's health, nutrition, and quality of life. Early identification and intervention are key to preventing complications and maintaining optimal function. By being proactive and supportive, you can help ensure that your loved one gets the care and support they need.

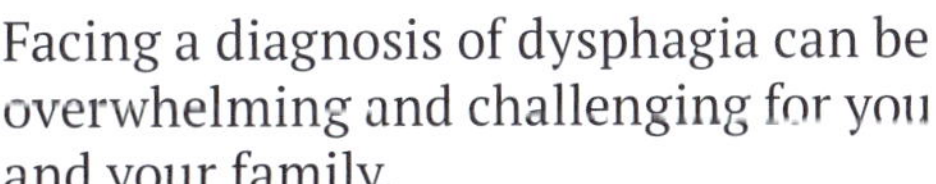

Facing a diagnosis of dysphagia can be overwhelming and challenging for you and your family.

However, by being informed, proactive, and advocating for person-centered care, you can work with your healthcare team to develop an individualized management plan that addresses your unique needs, preferences, and goals.

Remember, there is no one-size-fits-all approach to dysphagia management, and what works for one person may not work for another. The key is to stay informed, communicate openly with your healthcare team, and advocate for the care and support you need to maintain your health, safety, and quality of life.

You Have Dysphagia

What's Next?

KAREN SHEFFLER, M.S., CCC-SLP, BCS-S
Founder/Editor of SwallowStudy.com
and SwallowStudy & Associates, LLC

You have been given the diagnosis of *dysphagia (*difficulty swallowing). What does that mean for you? This may mean a transition to a new form of eating. Hopefully, you have medical guidance, and now you will need practical advice for the home healthcare environment. The principles in this book for the dysphagia kitchen may be applied in a healthcare facility. The content in this chapter will also help you advocate for yourself or your loved one.

Your primary care physician has created a healthcare team to gather more information about you and your dysphagia in order to devise a treatment plan for you. As part of this information gathering, a speech-language pathologist (SLP) will assess your swallowing capability.

Instrumental evaluations, as discussed in the prior chapter, are two types of swallowing tests by an SLP that use specialized technology and equipment. One is the videofluoroscopic swallow study (VFSS), also known as a modified barium swallow study (MBSS), and is an X-ray that is like a video or movie of your swallow. The other test, a fiberoptic endoscopic evaluation of swallowing (FEES), uses a thin endoscope inserted through the nose and into the throat to see the swallow.

Based on the problems found in testing by your SLP, and/or recommendations from your medical team, you may be referred to other specialists. For example, difficulty swallowing often happens across more than one phase of the swallowing process. You may have problems in multiple phases at the same time. *Oropharyngeal dysphagia* is when swallowing problems happen in both the mouth and throat phases.

Pharyngoesophageal dysphagia is when there are problems in the throat/pharynx and esophagus. Problems in different phases may require input from different specialists.

The following are some of the specialists who work closely with SLPs:

- An ear, nose, and throat (ENT) doctor, also called an otolaryngologist, can make sure that your voice box (larynx), which houses your vocal cords, is working well for airway protection and swallowing safely. The ENT also addresses issues with the upper esophageal sphincter, which allows material into the top of the esophagus.
- A gastroenterologist (GI) is a doctor who specializes in the entire digestive system and manages swallowing and eating issues of the esophagus and stomach.
- A neurologist evaluates and treats issues of the nervous system that may cause problems in sensation or motor movements related to eating and swallowing. A neurologist also collaborates with an SLP to evaluate thinking skills (cognition), memory, problem-solving, and attention, which can greatly impact the safety of your swallow.
- A psychiatrist addresses issues of medications for mental health that may cause difficulty swallowing, and treats any anxiety, depression, fear of swallowing, or food aversion issues that may impact your eating.
- A pharmacist may check to see if any of your medications are causing trouble swallowing, are causing dry mouth, or are making your reflux worse, for example.
- A registered dietitian nutritionist (RDN) helps you make sure you are getting enough nutrition and hydration (eating and drinking enough). They make recommendations about tube feedings if you are not getting all your nutrition by mouth or give you options for oral supplements.

After the examinations, make sure you understand all the findings. Did your care team explain clearly what happened and what you can do about it? What procedures and/or surgeries may help? Ask more questions if needed. It often helps to watch videos of your swallowing evaluation and review anatomy pictures with the specialists.

What Happened in the Swallowing Evaluations?

The swallowing evaluation tells you more than whether you *aspirated* (i.e., food, liquid, or pills went into your airway or lungs) or not. It is a motion picture of what is happening when you swallow.

What worked and did not work? What part of your eating/swallowing has problems? How can those problems be addressed? What are the risks to your health and quality of life?

SLPs consider swallowing problems from two different perspectives: safety and efficiency.

Safety (Severity of Aspiration Risk)

If you aspirate, you may respond by coughing or clearing your throat. However, sometimes things go down the wrong way and you do not feel it or show any obvious signs at all. That is called *silent aspiration*, which can be very concerning for you or for your caregiver at home. Silent aspiration is common in people who have reduced sensation due to dementia, Parkinson's disease, or radiation after head and neck cancer, for example. This further highlights the need for instrumental evaluations of swallowing.

Efficiency (Amount of Residue and Choking Risk)

The evaluation may also find that food, liquids, or pills are getting stuck in the mouth, throat, and/or esophagus. That is called *residue.* Residue could go down the wrong way after you eat. Also, if too much residue builds up in your throat, you could be at risk for choking.[1]

MORE ABOUT ASPIRATION

Aspiration can sometimes lead to a lung infection called pneumonia. However, it is not a simple path from aspiration to pneumonia. Not all people who have aspiration will get sick with pneumonia. A bacterial lung infection, called aspiration pneumonia, usually happens more often in someone who has poor mouth hygiene, with a lot of bacteria buildup in the mouth and around the teeth.

Other risk factors that make pneumonia more common include: dependence on another person for feeding, being bedridden, frequent aspiration in large amounts, reduced immune system response, and smoking. Discuss your own risk factors with your team.

See the end of this chapter for more about oral hygiene and prevention of aspiration pneumonia.

1 Choking is when food (or a nonfood object like a marble) drops into the top of the voice box (larynx) and blocks the airway. This prevents you from breathing. People who are able to do so may signal that they can't breathe with hands up to their throat and seek help immediately. The Heimlich maneuver, to clear the airway in an awake person, can be done by a trained person. Your CPR training will teach how to give chest compressions once the person who is choking becomes unresponsive. If you typically eat alone, ask your medical team to give you other options, as recommending suitable ones is beyond the scope of this book.

Dysphagia Treatment

What Can You Do About Your Dysphagia?

Once all the information is gathered from your thorough dysphagia evaluation, your healthcare team can develop a treatment plan.

Your SLP will teach you ways to reduce your risks of aspiration and residue. The SLP clinician will talk with you about your goals and preferences, share recommendations, and discuss options that you could try, such as the following:

1. **See other specialists.** The SLP will often suggest that you talk to other members of your healthcare team to see what they recommend. Sometimes these healthcare providers can suggest certain procedures, surgeries, medications, or other methods to help you swallow better and maintain good nutrition and hydration. It is important to follow up on those suggestions.
   - Registered dietitian nutritionists can make sure that you are taking in enough calories and liquids.
   - Physical therapists can help improve posture, body and neck strength, and positioning. They can give exercises to strengthen the body overall.
   - Occupational therapists can give ideas on how to feed yourself easily and with less effort, so that you can avoid getting tired quickly.
   - Ear, nose, and throat doctors may suggest procedures to improve your vocal cord closure (to protect your airway better) or to loosen a tight upper esophageal sphincter. They can test for and treat reflux, especially when the reflux is getting up high into your throat and may be giving you the sense that you have a lump in your throat.
   - Gastroenterologists can look directly at the esophagus to see if there is a narrowing that can be stretched. They can also test the muscles of the esophagus (a test called esophageal manometry) to see if they are squeezing in a good and coordinated way to clear the food into the stomach.

2. **Rehabilitation.** An SLP who specializes in swallowing can customize a set of exercises. These may vary greatly from person to person, as the SLP can develop specific plans to improve the timing, coordination, and strength of all the muscles involved in chewing and swallowing. Exercises must be targeted to the specific problems you are having with your swallow. In other words, if the problem is that the back of the tongue is not adequately pushing the food down, then the exercises may be intended to improve the effort of that push; however, if your problem is in the esophagus, tongue exercises may do you no good. Some exercises have the goal of improving your ability to cough and clear material that may go down the wrong way. You must have a full evaluation, including instrumental

evaluations, to target therapy to your needs. Specific exercise details are beyond the scope of this book.

3. **Strategies to compensate for dysphagia.** Compensatory strategies change how you eat and drink in order to make it easier and potentially safer to swallow. Examples include:
   - Safer[2] swallowing strategies.
   - Mealtime and environment changes.
   - Head or body positioning to make it easier to swallow.
   - Food and liquid texture changes (i.e., diet modifications).
4. **Infection control and prevention of aspiration pneumonia.** Some examples include:
   - Keeping your mouth and teeth very clean to reduce your risk of aspiration pneumonia. Aspiration cannot be prevented 100 percent of the time, despite all the safer swallowing strategies used. However, the goal is twofold: to reduce aspiration *and* to reduce the risk of getting sick with aspiration pneumonia. Good oral hygiene helps with the second goal.
   - Staying active and exercising to help the lungs become stronger and better able to clear out small amounts of aspiration.

The specific set of recommendations that you will be given is your treatment plan. Your treatment plan will be crafted with you to address your own goals, preferences, and wishes. Your healthcare providers may offer you referrals and rehabilitation methods to improve your swallow, but this book will not go into detail on those items.

Dysphagia Management at Home and in Healthcare Facilities

All of the following information applies whether you are at home or advocating for your care at any healthcare facility.

Simple Solutions

This book aims to give you simple solutions for your home. These focus on strategies to compensate for dysphagia and reduce risks of choking and

2 The term *safer* is used to describe swallowing strategies, as there is typically not one set of strategies that is perfect and will prevent all risks 100 percent of the time. Strategies are meant to reduce risks as much as possible; therefore, there may be no one "safest" option. A treatment plan needs to be customized for you. There is certainly no one-size-fits-all method that works for everyone—that point cannot be stressed enough. Please review with your medical team all the options that apply to you.

aspiration. While this book cannot recommend all the specifics of what is best for you, we can introduce the ideas of *safer* swallowing strategies and infection prevention.

If you understand the ideas and options better, you will be better able to review them with your specialists so that you can be active in crafting your treatment plan. This is person-centered care.

Before we get to some specific safer swallowing strategies, we need to cover person-centered care and your decision-making around your own eating and swallowing.

Person-Centered Care and Decision-Making

With all the information provided to you by your medical team, you are considering the options and *what may be right for you*. You are the center of your medical team. You are the driver of the team.

Person-centered care is certainly *not* the doctors telling you what they think is best for you. However, medical decision-making can be quite complex, and you may need help. The best decisions for you are based not only on all the facts and data but also on your goals, preferences, lifestyle, and wishes for yourself. Healthcare providers should see you not as a patient but as a whole person, who may come with a support circle that includes family members, friends, and other caregivers. When a person is no longer able to make their own decisions, they will have an appointed healthcare proxy to carry out their previously stated wishes.

Before this chapter dives into ways to change the texture and thickness (viscosity) of foods and liquids, it's important to say again that every person should discuss all options with their medical team. Ask yourself these questions:

- What is right for me and the goals I have for myself?
- Do I understand what is wrong at each phase of my swallow—mouth (oral), throat (pharyngeal), and tube to stomach (esophageal)?
- Do I need to learn more about what has worked and what has not worked?
- Do I need any more testing?
- Do I understand all my options and the risks and benefits (or pluses and minuses) for me?
- What other questions do I still have?

Treatment Plan for Safer Swallowing

Now that you and your care providers have the information you need, we will cover how to compensate for the dysphagia (including information about standardized diets for dysphagia), environmental changes you can make, tips for holidays and travel, and prevention of further issues. Part II of this book details changes you may want to make to your kitchen and food preparation, and Part III provides more than one hundred recipes.

Compensatory Strategies to Manage Dysphagia

The idea of *compensation* means that, instead of making the problem go away, you are working around it with some strategies. Swallowing strategies may have you eat and drink a little differently to make doing so easier and potentially safer. Of course, many people do not want to change what they are eating; everyone has their own preferences and habits. Therefore, these are options for you to consider when making decisions about your treatment plan.

Safer Swallowing Strategies

Right after the evaluation, the SLP may provide you with customized options to make eating and swallowing easier, such as by:

- Making sure you are eating in a good upright posture with any positioning supports that you may need. Typically, sitting up at a 90-degree angle is recommended, but sometimes your instrumental evaluation will suggest other positions (e.g., side-lying) to use as you eat and swallow.

- Changing *how* you eat and drink. These may include the following head positions (warning: do not try any of these before you have an instrumental evaluation by your SLP clinician, as some positions could make the problem much worse):
  - › Chin tuck
  - › Head turn
  - › Head turn and tuck down to the shoulder
  - › Head tilt
  - › Side-lying position or reclined position

  Your SLP may also recommend any of the following safer swallowing strategies:
  - › Slow down the rate of eating or drinking.
  - › Try to chew up your food better.
  - › Avoid distractions and talking with food in your mouth or before swallowing.
  - › Take smaller bites or sips (but sometimes taking larger bites/sips is found to be the best approach; ask your SLP).
  - › Take a sip of liquid after every few bites of food to help wash food residue through your throat and through the tube (esophagus) to your stomach.
  - › Use an effortful swallow, pushing harder with your tongue and squeezing with your throat muscles.
  - › Before attempting a swallow, bear down and hold your breath (this closes the vocal cords tightly), then sip and swallow, and finally release the breath with a cough and dry swallow. This method protects the top of the airway before you take the sip. The cough ejects any drops of liquid that

may have entered into the top of the airway during the swallow. This is called the *super supraglottic swallow* strategy (we share that mouthful of a name so that you can really impress your SLP).
  - Have small but more frequent meals and snacks (for example, six small meals a day instead of three larger meals).

- Changing how you take your pills, as the process of swallowing whole pills with thin liquid is one of the riskiest swallowing tasks. Try taking them one at a time with a sip of water. If that is too challenging, swallow pills in a pill-swallow gel (such as Gloup, formerly known as Phazix; see Resources, page 239). Talk with your pharmacist about food-drug interactions if you have been embedding pills in applesauce or dairy-based purees. Do not crush your pills unless you have cleared that with your pharmacist. You cannot put crushed pills in a thickened liquid or add thickener to any liquid medication.

- Making sure you are feeding yourself as much as possible, with assistance and cueing as needed. People who are completely dependent on another person for feeding can have a higher risk of aspiration and aspiration pneumonia. Your SLP and occupational therapist may provide you with further guidance on feeding.

It is important to note again that many of these strategies need to be trialed first with instrumental evaluations (using X-ray or endoscope) to see if they actually work. Both of these types of examinations can trial liquids, solids, and pills while you are doing specific postures, head maneuvers, and other strategies. Some strategies, such as the chin tuck (taking a sip of liquid, holding it in the mouth, tucking the chin, and then swallowing with the chin tucked), can actually make the swallow worse for some people, causing the liquid to go down the wrong way.

Diet Texture Modification (Diet Framework of IDDSI [International Dysphagia Diet Standardisation Initiative])

Changing the texture of your diet may be an effective compensatory strategy for dysphagia. These techniques include:

- Making sure that foods are soft and easy to chew.

- Reducing the size of food pieces, such as cutting food up into bite-sized pieces that are about the size of your thumbnail, mincing, or blending/pureeing foods).

- Adding sauce or other moisture to foods to make food more slippery.

- Thickening liquids.

- Cooking food with techniques that render it moist and tender, ideal for puree (much more on that in Part II of this book).

One excellent resource is the International Dysphagia Diet Standardisation Initiative (*iddsi.org*), the globally agreed-upon standardized framework for all solids and liquids (ranging from regular foods and regular liquids through dysphagia diets and thickened liquids), as well as detailed definitions and testing methods.

Please see the IDDSI Framework and IDDSI tutorial at the end of this chapter, starting on page 39.

Environmental Strategies to Manage Dysphagia

Now that we have talked about how and what you are eating and drinking, let's think about the environment around you. *Where* you are eating is important for the success of your meals.

For many people challenged by dysphagia, swallowing difficulties are accompanied by other difficulties that can impact your mealtime or social eating setting: hearing loss, impaired vision, difficulty attending in the presence of background noise, reduced memory, and reduced problem-solving ability or safety awareness.

Some of these may be especially the case for people with head injuries, stroke, dementia, or Alzheimer's disease. The following tips can be applied at home or in any eating situation.

Reduce Distractions and Supervise as Needed

- Make sure to turn off the TV or lower the volume on background music.
- Monitor the loudness, distractions, and conversations at mealtime or around the family dinner table. Find out what level is too much, causing difficulty in attention and concentration. You may need to make changes so that mealtime is quiet and free of distractions.
- Reduce the amount of food and drink items that are in front of you if you have difficulty with distractions. One plate, one utensil, and one cup may be enough.
- Small meals and/or small portions may be best, especially when at a large social event.
- Think about seating arrangements around the table, placing one or two people next to you who could provide subtle help and cues as needed.
- Request supervision as needed to keep you on task and doing your safer swallowing strategies (such as not eating too fast).

Lighting and Visuals

- Make sure to have good lighting in your dining area.

- Use plates that provide a good visual contrast between the plate and the food (e.g., solid white plate with darker-colored food).

Humidification

- Add humidifiers if dry mouth is a major issue at mealtime.
- Make sure your mouth is clean and moist prior to eating. If you have dry mouth, bring your artificial saliva substitute spray bottle. Spray, swish, and swallow before your meal to lubricate your swallowing pipes, and to better enjoy your meal.

Tips for Holidays and Travel

Managing dysphagia at home can be difficult and time-consuming at any time, but around the holidays it can be even tougher. You may be traveling away from home, joining large gatherings where food options may be limited, or spending time with family or friends who may not be as familiar with your eating/swallowing needs. In addition to the environmental considerations above, here are some more tips.

Enjoy Many Holiday Foods That Are Already Pureed

- Many foods commonly found at the table on North American holidays, like mashed squash, mashed potatoes, and smooth cranberry sauce, are already pureed.
- Pumpkin pie is mostly a pureed food. Rather than using a typical flour crust, search for a recipe with a graham cracker crust. Pulverized graham crackers are held together with loads of butter, making the whole pie smooth and moist.

Add Moisture to Make Foods Slippery

- Traveling can make dry mouth worse, as you are out of your routine and airplane travel will certainly exacerbate the problem.
- Holiday meals may be particularly difficult in colder environments with heat on, as that dries out the room.
- Adding gravies and sauces to purees and other soft foods gives a delicious flavor punch while making them moist and slippery for easier swallowing.
- As foods cool down, they will tend to become stickier. Watch out for mashed potatoes, as they can be quite thick and sticky. Add butter, gravy, and sour cream. Heat up foods as needed.
- A heart-healthier option is olive oil. You can find many delicious flavored olive oils (such as basil, rosemary, thyme, or other herbs and spices) that complement food beautifully. Many people with dysphagia find that olive oil really does the trick to make foods more slippery and prevent them from

getting stuck. Travel with a small sealable bottle.

Thickened Liquids on the Go

- Bring thickener packets (made by thickener companies) or your thickener in a sealable container. Don't forget your IDDSI Funnel or 10 mL syringe for the IDDSI Flow Test.
  - Bring your own teaspoon or tablespoon measuring device so that you can add your thickener without having to ask your host. Being prepared ahead of time helps you be discreet and focus on the fun of the holidays rather than all the technical issues.
- Bring your own thickened liquids in resealable bottles (follow thickener instructions, as each product is different and each liquid thickens differently).
  - Resealable bottles will allow you to prepare your liquids ahead of time or add thickener packets to any liquid just before serving. Just shake before serving to make sure the thickener powder or gel is still mixed in well. Then pour your beverage into a nice glass on the table. That makes it easy for your hosts to meet your thickened liquid needs.
- Check all soups and special drinks to make sure they are the appropriate thickness.
  - Eggnog will likely pass an IDDSI Flow Test as a Mildly Thick liquid (Level 2), but double-check with your 10 mL syringe or IDDSI Funnel.
  - If your host is serving a soup that has solids in a clear, thin broth, that is a mixed consistency, which may be harder to manage. Soups can be easily blended to a smooth and thick consistency by using a portable blender. There are small blenders that are easy to travel with (e.g., Magic Bullet). Potatoes will naturally thicken a soup when blended, or you may have to add a little thickening agent to your final product to meet your prescribed thickened liquid level.

Infection Control and Aspiration Pneumonia Prevention

As discussed above, we cannot prevent aspiration 100 percent of the time. Food, liquids, pills, saliva, or even refluxed stomach contents sometimes go down the wrong way. Aspiration can cause a lung infection, called aspiration pneumonia. Not all people who aspirate will get aspiration pneumonia; therefore, let's consider what puts someoneat a higher risk for getting sick with an aspiration pneumonia. Then maybe you can find ways to lower your own risk.

Risk Factors for Aspiration Pneumonia

As noted earlier in this chapter (in More About Aspiration), there is no simple path from aspiration to pneumonia. The development of aspiration pneumonia is more complex. The following outline makes this complex sequence easier to understand. Each step listed below has predictors or factors that increase a person's risk to develop an aspiration pneumonia infection. These predictors of aspiration pneumonia are based on foundational studies by Dr. Susan Langmore and colleagues in 1998 and 2002 (see Sources).

1. **High levels of potentially harmful bacteria in the mouth (pathogenic microorganisms).** Many bacteria colonize the mouth, throat, and stomach. Often when someone is ill and in a healthcare institution, the bacterial environment changes from good bacteria to bad bacteria. The following factors can increase the levels of harmful bacteria that can enter the lungs during aspiration and make a person sick:
   - Dependency on others to keep the mouth, teeth, gums, tongue, and palate clean.
   - Large number of decayed teeth and poor gums.
   - Taking a lot of medications (more than five is called *polypharmacy*). Many types of medications cause dry mouth (*hyposalivation* or *xerostomia*), which can cause poor oral and dental health.
   - Taking medications that reduce the acid in the stomach. This changes the stomach pH, causing it to become more alkaline, which can foster harmful bacterial growth.
   - Tube feeding: The tube feeding formulas can also make the stomach alkaline. People who are tube-fed may not eat anything by mouth (also known as NPO, which is the Latin abbreviation of *nil per os*). Therefore, they are missing the mechanical action of chewing and stripping the food bolus through the mouth and throat that helps to keep these areas clean. The mouth of a person who is NPO tends to have less healthy salivary flow, and the mouth can become coated with a sticky film of bad (pathogenic) bacteria.

2. **Aspiration.** Aspiration, as we have discussed, is when food, liquid, saliva, and/or stomach contents go down the wrong way and into the lungs. The following factors will increase the likelihood that aspiration will occur in significant amounts:
   - Being bedridden. Eating in bed in a poor position increases aspiration risk. Being bedridden also increases the risk of refluxing (bringing up) stomach contents and aspirating them.
   - Tube feeding. In the case of a nasogastric tube or gastrostomy tube (feeding tubes in the nose or directly into the abdomen), the liquid formula is pumped

into the stomach. This may increase your risk of aspirating tube feedings if you have poor positioning, reflux, and reduced airway protection. It is important to discuss formulas, rate, tube feeding scheduling, and positioning needs with your medical team.
   - Delirium or a confused and less alert mental status.
   - Dependency on others to be fed, as the rate of feeding may be too much and too fast.
   - Dysphagia with recommendations for a dysphagia diet or mechanically altered diet (which may indicate that the swallowing problem is more severe).

3. **Poor pulmonary clearance.** When the lungs have difficulty raising up and expectorating aspirated material and secretions, this is called *decreased pulmonary clearance*. The following predictors make it more likely that this aspirated material mixed with bad bacteria will then stay in the lungs:
   - Requires suctioning to clear secretions.
   - Smoking, which harms the lungs' ability to clear out material and prevent infection.
   - Diseases like chronic obstructive pulmonary disease (COPD), congestive heart failure (CHF), and other respiratory problems.
   - Being bedridden. The lungs will have a harder time clearing out aspirated material when a person is in bed and not able to move on their own.

4. **Poor immune system response to resist an infection.** The following predictors contribute to a decreased ability to fight off infection (also called *decreased host resistance, reduced systemic immunologic response,* and *immunosuppression*):
   - Weight loss, generalized weakness, and frailty.
   - Multiple medical diagnoses.

Final Take-Home Prevention Tips

You may not be able to immediately improve all your eating and swallowing challenges. However, you are taking a big step forward. You are reading *Cooking for Dysphagia* to reduce the effort that you have with eating/swallowing, while still enjoying your favorite foods and drinks. That can reduce choking risks, aspiration risks, weight loss, and dehydration/malnutrition risks, while hopefully improving your quality of life.

Finally, here are three key tips that can make a big difference:

1. **Stay active and out of bed as much as possible.**
   - Stay active to help the lungs become stronger and better able to clear out small amounts of aspiration. (Activity is based on recommendations by your medical team, of course.)

- A physical therapist and occupational therapist can provide a safe treatment plan for how to stay active, with exercises for the body and lungs.
- When you strengthen the body overall you can prevent muscle loss and frailty.

2. **Improve your cough.**
   - Coughing clears material out of your airway and out of your lungs. That cough is your secondary line of defense against aspiration pneumonia. You may have some aspiration, but if your lungs are healthy and you have a strong cough, your overall risks are lower.
   - Ask your medical team about ways to evaluate and improve your cough (e.g., pulmonology testing or otolaryngology [ENT] testing to assess whether any vocal cord impairments are weakening the cough).
   - The speech-language pathologist, occupational therapist, and physical therapist can provide cough assist tools or cough strengthening devices to improve your cough.

3. **Keep your mouth very clean.** This helps reduce buildup of the bad (pathogenic) bacteria that can make you sick with aspiration pneumonia.
   - This is sometimes called oral care, but it needs to be more important than a task like combing hair. Good oral hygiene practices should really be called "oral infection control," as keeping the mouth clean can help prevent you from getting sick (i.e., aspiration pneumonia prevention).
   - See a dentist every six months or more frequently based on your needs.
   - Brush your teeth, floss, use a water flosser, and rinse with mouthwash. Get an evaluation by your dentist and ask for training in using these tools. Schedule your next checkup today.
   - Brush your teeth first thing in the morning, after you eat, and before you go to bed at night. Make sure there is no food

In "The 3 Pillars of Aspiration Pneumonia" by John R. Ashford, Ph.D., CCC-SLP (*www.sasspllc.com/three-pillars-of-pneumonia*), Dr. Ashford identifies three factors that lead to someone getting sick with aspiration pneumonia:

1. **Aspiration** (saliva, liquids, and/or food particles going down the wrong way, into the lungs).
2. Bad **bacteria** in the mouth.
3. Weakened immune response and **frailty**.

pocketed in your cheeks or stuck around your mouth.

- If you wear dentures or partial plates, it is important to remove them after meals to brush away food that is stuck around them. Soak them at night according to your dentist's instructions.
- Mouthwash. Avoid mouth rinses with alcohol. If you have good control in your mouth, you can rinse with a mouthwash that is a thin liquid. Hang your head over the sink, swish, and spit out. Do not swallow the mouthwash. If you have difficulty keeping the liquid controlled in your mouth, dip your mouth sponge or toothbrush in the mouthwash and sweep it around your mouth and scrub your tongue. Spit out all excess. Have a home suction machine available as needed. There are products that you can purchase for safer brushing and rinsing actions, including suction toothbrushes and suction swabs. Do not add thickener to mouthwash.
- After thorough mouth cleaning, use an oral moisturizer that protects your teeth and gums. There are several artificial saliva substitutes on the market (similar to artificial tears for dry eye). You can get these in a gel, mouth spray, or oral-adhering wafer. The mouth spray bottles are so convenient to carry with you throughout the day and when traveling. Keep one at the bedside for overnight dryness that may disturb your sleep. You can spray, swish, and swallow these products.
- Also, clean your mouth before you eat, especially if you have dry mouth, which increases the risk for bad bacteria buildup. Brushing will stimulate saliva flow. Use the oral moisturizer to "lubricate your pipes" before eating.

This information has been provided to supplement and support the information you have received from your full medical team. All this dysphagia content can be helpful as you navigate your healthcare, from the hospital through the rehabilitation and skilled nursing settings. It may also help your caregivers and loved ones become strong advocates for you. Then, hopefully, the rest of this book will provide a bridge from healthcare to home, as you create your dysphagia kitchen and return to enjoying your favorite foods and drinks.

For further information and reading, see Resources (starting on page 237) and Sources (starting on page 241).

IDDSI

The International Dysphagia Diet Standardisation Initiative

The International Dysphagia Diet Standardisation Initiative (IDDSI) was formed in 2013 as a volunteer-run initiative with scientists, researchers, and clinicians from around the world collaborating to create a new globally standardized diet framework and testing methods, because standardization fosters patient safety. See *iddsi.org* for the latest version of the IDDSI Framework, detailed definitions of each of the IDDSI levels, and the IDDSI testing methods. Please refer to the IDDSI website for all its resources, including patient/caregiver handouts. This chapter is meant to be an educational summary only.

IDDSI Framework

The world has agreed on how to categorize, label, describe, and test all foods and liquids with regard to eating, chewing, and swallowing. All foods and liquids have been assigned to a level based on standardized testing procedures, and the levels are easily identifiable by name, color, and number, as in the diagram on page 41.

The IDDSI standards mean that healthcare providers and consumers can finally speak the same language. A standardized system makes it possible for people around the world to order, prepare, and serve similar textures of food and consistency of liquids for people with dysphagia.

In the image, you can see that the categorization of foods ranges from Regular solids (Level 7) through the "dysphagia diets" of Easy to Chew (Level 7), Soft & Bite-Sized (Level 6), Minced & Moist (Level 5), Pureed (Level 4), and Liquidised (Level 3). The drinks move up from thin liquids like water (Level 0) to thicker and thicker liquids, all the way up to Level 4 (Extremely Thick), which would have to be consumed using a spoon. The category of *transitional foods* includes foods that change from one texture to another (such as popsicles) or dissolve in the mouth (such as teething wafers).

IDDSI Testing Methods

The IDDSI testing methods are used to make sure a specific food is right for you. The focus is on testing individual foods and liquids, rather than giving you a list of what to eat and what not to eat. You can use IDDSI testing methods to test any food across any culture. For example, imagine how a ripe banana is much softer than one that is still green; therefore, we cannot simply say that all bananas are "soft." IDDSI likes to remind users: "When in doubt, test it out."

IDDSI provides simple food-testing methods that can be done in any kitchen with common tools: fingers, spoons, forks, and/or chopsticks. In this chapter we focus on testing methods that utilize forks and spoons; however, information about adapting testing methods for use with chopsticks and fingers can be found on *iddsi.org* and IDDSI's YouTube channel (*youtube.com/@iddsi2903*).

Testing helps us avoid vague terms such as "bite-sized," "cut-up," "soft," "easy to chew," and "smooth and moist" that could be interpreted in different ways by different people.

These concepts are defined with the IDDSI testing methods (summarized on pages 42–48). For example, we know that if we use testing methods for Soft & Bite-Sized, Level 6 (such as the Fork Pressure Test for "soft" and particle-size measurements for bite-sized), we can significantly reduce choking risks. A piece of soft food that is cut into a cube roughly the size of an adult's thumbnail (1.5 cm on each side) is smaller than your airway. Therefore, that bite of food will most likely fall through your adult airway without blocking the airway and making it difficult or even impossible to breathe. That will reduce the risk of death from choking. See *iddsi.org* for pediatric bite-size requirements.

IDDSI Progress

IDDSI has already been implemented in many places across the United States, as multiple professional organizations supported the IDDSI implementation and rollout in May 2019. Some countries have benefited from faster IDDSI adoption due to smaller size and governmental mandates.

When all healthcare facilities adopt this standardized framework, there will be less confusion when a person goes from the hospital to a rehabilitation facility to home. The hospital should provide a diet order at discharge that uses the same naming system as the skilled nursing facility or the visiting nurse association that is admitting the person. That allows for clear and standardized communications and trainings.

However, facilities in your area may be at different stages in the implementation of IDDSI. While you can certainly advocate for IDDSI implementation in your local healthcare facilities, you can also learn and use IDDSI standards for food and drink preparation at home. All the recipes in Part III of this book use the IDDSI standards. IDDSI aims to improve patient safety everywhere.

IDDSI and Person-Centered Care

IDDSI does not tell you what you are "allowed to eat" or "not allowed to eat." Rather, IDDSI will promote better person-centered care, as it provides a set of standardized labels and descriptions to allow for clear communication among healthcare providers and the people they serve. Good communication helps people understand their options and make better healthcare decisions.

The IDDSI Framework

Providing a common terminology for describing food textures and drink thicknesses to improve safety for individuals with swallowing difficulties

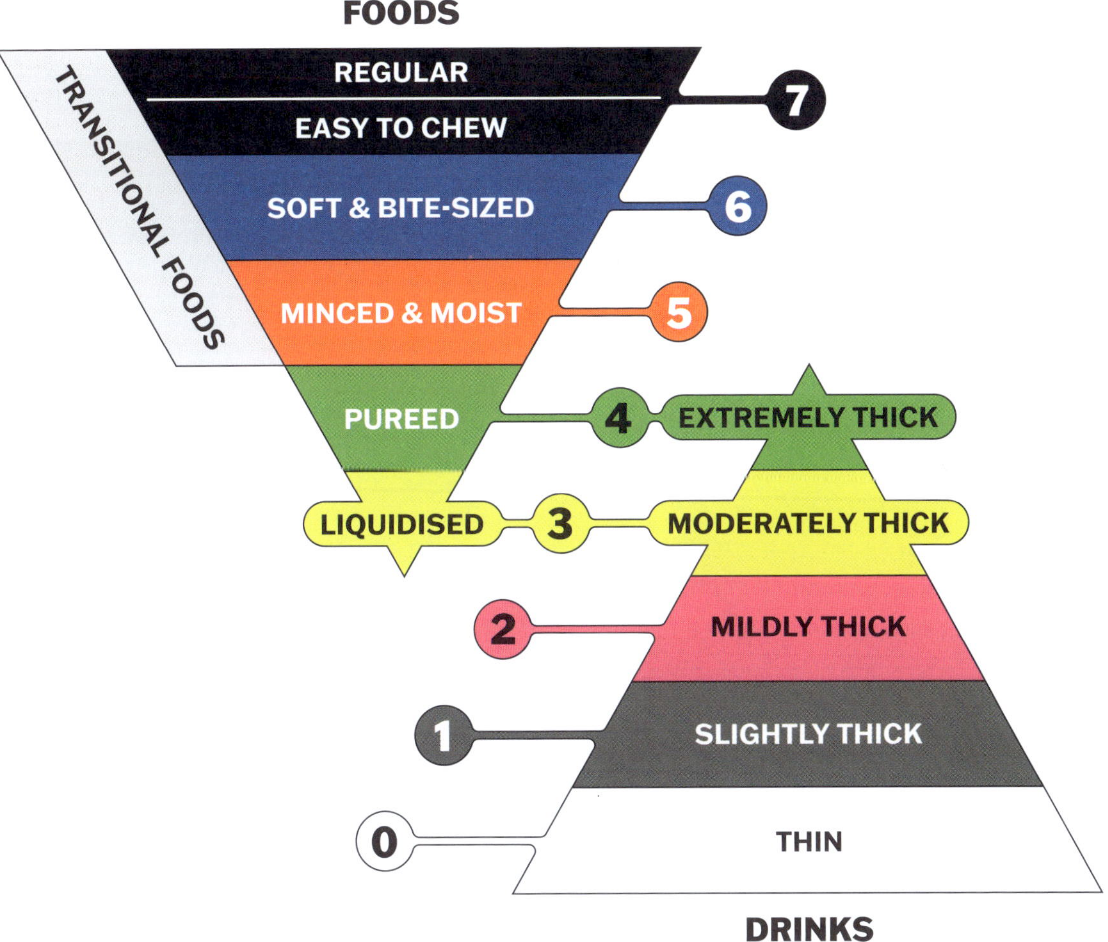

This diet framework is for all ages and all settings. The IDDSI Framework is being translated into many different languages.

IDDSI Levels and IDDSI Testing: Summary Chart

The following chart summarizes IDDSI levels, descriptions, reasons for this texture (rationales), and testing methods. For complete information, please refer to the IDDSI website's "Standards" tab for the following documents: "IDDSI Framework and Detailed Definitions" and "IDDSI Testing Methods" (available at *iddsi.org/*).

For more details on IDDSI testing methods for the home and for healthcare facilities, see page 50.

IDDSI LEVELS AND TESTING SUMMARY CHART	
SOLIDS	**DESCRIPTION**
REGULAR, LEVEL 7	• All regular foods. • No restrictions.
EASY TO CHEW, LEVEL 7	• Soft, tender foods. • Food pieces and bite sizes are not restricted. Does not reduce risk for choking. • Avoids hard, dry, crumbly, tough, chewy, stringy, fibrous foods; foods with gristle, seeds, husks, or bones. • May have mixed-consistency (e.g., liquid and solid in same bite) and soft breads per clinical testing and decision-making. **Examples:** Salmon, lasagna
SOFT & BITE-SIZED, LEVEL 6	• Soft, tender, and moist foods. • Mashable with fork pressure. • Reduce choking risks: Cut food into bite-sized pieces no bigger than 1.5 cm x 1.5 cm x 1.5 cm (for adults) or 8 mm x 8 mm x 8 mm (for children). • No mixed-consistency foods (e.g., thin liquid separating from the food). • Avoid bread because of choking risks. Per clinical testing and decision-making, soft bread products may be included as exceptions. **Examples:** Small pasta or cut-up pasta with well-cooked bite-sized pieces of vegetables, meatballs, or tender pieces of chicken. Made moist and cohesive with a smooth sauce.

WARNING: The IDDSI Framework is a "living document"; it may go through revisions after publication of this book. Please always refer to *iddsi.org* for the most up-to-date information.

WHY THIS TEXTURE?	HOW TO TEST?
No difficulty chewing or swallowing; no decision-making needed to continue with regular diet.	IDDSI Testing Methods are not needed for this level.
Some difficulty chewing harder foods. May get tired or have pain when chewing. Dry mouth or new dental problems. No significant choking or dysphagia risks, but may favor softer foods if recovering from illness.	**TEST SOFTNESS WITH:** • **Fork Separation Test:** Food breaks apart easily wlth side of fork. • **Fork Pressure Test:** Press fork into food with enough pressure so that the thumbnail lightens. Food mashes and does not return to original shape or stick to fork.
Cannot bite off pieces of food, but is able to chew when food is soft. May have difficulty chewing and forming ball if food is harder, drier, or in a larger amount. Can chew and manage when food is softer, moister, and in a small bite size. Make sure to add sauces or gravy, especially if dry mouth is a problem. The bite-sized limitation reduces choking risks, as that size will fall through the airway rather than block the airway. May eat too fast or take impulsive large bites. May need supervision.	**TEST SOFTNESS WITH:** • **Fork Pressure Test:** Press fork into food with enough pressure so that the thumbnail lightens. Food mashes and does not return to original shape or stick to fork. **TEST BITE SIZE WITH:** • **Metric ruler:** No more than 1.5 cm x 1.5 cm x 1.5 cm pieces for adults; no more than 8 mm x 8 mm x 8 mm pieces for children. › **Estimate:** Use adult thumbnail for adults and child pinky nail for children as rough estimate of bite-sized.

IDDSI LEVELS AND TESTING SUMMARY CHART

SOLIDS	DESCRIPTION
MINCED & MOIST, LEVEL 5	• Soft, minced, moist, and cohesive. • Can be scooped and shaped into a ball, but no separate liquid. • Very small pieces of food, no bigger than 4 mm × 4 mm × 15 mm. This is the size of food that has been chewed and is swallow-ready. • Food has some texture with small lumps that can be squashed with the tongue. • Must add moisture into recipes and add sauce or gravy. • Food should not separate into individual dry pieces when cooked and served. • No dry crumbles. • No challenging textures, such as mixed consistencies or bread. **Examples:** Risotto with sauce, lentil stew, scoop of tuna fish salad without raw vegetables.
PUREED, LEVEL 4	• Blended smooth, with no lumps and minimal granules. • Does not require chewing. • Holds its shape on a spoon. Sits in a mound on a fork with no liquid dripping through the tines of the fork. • Not sticky (puree can still be a choking risk if too sticky). **Examples:** Pureed squash; mashed potatoes with enough butter, gravy, or sour cream to make sure the texture is smooth and moist.
LIQUID-ISED, LEVEL 3	• Blend or liquefy in blender until smooth-liquidy puree. • Cannot be eaten with fork. Best to use spoon or cup. • Thinned-out, liquidy puree has moderately thick texture with no lumps. • Does not hold shape on fork. Drips slowly through tines. **Examples:** Tomato soup or any liquefied soup without chunks; cream of wheat or cream of rice cereal.

WHY THIS TEXTURE?	HOW TO TEST?
Significant difficulty chewing. Minced pieces require minimal chewing. Significant pain, fatigue, and dental problems with chewing. *Be careful with this texture, as minced pieces can dry out easily if no sauce/gravy is mixed directly into the food. Moisture needs to be added to the recipe; cannot just add gravy to the top when serving food. Presents a risk of inhaling dry, crumbly pieces, especially if dry mouth is a problem.*	**TEST MINCED PIECES OR LUMPS WITH:** • **Metric ruler:** No more than 4 mm x 4 mm x 15 mm for adults; 2 mm x 2 mm x 8 mm for children. › Lumps will fit between tines of dinner fork. **TEST SOFTNESS WITH:** • **Fork Pressure Test:** Use a little pressure from fork (thumbnail should *not* lighten). Pieces squash and come through tines of fork. **TEST STICKINESS WITH:** • **Spoon Tilt Test:** Spoonful slides off spoon when tilted but will hold shape on fork. **TEST FOR LIQUID SEPARATING WITH:** • **Fork Drip Test:** Scoop food into a mound on fork. No or minimal liquid drips through tines.
Unable to bite or chew; AND/OR Significant pain and fatigue with effort of chewing and preparing food in mouth to swallow. Tongue strength and control are very reduced. Puree needs less tongue effort and control to move it to the back of mouth (versus Levels 5-7). May be at risk for food sticking and/or choking on non-pureed foods. High aspiration risk with dry food particles. If dry mouth is a problem, add extra moisture to food to prevent sticking around mouth and throat.	**TEST SOFTNESS AND SMOOTHNESS WITH:** • **Fork Pressure Test:** Use minimal pressure from fork (thumbnail should *not* lighten). No lumps seen. Fork makes clear markings on food. **TEST STICKINESS WITH:** • **Spoon Tilt Test:** Food holds shape on spoon. Easily plops or slides off spoon when spoon is tilted, with very little food left on spoon. **TEST FOR LIQUID SEPARATING WITH:** • **Fork Drip Test:** Scoop food onto fork and make sure no or minimal liquid drips through tines.
Unable to chew. Pureed foods are still too thick and may get stuck. May have minimal tongue/mouth movement or strength to form ball of food and push it to back of mouth. May have missing structures in mouth due to surgery (e.g., removal of part of tongue [glossectomy]). Will require liquid smoothies/liquid supplements.	**TEST FOR LIQUID SEPARATING WITH:** • **Fork Drip Test:** Scoop food onto fork and make sure liquid drips through tines slowly, in strands or dollops. **TEST LIQUID THICKNESS:** • **IDDSI Flow Test:** Liquid flows through a 10 mL syringe, leaving 8 to 10 mL in the syringe after 10 seconds.

IDDSI LEVELS AND TESTING SUMMARY CHART

LIQUIDS	DESCRIPTION
EXTREMELY THICK LIQUID, LEVEL 4	• Drink from spoon. • Smooth texture. • Has same thickness properties as Pureed food, but is a drink/liquid thickened with thickener products. **Example:** Some thick sauces. *Note: The words* drink *and* liquid *are used interchangeably.*
MODERATELY THICK LIQUID, LEVEL 3	• Drink from spoon or cup. • Effort needed to sip from a wide-bore straw. • Spoon will stand up in full cup. • Flows off spoon slowly. • Flows even slower than Mildly Thick liquid. • Has the same thickness properties as Liquidised food, but is a drink/liquid thickened with thickener products, instead of food that is liquefied in a blender. **Example:** Smoothie made in blender with banana and yogurt to thicken.
MILDLY THICK LIQUID, LEVEL 2	• Drink from spoon, cup, or standard straw. • Mild effort to sip from standard straw. • Flows at a slower rate than Thin or Slightly Thick liquid. • Some nutrition supplements may be labeled as Mildly Thick, but they need to be tested with Flow Test. **Examples:** Some fruit nectars, some nutrition supplements.

WHY THIS TEXTURE?	HOW TO TEST?
Rarely recommended or ordered. Long-term use could cause severe dehydration risks. If testing shows no thinner liquid is safe, the person is often still on intravenous liquids, or receives tube feedings via a thin tube through the nose or via feeding tube surgically placed to the stomach.	**TEST LIQUID THICKNESS:** • Too thick to use the IDDSI Flow Test. • **Spoon Tilt Test:** Spoonful plops or slides off spoon when spoon is tilted, with very little food left on spoon. • **Fork Drip Test:** Scoop liquid onto fork and make sure minimal liquid drips through tines.
Significantly reduced tongue control and/or other swallowing problems. Needs Moderately Thick liquid to allow more time to control liquid and move it to back of mouth. Reduced safety of swallow and aspiration risk present with Thin, Slightly Thick, and Mildly Thick liquids. May be used as a last resort when no strategies work to make thinner liquids safer. *Be careful with this level of thickness. Thicker is not always better. This moderate amount of thickness needs more tongue and throat effort than thinner liquids. Could get stuck in mouth, throat, esophagus. Have swallow testing done before use.* *CAUTION: High risk for dehydration if not drinking enough liquid.*	**TEST LIQUID THICKNESS:** • **Fork Drip Test:** Scoop liquid onto fork and make sure liquid drips slowly in dollops through the tines of the fork. • **IDDSI Flow Test:** Liquid flows through 10 mL syringe, leaving 8 to 10 mL in syringe after 10 seconds.* **It is also important to test liquid medications and supplements.*
Mildly reduced tongue control and/or other swallowing problems. Needs Mildly Thick liquid to allow more time to control liquid and move it to back of mouth for swallow (versus Thin or Slightly Thick liquid). Reduced safety of swallow and aspiration risk present with Thin and Slightly Thick liquids, even when using safer swallowing strategies.	**TEST LIQUID THICKNESS:** • **IDDSI Flow Test:** Liquid flows through a 10 mL syringe, leaving 4 to 8 mL in the syringe after 10 seconds.* **It is also important to test liquid medications and supplements.*

IDDSI LEVELS AND TESTING SUMMARY CHART

LIQUIDS	DESCRIPTION
SLIGHTLY THICK LIQUID, LEVEL 1	• Drink from spoon, cup, or standard straw. Still flows through a teat/nipple. • Flows at slower rate than Thin liquid. • Slight effort needed to sip from standard straw. **Examples:** Some fruit nectars; tomato juice; some nutrition supplements; breast milk; infant formula. *Note: Nutritional supplement brands and other products may vary greatly. They need to be tested with the Flow Test.*
THIN LIQUID, LEVEL 0	• Drink from spoon, cup, or standard straw. • This is a regular liquid with fast flow. Flows like water. • Flows quickly, needing good control, speed, and airway protection. **Examples:** Any water; juice; milk; tea; coffee; etc.

WHY THIS TEXTURE?	HOW TO TEST?
Slightly reduced tongue control and/or other swallowing problems. Needs a Slightly Thick liquid to allow a little more time to control liquid and move it to back of mouth for swallow (versus a thin liquid). Reduced safety of swallow and aspiration risk present with thin liquids. Based on testing results, maybe just a very small amount of additional thickness is enough to reduce aspiration risk (thicker is not always better). Slightly Thick liquid may provide a solution to meet hydration needs and quality-of-life wishes while still reducing aspiration risks.	**TEST LIQUID THICKNESS:** • **IDDSI Flow Test:** Liquid flows through 10 mL syringe, leaving 1 to 4 mL in syringe after 10 seconds.* **It is also important to test liquid medications and supplements.*
No difficulty swallowing and protecting airway with or without safer swallowing strategies; *OR* After discussing options, wishes, risks, and benefits with team, a decision is made to continue with Thin liquids.	**TEST LIQUID THICKNESS:** • **IDDSI Flow Test:** Liquid flows through 10 mL syringe in 6.5 to 7.2 seconds.* **Testing a Thin liquid like water is a good way to make sure your syringe or IDDSI funnel is working properly.*

This chart is a summary by this author to help visually categorize all the IDDSI levels and introduce the formal IDDSI Testing Methods. It is based on 2019 IDDSI documents. Please refer to iddsi.org, *www.iddsi.org/standards/framework,* for complete details and up-to-date information.

For more details on IDDSI testing methods for the home and for healthcare facilities, see page 50.

Using IDDSI Testing Methods in Your Kitchen

Make sure you understand the IDDSI testing methods listed in the chart. This section will cover four key tests, but for all IDDSI testing methods, please see: *www.iddsi.org/standards/testing-methods*. You will be using these in your kitchen as you prepare and serve foods. The first two tests listed below are great for solids. The last two tests are for all kinds of liquids, soups, and sauces.

IDDSI Fork Pressure Test

This is a favorite test. It is so clear and useful because it defines "soft" food. Here are the steps:

1. Use a standard dinner fork (metal is better than plastic). If no fork is available, you can use a spoon, chopstick, or finger.

2. Put a piece of food on the plate. (When testing for Level 6, Soft & Bite-Sized, use a piece no bigger than 1.5 cm x 1.5 cm x 1.5 cm.)

3. Hold the fork with your thumb pressing into the bowl of the fork (just above the tines and below the handle).

4. Use the amount of pressure needed to make your thumbnail lighten. (That is the amount of pressure we use with our tongue to push food down with the swallow.)

RESULT: The food should squash or mash and not return to its original shape. You may see fork marks in the food. That means that the food is "soft" and passes the Fork Pressure Test. It should not stick to the fork.

PRO TIPS | Fork Pressure Test

- This test measures softness. But you can really reduce choking risks in adults by also cutting food into bite-sized pieces no bigger than 1.5 cm × 1.5 cm (roughly the size of an average adult thumbnail).

- If you are using this test for Level 4 (Pureed) or Level 5 (Minced & Moist), your thumbnail should not lighten. The food is softer and should be able to be mashed without much pressure.

IDDSI Spoon Tilt Test

This is an important test for making sure your pureed food is smooth and moist. Imagine a sticky mashed potato, especially when it gets cold. You could throw it at the wall, and it will stick! You don't want pureed foods to stick to the tongue, the roof of the mouth, or the throat. This simple test with a spoon (or fingers) will help. This test is also used for Level 4 (Extremely Thick liquid) and Level 5 (Minced & Moist). Here are the steps:

1. Scoop up a full spoonful on a spoon.

2. Check to see if the food holds its shape on the spoon. We call that

moist and cohesive, meaning that the food holds together in a mound. You do not want a sticky, dry, or crumbly texture.

3. Tilt or turn the spoon sideways. You may use a gentle flick of the wrist.

RESULT: Food slides or plops off the spoon. Only a thin film or coating of food is left on the spoon. That is a pass for the Spoon Tilt Test. You do not want a lot of food still stuck on the spoon. If the puree is stuck to the spoon, it could also stick in the mouth and throat.

PRO TIPS | Spoon Tilt Test

- If testing for Level 5 (Minced & Moist), the result should be a moist and cohesive mound that slides off the spoon. There are no separate dry crumbles. It is important to avoid dry, crumbly food textures that could get stuck in the mouth or even go down the wrong way.
- If the food sample did not pass the Spoon Tilt Test, change the recipe and/or add more sauce, gravy, or condiments to make sure the food is smooth and moist all throughout. It should be slippery enough to slide off a spoon.

IDDSI Fork Drip Test

The IDDSI Fork Drip Test measures how quickly thicker liquids flow through the tines of a fork. Level 3 foods and liquids (Liquidised foods and Moderately Thick liquids) drip slowly through the tines in dollops or strands. By contrast, Level 4 foods and liquids (Pureed foods and Extremely Thick liquids) sit in a mound on the fork with very little poking through the tines (maybe a little pokes or peeks through, but it does not drip or flow). This is a great test when making sauces, gravies, and soups at a Moderately Thick level. You can make sure it is fully liquidized and does not have lumps or chunks. This can also be useful to make sure thin liquid is not separating out of a sample of Level 4 food (Pureed) or Level 5 food (Minced & Moist). Here are the steps:

1. Scoop a sample onto a standard dinner fork.

2. Check to see if it sits in a mound on the fork. Level 4 foods and liquids (Pureed foods and Extremely Thick liquids) will mound, but Level 3 foods and liquids (Liquidised foods and Moderately Thick liquids) will not form a mound on top of the fork.

3. Hold the fork up to your eye level to look under the fork.

RESULTS: Level 4 foods and liquids (Pureed foods and Extremely Thick liquids) will only poke or peek through the tines of the fork, with no dripping. Level 3 foods and liquids (Liquidised foods and Moderately Thick liquids) will only slowly flow or drip in dollops or strands through the tines of the fork; they will not flow continuously like a thinner liquid.

IDDSI Flow Test

The IDDSI Flow Test uses a standard 10 mL syringe (measuring 61.5 mm from the 0 line to the 10 mL line), which can be found in any health-care facility in the United States. Alternatively, you could use a special IDDSI Funnel that is conveniently marked with each liquid level (*iddsi.org/resources/funnels*). The test measures how much liquid flows through a syringe or IDDSI Funnel in 10 seconds.

Here are the key points to remember:

- It is so important to measure the thickness of the liquid you are drinking to make sure it matches the level you were recommended (based on your evaluations).
- Test the liquid after making it and before taking it. Liquids thickened with powder thickener products may thicken up more over time.
- There are other uses for this flow test besides just for the liquids that you drink. Don't forget to test liquid medications too, as you do not want to aspirate a liquid medication! Sauces, gravies, and smoothies/supplements can also be tested with this flow test.

IDDSI Flow Test Instructions:

1. If using a syringe, remove the plunger. If using an IDDSI Funnel, there is no inner plunger.
2. Hold the syringe or IDDSI Funnel upright in one hand with thumb and index finger.
3. Cover the opening at the bottom of the syringe/funnel with another finger on the same hand (usually pinky finger or ring finger).
4. Hold the cup of liquid in your other hand and pour liquid into the syringe or funnel up to the 10 mL mark on the syringe or the fill line on the IDDSI funnel.
5. Remove finger from the bottom opening at the same time as you start a stopwatch with the other hand.
6. After exactly 10 seconds, return finger to bottom opening, stopping the liquid flow.

RESULT: How much liquid remains in the syringe or IDDSI funnel after 10 seconds of flow?

Slightly Thick, Level 1	=	1 to 4 mL
Mildly Thick, Level 2	=	4 to 8 mL
Moderately Thick, Level 3	=	8 to 10 mL

You cannot test for Level 4 (Pureed foods and Extremely Thick liquids) with this IDDSI Flow Test. Use the Spoon Tilt Test instead.

PRO TIPS | Flow Test

- You don't want a result that falls right on the boundary between two levels—1 mL, 4 mL, 8 mL, or 10 mL. For example, if you want a Mildly Thick (Level 2) liquid, thicken up the liquid a little bit if the Flow Test result is exactly 4 mL. You want the amount remaining after 10 seconds to be between 4 mL and 8 mL, not a borderline result.
- If you need Mildly Thick (Level 2) liquids, then your sauce, gravy, broth, and liquid medications should also be at that level, not Thin liquid (Level 0).
- Keep in mind that thicker is not always better. If you are trying to moisten thick and sticky pureed potatoes with an Extremely Thick (Level 4) gravy, that may not work—the puree will not become moist enough. You may only need to thicken your gravy to Mildly Thick (Level 2). When you mix that into the already sticky pureed potatoes, that will thin out the puree, producing a slippery, moist, and smooth puree.

Thickener Variability

The IDDSI Flow Test is extra important due to the variability in thickener products on the market. Premade packaged thickened liquid products can vary greatly from one company to another and from one type of liquid to another. For example, the container may claim that the product is Mildly Thick (Level 2), but the IDDSI Flow Test may reveal that the label is not so accurate.

Also, when you thicken liquids with powders or gels, the result can vary depending on the type of liquid. For example, orange juice tends to thicken faster and need less thickener added than other juices. Also, liquids can continue thickening up over time—you may think your liquid is too thin, but when it sits for a few minutes, it may thicken more.

Thick liquids also change based on temperature. When a liquid is cold, it is thicker than when that same liquid is at room temperature or hot. So, if you prepare a cold juice to a Mildly Thick level, it may thin down to a Slightly Thick level as it warms up.

The type of thickening agent you use will produce varying results, too. If you use cornstarch-based or modified-food-starch-based thickener powders, the liquid can thin down too much when it combines with your saliva. Xanthan gum or other gum-based clear thickener powders and gels are preferable and recommended because they are the most stable, mix clear in the liquid, and have a better mouthfeel. Cornstarch-based or modified-food-starch-based thickener powders can feel very gritty in the mouth and make the drink cloudier.

More information and tips can be found at *iddsi.org* and on IDDSI's YouTube channel (*youtube.com/@iddsi2903*).

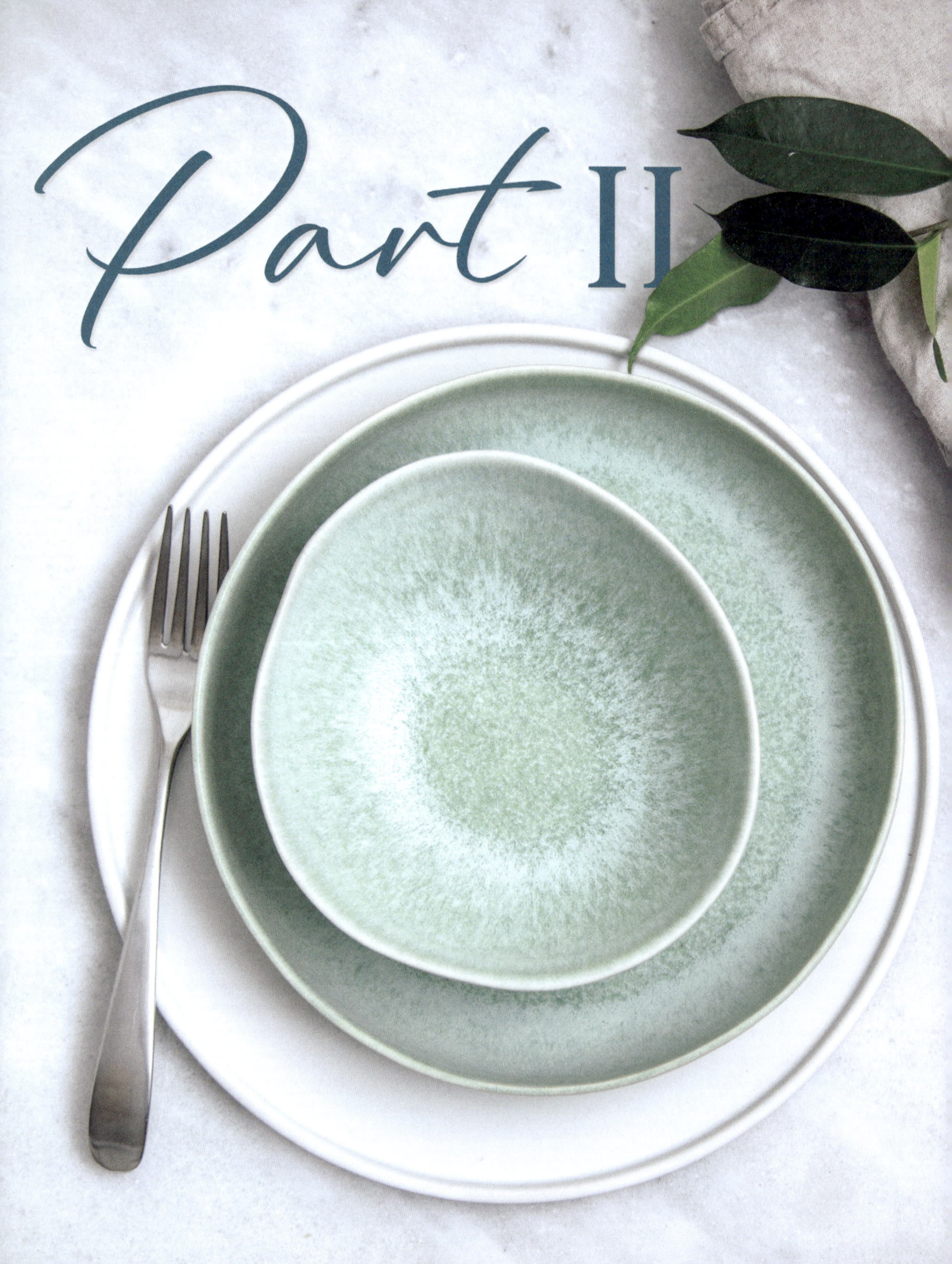
Part II

The Puree Kitchen System

As the cost of healthcare facilities rises, more people are choosing to age in place or to live on their own. If you are living with dysphagia or caring for someone who is, this means that making pureed food efficiently is a concern, as it was in my household. I wanted to make delicious pureed foods, so I experimented with different techniques, ingredients, and cooking methods to arrive at the most efficient ways of preparing tasty purees at home.

What worked for me was a combination of a restaurant-style setup in my kitchen and classic cooking techniques that are perfect for the puree kitchen. The basic idea is to cook once, puree and store, and then eat multiple times. If you cook one day a week, this frees up time during the rest of the week.

For the first two years that I cooked for my mother, I used my home kitchen as is—a cooktop, an oven, and regular pots and pans. Then I discovered that the most efficient way to create delicious purees was to set up a basic cooking and puree station on the counter. Because I did not have to take it down every day, it was convenient and easy to use several times a day.

Batch cooking—making multiple servings at one time—lightens the cooking load, as there is always a meal on hand ready to serve. This is especially helpful if you are busy, are likely to get home late, or need to be away for a period of time, as meals can continue on schedule without someone needing to cook every day. All the recipes here make four to six servings, so you can keep the refrigerator and freezer well stocked.

After I cooked a dish, I found the most helpful technique was to puree one serving for same-day service, put one serving in the fridge labeled for service within 48 hours, and label and freeze the remaining servings for use in the time specified in individual recipes.

Setting Up the Puree Kitchen

Setting up your kitchen for success will make the process of creating meals run smoothly.

One of the most important aspects of making that process easier is acquiring the right time- and labor-saving appliances. The two most important appliances you need are a blender and a mini food processor that processes at least one or two servings, 3.5 cups. Once you have them, set up a puree station by placing them side by side on your counter so you can easily access them. This is your basic working setup—but for versatility, I recommend investing in some additional appliances and tools, depending on your budget and space considerations. The list below is a starting point and general guide. Also keep in mind that new products are always becoming available.

HOW TO SELECT APPLIANCES

There are a number of factors to consider in the purchase of kitchen appliances. Reliability and ease of use are the two top qualities you need to think about. Will the machine do the job that needs to be done? Is it too difficult to figure out? A third factor is whether you like the machine; sometimes it is worth making an additional investment so that you are not irritated every time you use it. In the puree kitchen, you may use a machine three times a day or more, making this an important factor to consider when purchasing. My guiding principles for product selection are performance, design, ease of cleanup, and ease of storage. You can buy your appliances all at once, or add them one at a time.

The Two Most Important Appliances You Will Need

Food Processor

Mini food processors are available in a range of capacities, from 2 to 5 cups. Regular-size food processor capacity ranges from 8 to 14 cups, for family-size servings. Some brands are also available in fun colors that brighten up the kitchen. The major brands are available at discount retailers, at department stores, at specialty stores, and online. I would avoid the least-expensive models, because you will use this appliance many times a day. A cheaper model is more likely to burn out sooner, and you will spend more replacing it than if you had bought a higher-quality one to begin with.

Blender, High-Speed Blender, or Nutrient Extractor

A regular blender is standard equipment for your puree station. You will use it two or three times a day, so go to a brick-and-mortar store and look at what's on display. Choose a machine that you like to use and that is easy to clean. I highly recommend that you stay away from the type of blender with a bottom that screws off and blades that need to be cleaned separately. These are a pain for repeated daily use, as screwing the bottom on and off just so you can clean the blades is irritating in the extreme.

My favorite high-speed blender is the Vitamix; it is expensive, but it offers a very good warranty. On the downside, except for one or two smaller models, a Vitamix blender takes up a lot of space and makes a lot of noise. That said, they have variable controls, and they blend like no other. In fact, they are so powerful that their spinning blades create enough friction to heat the mixture while it blends; that means you can serve a hot soup right from the blender in just seven minutes. Plus, they are easy to clean—you add a little dishwashing liquid to the container, turn the machine on for a few seconds, then rinse. QVC frequently has the best buys on the Vitamix and a wealth of information online. Amazon sells the Vitamix, and it offers the option of ordering a refurbished Vitamix at a lower price. They are also available directly from Vitamix online, with special offers for refurbished machines and payment plans.

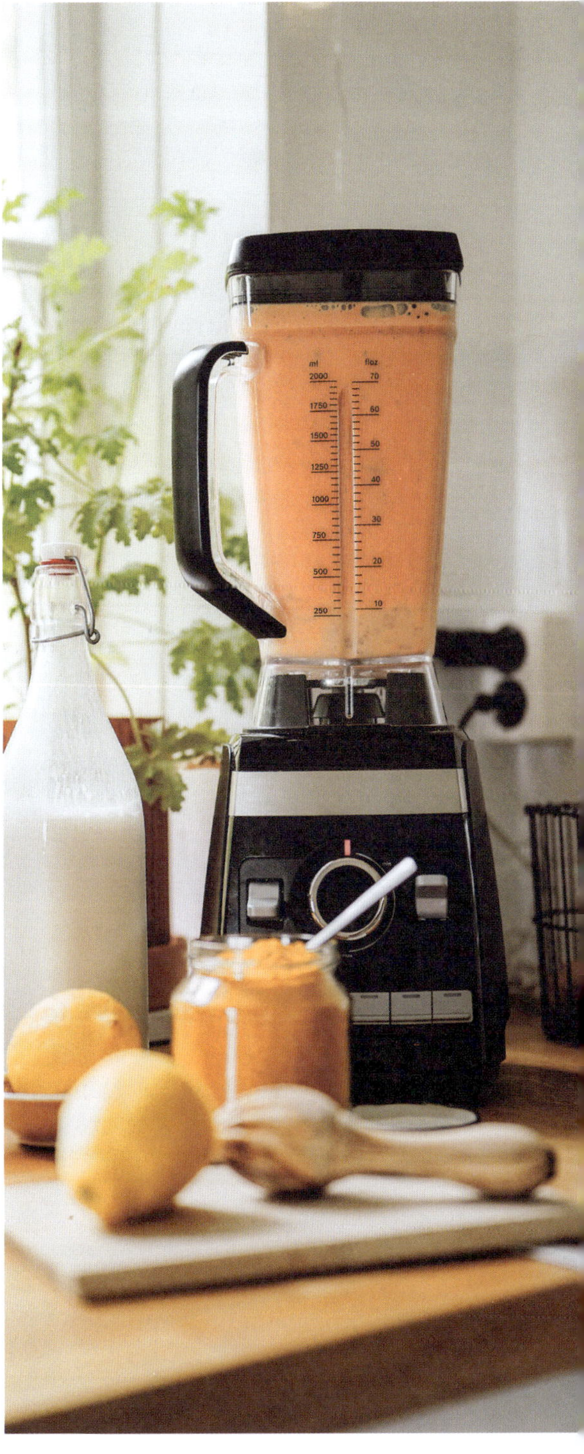

My second-favorite high-speed blender is the Ninja. It has a flat bottom and a multitiered blade system. I was able to buy a set that included both a small Ninja and a pitcher-sized Ninja with a vented lid. It is best to visit a store and take a look, as new models are always coming on the market. There are many different sets of Ninjas to be found in brick-and-mortar stores as well as online.

The Ninja Nutri-Blender and the similar Nutribullet are not technically blenders; they are high-speed nutrient extractors. A nutrient extractor has such a powerful motor that it will liquefy raw fruits and vegetables by breaking down the cell wall. This type of appliance gives you control over the botanical world. If you or the person you are caring for thrives on fresh fruits and vegetables, this is an appliance to consider adding. They are fantastic for making smoothies with fruit, including fibrous fruits like pineapple. I also make use of these when pureeing salads. They puree the cell wall.

The Nutribullet Rx is a nutrient extractor with a heating function, able to make soup from raw vegetables in seven minutes. It competes with the Vitamix at less than half the price. It has a vented lid for safety. It does not have the variety of settings that the Vitamix does, but it is less noisy than the Vitamix. This is definitely a convenience appliance. It is excellent for making a small amount of a dessert, such as pudding (see pages 232 and 233), oatmeal, or Cream of Wheat or farina. I also like to use it for making shakes or soups that will be served warm.

An immersion blender is convenient for pureeing in the cooking pot without having to transfer hot liquid to a blender.

WHY YOU NEED A VENTED LID

It is extremely important when blending hot liquids to fill the appliance at most two-thirds full and have a lid that can vent the steam. Otherwise pressure builds up and can blow the top right off the blender or spew the contents all over once you remove the lid, potentially causing serious burns. It is best to let liquids cool before attempting to puree.

› **TIP:** Do not puree hot liquids in a nutrient extractor such as a Nutribullet. It does not have a vented lid.

Other Useful Appliances

An electric or stovetop pressure cooker is a big timesaver, as it can cook food to a smooth, moist texture in a very short amount of time. Electric pressure cookers (including the popular Instant Pot) are computerized and completely safe. The stovetop models are not quite as convenient, but they too are easy to use and not as costly.

A slow cooker (or a multicooker with a slow-cook function) is best used for braising, for making soups and stews, and for anything that needs low heat and a long cooking time.

An indoor grill is good for safe grilling, low and slow, for the iconic meals of summer. An outdoor barbecue grill operates at such a high temperature that it produces charring of food, and charring is not safe for the swallow. With an indoor grill, you get the flavor and the atmosphere of a cookout, in modified form.

A steaming appliance or a multitiered steamer can be used in multiple ways. It is great for steaming an entire head of broccoli or cauliflower evenly—it gives the best result I have ever had in steaming these veggies. Steamed vegetables retain their color and nutrients, and are perfect for making eye-catching purees, such as a carrot soup that is really orange, a borscht that is really red, and broccoli puree that is bright green. And don't forget the parsnip, an overlooked vegetable (a relative of the carrot) that is quite tasty. When you use a steamer with the parchment parcel technique (see page 78), cleanup is quick and easy, with separate servings prepared in a single cooking session. Steaming is the way you will heat frozen meals. A multitiered stainless steel steamer, stovetop or electric, is a good choice.

A steamer can be made using a pot fitted with a colander. Not recommended are steaming baskets with center handles for lifting. Many companies make steaming appliances. The Instant Pot and other electric pressure cookers as well as many multicookers come with steaming trays. Bamboo stacked steamers are *not* recommended for the dysphagia kitchen for food safety reasons as they are made of organic material; the combination of moisture from steaming and organic material can provide the conditions for bacteria to grow. The steamer is an important tool, so select the one that is best for your kitchen. Whichever steamer you choose, ensure that your glass storage dishes can lie flat within it.

When considering which appliances to purchase, try to go to a store that has the machines on display. You can check out a machine's size and its suitability for your space. I also suggest handling the machine to see how it feels and if it is easy to use. Some stores will even let you plug in a machine and give it a test run, to see if it is quiet. It is also a good idea to determine whether you have a place to store the machine when not in use, or enough counter space for it if you plan to keep it out.

Tools and Utensils

There are quite a few gadgets that can be very helpful in the puree kitchen.

Potato ricer. Once a potato is cooked by any method, it can be put through a potato ricer. This creates small, grain-like particles that can be mashed with milk, broth, or cooking liquid to make a smooth puree. You put the potato in the holder and press the handle down. With a potato ricer, you can produce velvety mashed potatoes with butter and milk or cream.

Food mill. A food mill can be used with vegetables, soups, and sauces to produce a very smooth texture with no lumps. You put a small amount of food in the well of the cone shape and turn the handle. A blade circulates, forcing the food through the mill, leaving behind the larger particles. This produces the most glorious gravies and sauces.

Mesh strainers and silicone spatulas. Push any food pureed in a food processor or a blender through a strainer using a spatula, and any and all particles not suitable will be left behind. The strainer can also be lined with cheesecloth beforehand, which works well for removing the tiny seeds from fruits like strawberries, raspberries, and kiwis.

Cheesecloth. Useful for lining the mesh strainer.

Whisks. Useful for blending instant thickeners and other flavorings into liquids or purees.

Vegetable peelers. Both the Y-shaped peeler and the traditional straight variety are great for prepping fresh fruit and vegetables.

Other tools you may find helpful

- A good kitchen scale
- Instant-read thermometer
- Kitchen tongs
- Measuring cups and spoons
- A set of stainless steel mixing bowls, with lids for storage in the fridge
- Electric hand mixer
- Citrus juicer
- Sharp knives—a chef's knife, a paring knife, and a serrated knife are the three basics
- A mandoline for even slicing
- Souper cubes for freezing a single serving of soup, gravy, or broth for later use
- Glass storage containers with lids for storing food in freezer and reheating by steaming or boiling
- Zip bags, freezer-proof and tightly sealed for heating a serving in boiling water. Space-saving for storing single servings of whole grains, beans, and vegetables, because they lie flat
- Whiteboard for keeping track of food on hand.

Batch Cooking Method

The best way to maximize your time is by preparing recipes that make four to six servings. You can serve one meal right away, put one or more servings for follow-on service within 48 hours, and/or freeze extra servings so that you'll have a good meal on hand for up to 3 months. You or your loved one will eat deliciously with time freed up. The big secret of batch cooking: A backup caregiver, whether professional or family member, can heat and serve a delicious meal for the person with dysphagia. The principal caregiver gets a night off. The second big secret: The recipes in this collection may be served to the person who needs a dysphagia diet as well as other family members. The system is excellent for caregivers.

› **Tip:** Soups, stews, vegetables, grains, and protein dishes (whether animal or plant-based) all freeze well. Follow the freezing instructions for each dish. Label each dish with the day the dish was created and the USE BY date.

Here is my suggested approach:

1. As suggested previously, ask your loved one with the swallowing disorder to name ten dishes, their favorites. This list will be the basis of your cooking schedule. If you are the person with the swallowing disorder, and you do your own cooking, make a list of your favorites.

2. Plan for one cooking day each week when you make one or two dishes. This could be an entrée and a side, two sides, or a side and a sauce. Make different dishes each time you cook, so that you begin to have a selection in the freezer—for example, pea soup, stuffed cabbage, chicken pot pie, meat loaf with mashed potato, eggplant parmesan, and tortellini with pesto. If you cook two dishes one day a week, after five weeks you will have servings of all ten favorites on hand.

3. Shop for several meals at one time. This may be done a day in advance, so you have everything on hand and don't have to run out to the store right before you start cooking.

4. Once the food is cooked, allow it to cool, then store servings in glass containers, labeling them as suggested below. As noted, you can serve one meal right away, store a follow-on meal in the fridge for use within 48 hours, and store the remaining servings in the freezer for use within 3 months.

5. Keep track of the dishes and the number of meals frozen and in the fridge. When you notice that a particular dish is running low, make more of it, so that there's always some on hand. See "Keeping Track of Meals on Hand" on page 63.

Tips for Batch Cooking Day

- Cook what you like to cook. Do what works best for your household. Every household is different.

- Don't worry if you make a mistake, especially if a dish is new to you. You can always save a dish in some way.

- If you need help, get someone to peel the carrots or chop the onions, for example. Use a food processor as an assistant if necessary.

- Play music while you cook! A playlist enlivens the atmosphere in the kitchen. Whatever music you like—in my house, some days it's soul, some days it's classical, some days it's country. To relieve stress, dance in the kitchen while you cook.

- After initial cooking and cooling, entrees may be pureed and thickened first, and then frozen. Or they may be frozen in the unpureed state and then pureed and thickened after defrosting. I prefer the latter because it preserves the flavor. This is an individual choice, tailored to each household.

- Keep extra soups and sauces on hand in case a dish needs extra moisture for the puree. Extremely thick stock may also be used to thicken a serving. See SimplyThick CEO John Holahan's TikTok video for creating Extremely Thick Stock @simplythickjohn. The thickened liquid cannot be drunk from a cup or sucked through a straw.

FOOD SAFETY

The guidelines for food safety given in this book are drawn from the Food and Drug Administration website. When the use-by date has gone by, the food is thrown away, no questions asked. See the Resources section (pages 237–240) for FDA links.

Food Storage and Labeling

For storing, use glass storage containers with lids. Sets are available in discount stores like Walmart, Target, and Costco, and online from Amazon. Best to buy at the holidays when they go on sale in large quantities. Glass storage containers such as those from Anchor Hocking can go from the freezer and fridge to the oven and the dishwasher without shattering. Glass won't get stained by sauces or absorb strong odors from food, the way plastic does.

For labeling, some of the newer glass containers have lids that you can write on. Otherwise, use ruled Post-It labels, writing the name of the dish, the contents of the dish, and the number of servings (one, unless planning a family meal). Write whether the dish needs to be pureed or if it has already been pureed.

Generally, I prefer to store in single servings for food safety. That way there are no partial servings left over in the fridge that might be overlooked and allow bacteria to grow.

On the label, also add the date of preparation. For food that will be stored in the freezer, add a use-by date that is different for every recipe (with seafood, use a two-week use-by date for servings you freeze).

When freezing baked goods, wrap the baked goods first in plastic wrap and then in aluminum foil, and put them in a plastic or glass container. I also do this with purchased cupcakes and birthday cake. (Donna from the bakery at my local Publix supermarket gave me that tip.)

Keeping Track of Meals on Hand

To keep track of meals, I suggest using two small whiteboards. Put them on the fridge or freezer door. Mine attach with magnets and have a holder for the marker (keep erasers close by). I suggest updating the boards every time you cook and store food, and every time you use food stored in the fridge or freezer.

On one board, list each main dish, soup, and veggie side dish you have on hand, and the number of servings. On the other board, list salads, desserts, savory sauces, and fruit sauces, also with the number of servings. If you keep it up to date, you and any caregivers will always know what is on hand and can select from the items available. Everyone's job is made easier. Organization is the key to saving labor, time, and money.

When I did a dessert tasting at the New York charity God's Love We Deliver, I was pleased to notice that the director of nutrition services, my host, Lisa Zullig, used the same system of whiteboards to run her amazing professional kitchen that serves five thousand meals a day to people who are too sick to cook for themselves. Their motto is "Food Is Medicine, Food Is Love." This is an excellent charity and worth your support.

Shopping and Cooking Schedules

Use the whiteboards (mentioned above) to plan your cooking and shopping schedules. When cooking for my mom, with a glance at the board I could tell if I'd run out of Split Pea Soup (see page 84), my mother's favorite, and knew that I should plan to make a batch. This system prevents the wasting of food and money, since you don't cook too much and you don't cook too little. You can see what is on hand and can use the meals that are already cooked before needing to cook more. This saves time and energy running to the market.

The Pantry and Freezer

A guiding principle of mine is to always have the makings of a meal on hand. The way to do this is to keep a well-stocked pantry and a well-stocked freezer. When you need to get a meal ready in as little as half an hour, having good-quality store-bought convenience foods available in your pantry makes a huge difference and helps ease the pressures of a busy work life. Some of my newer recipes are ready in fifteen minutes. I like making things from scratch, but sometimes I am just too pressed for time. Even Julia Child admonished that it is best not to be a food snob!

The pantry is also important should there be an emergency. For example, I live in the land of hurricanes, and emergency management agencies suggest that households whose members have medical needs should keep two weeks' worth of food, water, and medicines on hand, in case the power goes out in a storm.

Pantry Checklist

Tomato products. Canned or jarred tomatoes are a must. Many of the recipes in this book call for tomato paste, tomato puree, tomato sauce, or diced tomatoes. I suggest having some of each on hand—the low-sodium varieties are best. I also suggest looking for the tubes of tomato paste rather than the cans. Some supermarkets offer a house brand of delicious organic tomato products, including fire-roasted tomato paste and diced tomatoes. These can be used to add a lot of flavor to dishes. Also look for jars of your favorite premade tomato sauce when they are on sale and stock up, as well as jarred Alfredo sauce to use as a base for the lemon sauce for the Salmon in Puff Pastry (see page 124). When buying store-bought tomato sauce, I look for one that lists tomatoes as the first ingredient, as I find they have better flavor than the ones that list tomato puree as the first ingredient. I like to make a big pot of homemade tomato sauce on Sunday that I can freeze or use during the week. (I am developing a recipe for an easy homemade Alfredo, made without butter and cream.)

Pasta. Keep a variety of pasta shapes—for example, thin spaghetti, linguine, penne, and elbow macaroni. I prefer whole-grain pasta. A new discovery of mine is black bean pasta and adzuki bean pasta. Both are flavorful additions

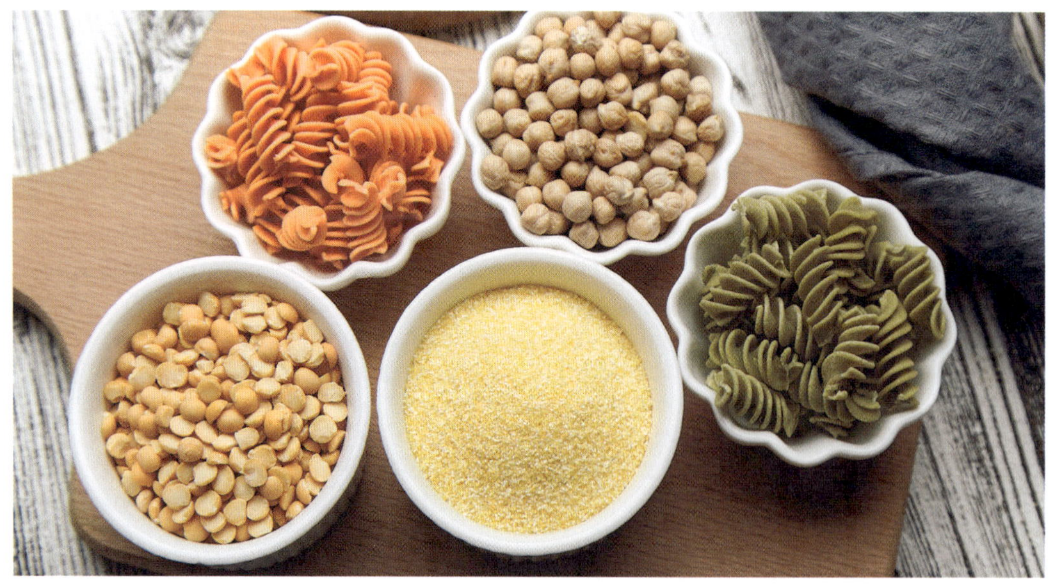

to pasta dishes and are gluten free. Japanese soba noodles can be used in soups flavored with dashi (an instant granulated form is available for making this traditional Japanese broth). Soba noodles are made from buckwheat. They puree beautifully and can be served with steamed vegetables and a protein like shrimp, chicken, or tofu.

Legumes and beans. I keep dried peas and French lentils on hand for making my mother's favorite pea soup. I also like to stock up on packages of nine-bean soup mix from the health food store. Keep a variety of canned beans on hand—they are useful additions to meals and soups, and are easily combined with rice, as in red beans and rice, for a healthy side or main dish. The best beans to keep on hand are cannellini or white beans, red kidney beans for chili, black beans for tacos, and chickpeas for soups and even making falafel. Dried chickpeas can be cooked easily in a pressure cooker, then used as needed or made into hummus.

Whole grains. Long-grain brown basmati rice is my go-to rice because

USING READY-MADE MEALS

My friend Betsy is a member of the "sandwich generation"—someone with aging parents, growing children, and a full-time job. She called me in a panic when her mother had to go on a pureed diet as a result of a neurological disorder related to aging. Betsy was the manager of the health food store where I shopped, and she and her staff had helped me with selecting food for my own mom. Betsy knew that I was the queen of puree. She had siblings who were willing to help but she needed a simple solution.

Here are a few of the ideas I suggested to her:

- Buy the nutritionally best available prepared frozen food items. Thaw, prepare, and puree them.
- Buy ready-to-prepare meal kits (fresh or frozen) from the grocery store or a delivery service. Thaw if needed, prepare, and puree.

Today many people have prepared meals delivered to their homes. These services are more expensive than cooking meals at home, but for some households, they are a necessity. Many meal plans are competitive with or cheaper than grocery store prices and may fit some family budgets. The convenience can free up extra caregiver hours. If you have a lower income and are eligible for Medicaid, you may be eligible to receive home-delivered pureed meals on a monthly basis.

of the flavor, and because it gets very tender after cooking. It does not have a tough husk, as short-grain brown rice does; short-grain brown rice can be difficult to digest. I keep kasha (buckwheat groats) on hand, too, along with quinoa, a high-protein whole grain native to South America that can be used in place of rice as a side dish or to stuff peppers or cabbage. Farro is a new favorite of mine. I prefer steel-cut oats for oatmeal (the 5-minute variety as opposed to the 30-minute variety). Barley is an excellent grain to use as a side dish or in soups.

Prepackaged mixes. Pancakes are easy to make from scratch, but sometimes you don't have time. Packaged buckwheat pancake mixes and instant pudding mixes can be kept on hand. Please see the recipe for Homemade Vanilla Pudding Mix (page 232).

Baking supplies. Unbleached flour, cornstarch, arrowroot, and Wondra flour can all be used for thickening sauces and gravies. Prepared breadcrumbs (my choice is organic whole wheat with Italian seasoning), matzo meal, and panko (Japanese-style breadcrumbs) can be used for light breading. These all puree well without granules that irritate the throat and make swallowing difficult. Jacques Pépin has a secret ingredient for thickening soups—potato starch. Easier than making a roux or a slurry.

Spices, seasonings, herb pastes, and condiments. It's nice to have a variety of spices on hand, including cumin, oregano, thyme, tarragon, sage, turmeric, curry powder, and chili powder. For desserts, real vanilla extract, cinnamon, cloves, nutmeg, and allspice are great to have. The dysphagia kitchen uses white pepper. Black pepper is to be avoided, as it has sharp edges and is not safe for the swallow. I use Adriatic sea salt because it is available online and in some natural foods stores, has great flavor, and is reasonably priced. The reason I choose sea salt, generally, is because it has a fine texture, unlike kosher salt and other chunky salts, and it dissolves easily. It is excellent for the puree kitchen.

Old Bay Seasoning is a must for fish and shellfish. Worcestershire sauce, Tabasco sauce, and low-sodium soy sauce are flavor powerhouses. Herb pastes like those made with parsley, basil, and ginger are easy to use and good to keep on hand in the fridge. I like having several varieties of mustard in the pantry—yellow mustard, Dijon mustard, and Chinese mustard (avoid grainy mustard for safe swallow reasons). Low-fat mayonnaise, Lemonaise, or any mayo substitute is useful to have. For ketchup, I prefer the organic kinds that are low in sugar. These are easy to find in a supermarket. Stubb's Bar-B-Q sauce is also low in sugar; there are four varieties and all of them are good. Annie's brand is also low-sugar.

Oils and vinegars. Keep good-quality olive oil and extra-virgin olive oil on hand for salads and sauces. I use extra-virgin olive oil for cooking; it is a bit more expensive but the nutritional profile is good. (See Dr. Willett's book for a thorough discussion of oils.) The reader may use regular olive oil, however. For other oils, I prefer cold-pressed (avocado and sunflower are good; grapeseed oil has a high smoke point). Rice vinegar is light and has a clean taste without the acidic after-burn. Red wine vinegar and sherry vinegar are good to have on hand, too, but use them in moderation, as acidic foods may cause aspiration.

Sweeteners. My favorites are the following: any local honey, real maple syrup, barley malt syrup, agave syrup, and stevia—but consult with your healthcare provider about what would be preferred choices for you.

Freezer Checklist

Fruit. Stock up on packages of frozen fruit like blueberries, strawberries, raspberries, pineapple, black cherries, and mango—all great to have on hand for making fruit purees. You can use just a few pieces at a time. As frozen vegetables and fruits are picked at the height of ripeness and flash frozen, they make an excellent choice when fresh is not available, or when you don't have time to go to the market.

Vegetables. Packages of chopped spinach, corn, and peas, plus pureed vegetables like butternut squash and turnips (I like the Birds Eye Southland brand) are good to keep stocked. Choose the ones that work for your family.

Meat and seafood. Cooked peeled shrimp (sold with the tail on, but remove the tail before pureeing), scallops, wild salmon fillets, ground turkey, chicken breasts, and chicken sausage (mild Italian-style) are good choices. Pork loin keeps well and is handy to have in your freezer.

Desserts. There is a need for imagination when it comes to desserts in the dysphagia kitchen. See the recipe for Instant Pudding Mix (page 232). Plain ice cream is the easiest dessert, but the same old flavors get boring. For variety, see How to Thicken Ice Cream (page 228) and eliminate items that are not safe for the swallow.

Part III

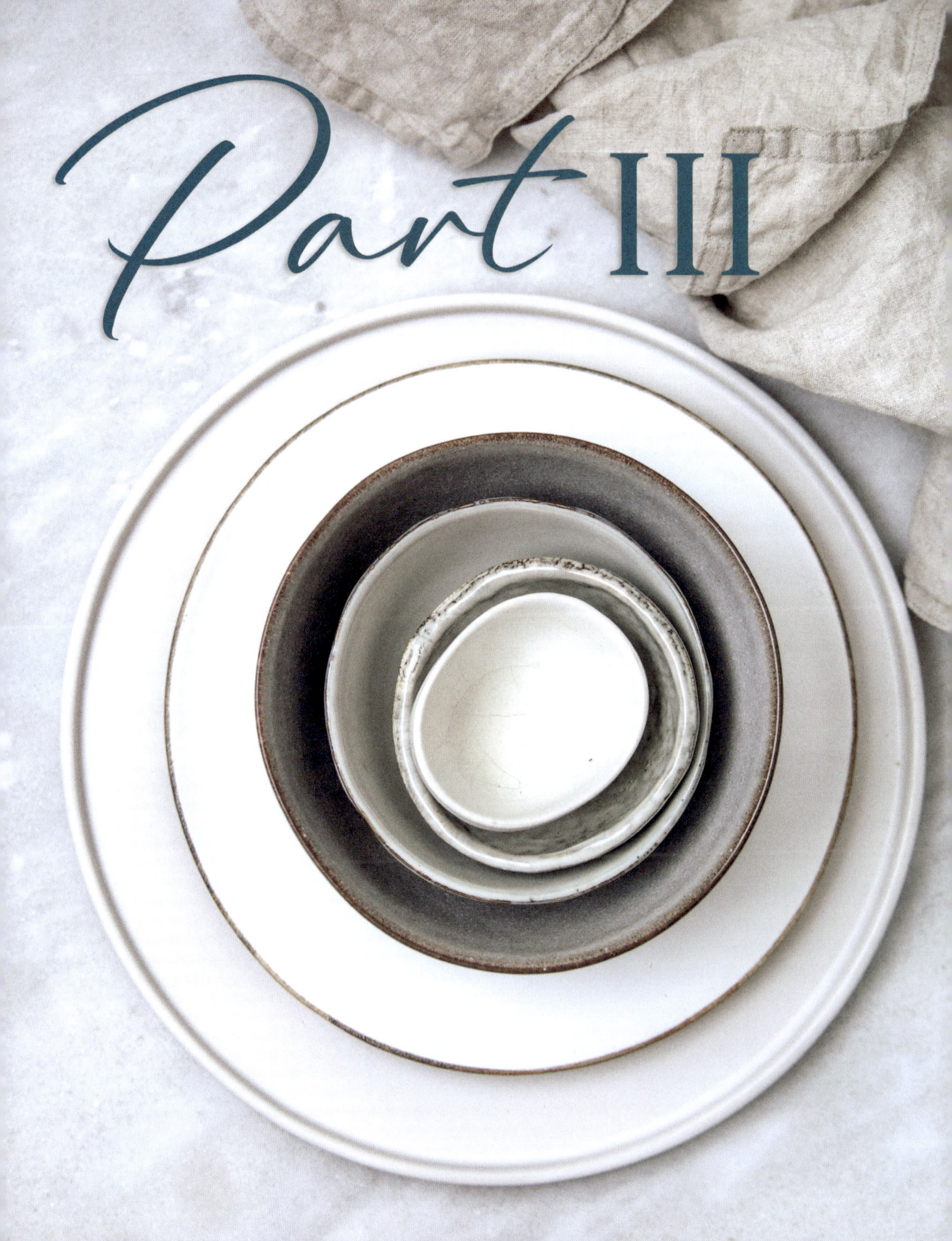

Before You Start

Introduction

The recipes that follow are updated family recipes developed over the years that I was taking care of my mother. Providing food that tasted good and allowed her to maintain a healthy weight was one of my main goals. Now my hope is that sharing what I learned and the recipes I developed will give you guidelines and inspiration for making delicious food when you or a family member is faced with swallowing difficulties: Food that offers quality nutrition to help maintain a good immune system. Food that improves your mood. Food that can be made in the home kitchen.

The recipes in this book are suitable for Pureed, IDDSI Level 4, through Regular, Level 7 (the Shakes are suitable for Level 3, Moderately Thick Liquid). For detailed instructions on how to create and test for each level, please see the IDDSI materials, text, and charts in Karen Sheffler's chapter, pages 24–53.

To achieve IDDSI Level 5, Minced & Moist, chop items to the right particle size (particle size compliance) and ensure that the pebbly particles are moist/cohesive enough to pass the IDDSI tests (see pages 42–47) and bind together.

Before we get to the actual recipes, here are a few helpful ideas, reminders, and procedures for making them as safe as possible, as appetizing as possible, and as appealing as possible.

Thickeners

Any individual diagnosed with dysphagia requires a healthcare plan that is tailored to the results of a swallow test. Your healthcare provider will identify the level of the IDDSI framework for food and beverages that is suitable for your particular situation. To use the recipes that follow, create the dish, thicken to the prescribed IDDSI level if needed, and run the IDDSI test for the dish. For detailed information, refer to the IDDSI section (starting on page 39).

The thickeners used for food and beverages are available in powdered and gel forms. They are sold in pharmacies or can be bought online directly from the manufacturer, from other sources like Carewell Home Health Products, or from major online retailers.

WHEN USING THICKENERS, KEEP IN MIND

Closely follow the directions on the label of your chosen thickener.

Use glass containers for storage when possible, because thickened liquids cling to plastic containers.

Gum-based thickeners work in all liquids and do not add a starchy, pasty flavor.

Powdered thickeners take time to hydrate and to make your beverages safe for consumption. After mixing, allow them to stand for three to five minutes to achieve full thickening potential.

As noted earlier, I recommend storing food in individual servings for convenience and for safety. There will be no leftovers to store and less chance of developing bacteria. And since loss of appetite may occur with dysphagia, there will be less waste.

› **TIP:** Thicken the dish and then store in individual servings. The idea is that a backup caregiver may serve a meal. To get a night off for the primary caregiver, it helps to have a dish that either a professional caregiver or a family or friend who is serving as caregiver can heat and serve. In my own case, certified nursing assistants (CNAs) sent from an agency were not allowed to do any cooking, but were allowed to prepare a heat-and-serve meal.

Additionally, manufacturers have created educational materials and posted them on their websites. These materials include well-researched and illustrated webpages and instructional videos showing how to use the products (see Resources, page 237).

There are other items that you can use to thicken dishes in addition to a commercial thickening agent, such as flour, regular cornstarch, pureed potatoes, sauces, or gravy.

The Importance of Sauces: Making Great-Tasting Purees

Good-tasting sauces, homemade or store-bought, are the key to delicious pureed food. Why? The surface area of the ingredients is greatly increased when the food is pureed, and that can result in a loss of flavor; suspending the pureed food in a sauce adds more flavor back. The sauce also adds color, nutrients, and texture to the final dish. My mother liked sweets, so I discovered that using ice cream as a sauce in pureeing desserts like cake worked nicely, as did using fruit sauces for pureeing pancakes and pies. The idea is to maximize flavor and visual appeal.

The Importance of Snacks

Healthy snacks with nutritional density are important additions to the diet if you have a swallowing disorder. You need calories, because if you do not maintain a healthy weight, you may be less able to fight off infections. Those on a pureed diet can lose weight because some of the functions of digestion, such as the breakdown of the food by mastication, are performed by the pureeing of the food. Also, a person with a diminished appetite may only want to eat small meals, so snacks can be useful. There are a variety of shakes suitable for sweet snacks (see pages 216-220). For savory snacks, I suggest soups (see pages 80-88), especially quick soups that can be made with a high-speed blender. You can also thicken servings of store-bought soup.

Cooking Tips for Making Favorite Ethnic, Family, or Regional Recipes

The IDDSI system of describing the texture of modified foods and thickened liquids for people with swallowing disorders is used all over the world, for every ethnic cuisine. An amazing variety of cuisines make up the food landscape. All of them may be modified and pureed using the system in this book. The source of the recipe may be a family recipe, a well-reviewed cookbook on the cuisine, or takeout food. A discussion with your healthcare provider is recommended so that you can review the ingredients and cooking techniques. Additional materials on ethnic cuisines may be found on the IDDSI website.

The standard rules for puree apply to cooking techniques in other ethnic kitchens. Here, for example, I show how you can create purees for classic southern food family favorites. These techniques can also be used for other family-favorite cuisines.

HOW TO MAKE A SUPER SHAKE USING SUPPLEMENTS

To boost nutrition, a snack shake may be fortified with supplements—super ingredients. Check with your healthcare professional before adding supplements to make sure that the supplement does not conflict with any medications. Among the nutrients most often missing are minerals, but you must be able to tolerate them, and they must not interfere with other medications—be sure to discuss with your healthcare team. Some supplements to consider are liquid vitamins, liquid colloidal minerals, protein powder (whey or plant-based), and probiotics for digestive health.

If you use supplements, add them when blending the shake. At the suggestion of my mother's primary care physician, I added one supplement at a time, generally vitamins in the morning and minerals in the afternoon, for ease of absorption.

I have just taste-tested a product called Thrive Ice Cream that is already fortified and is shipped on dry ice. Made of excellent ingredients, the ice cream comes in three flavors as well as a no-sugar-added vanilla suitable for diabetics. It has great flavor and may be added to a shake without mixing in supplements separately. See *thriveicecream.com/products/thrive-ice-cream/*. Thrive also makes four flavors of Thrive Gelato. These have excellent flavor and texture.

1. **Choosing a recipe.** Choose a recipe with a tender protein and a sauce or liquid. Oxtail soup is a great example. The perfect recipe for puree renders food moist and tender while preserving nutrients. In the case of oxtail soup, long cooking renders a less expensive cut of meat soft and tender. Another example is barbecued ribs—cook them first in an electric pressure cooker with a mild sauce following directions for your appliance. Once the protein is cooked, go to step 2.

2. **Prepping proteins.** After cooking, prep the protein for pureeing. Make sure when removing the meat from the bones to eliminate any sinews, tendons, or connective tissue, as these do not puree. For this process, use a mesh strainer and a silicone spatula. Sometimes you can dig a little marrow out of the bones. This provides not just nutrition but also flavor and richness, so add it to the puree. Legumes can be a great protein source, too—a holiday favorite for New Year's is black-eyed peas that have been simmered for a long time, until they are soft and perfect for the dysphagia kitchen.

3. **Prepping veggies.** All skins, seeds, and fibrous parts of any vegetable must be removed from the final puree. The best way to do this is to run the puree through a mesh strainer with a silicone spatula to eliminate any parts that might not be safe for the swallow. If your sweet potatoes are fibrous, for example, run them through the strainer. Prep collard greens by removing the ribs and tough stems, as these will not puree. Use a high-speed blender or a nutrient extractor for vegetables that are more resistant, like green beans or lima beans. This will liquefy the veggies, which can then be thickened. Be sure to strain out whole spices used in cooking. Corn needs special treatment, as the outside of the kernels is very tough. If using fresh corn, remove the kernels from the cob and cook them until soft, then place in a high-speed blender to break down the kernels. Remove from the blender and push through a mesh strainer using a silicone spatula to remove any remaining tough bits. A substitute for corn is polenta.

Eating with Your Eyes

To make pureed food look good, I recommend serving it on colorful plates in interesting shapes—look for fun plates at retail outlets, garage sales, flea markets, consignment shops, and thrift stores. You can make a plate of food even more visually tempting by piping (a technique used in pastry-making) the pureed food to make different shapes or designs (see page 74).

Integrative Medicine and Nutrition

Integrative medicine, or functional medicine, is based on the idea that nutrition can promote health. In recent years Western medicine has begun to recognize some of the principles of Eastern medicine, like traditional Chinese medicine (TCM), which has a clinical history of several thousand years, and Ayurvedic medicine.

TCM recognizes three categories in relation to food, all of which are equally important:

1. The science of nutrition, meaning what is in the food should be good for you. In this system, ingredients are selected for nutritional healing.

2. The preparation of food, which includes cooking, plating, and serving. One technique is to engage the senses to compensate for the loss of the swallow. I used to show my mom the beautiful vegetables selected for her meals. She could smell the dish while it was cooking. I showed her the whole dish before it was pureed. The meal became something she could see unfolding, rather than the presentation of a pureed dish.

3. The context in which the meal is eaten—the people with whom a meal is eaten, the conversation during the meal, the environment in which the food is eaten. From the standpoint of the Western tradition, this is the most unusual of the three categories. A friend who is a practitioner of TCM told me, "One of the teachers I have known and respected for a long time emphasizes the importance of context from a standpoint of health benefits in a meal. This teacher often stated that context was as important or more important than the food itself. The idea of connecting with family and friends, of having conversation, of the environment and surroundings of the meal is as important or sometimes even more important because these elements of a meal are nourishing too."

The meal is not only what is on the plate. We take in our surroundings and what we know about the ingredients and the preparation. We eat with our minds and hearts. This approach is welcome when dealing with swallowing difficulties. Creating an environment of health and healing does not take much. It is an attitude.

TO CHEFS AT HEALTHCARE FACILITIES:

These recipes may be used for healthcare facilities in the following manner: Using a standard conversion chart, convert the recipe to be used to metric measurements. Scale up the recipe to the desired size by multiplying the metric measurements by the number of servings you want. The chef should then modify the temperature and time for cooking. A freelance chef from a cooking school could also be hired to do the upscale or simply to figure the temperature and time of cooking and the cooking vessel to be used.

How to Make a Beautiful Plate Using Piping Techniques

BY ANDREW CULLUM
The iddsi Guy

Why is it so important to make IDDSI-modified meals smell and taste wonderful?

Here's the answer. When we eat or think about eating, our brain and senses kick in. Recognizing foods and smells can spark memories of enjoyable meals had with family or friends.

When we eat, our senses come into play. The smell of food cooking stimulates the brain and taste buds before we even see the food. We can all remember the smell of freshly baked bread.

Visual appearance gives the brain information about the food and what we should be expecting. Not recognizing a food may be confusing and may have a negative impact on eating. As the saying goes, we eat with our eyes.

Color helps us recognize a dish, but we try not to make color distracting. For example, mixing colors can lead to disaster even if the taste is lovely. So while color is important, we must get the balance right so we can focus on what is in front of us.

Shape is a hallmark for recognition. A round shape for meat, for example, is reminiscent of a hamburger. Making shapes is easily done, but you will need to put some thought into your presentation.

As for taste, the first mouthful is so important. When modifying foods, always taste the food for seasoning. If the food is bland, the person with the swallowing disorder will probably lose interest, as anyone would.

The meal should be presented with attention and care. You do not have to be the best cook in the world if the person can feel the love you have put into the meal. This will then make the dining experience memorable.

Finally, mealtimes are important not only for the nutrition they provide. Meals are also social occasions (with attention to safe practices).

How to Pipe

Piping is done by squeezing the puree from a thick disposable pastry bag to create shapes on the plate or bowl. For example, you can pipe rose shapes for mashed potatoes or pureed vegetables, dots of pureed peas, rectangles of pureed sweet potato, and lines of sauces and gravy for dipping.

You can pipe using metal tips, available in cooking stores, or you can mold food into shapes, but piping with a zip bag is the easiest, especially for beginners.

Equipment

You need a heavy-duty pastry bag suitable for warm food. These bags are available in cooking supply stores, restaurant supply stores, craft stores, and online. Amazon is a good source for bulk buying. You can use the piping bag with the corner snipped off to pipe. You can also buy tips that create different shapes.

A good brand of metal tips and other equipment, such as a rack for holding the plastic bags and tips bought separately or in a Decorator Set, is Celebrate It, available at Michael's in the cooking section (*www.michaels.com/product/disposable-decorating-bags-by-celebrate-it-10051561?michaelsstore=9946&inv=4*). Other brands are available online at Amazon.

Having the tools on hand is a great way to involve children and young adults in meal prep for family members.

Technique

Fill the pastry bag with the puree to be piped. To fill the pastry bag, lower it into a tall glass or vase and fold the edges of the bag over the rim. This will hold it in place for hands-free filling.

Before piping, cut the tip off the pastry bag. Create puree shapes on the plate by gently squeezing the bag.

Suggestions for Shapes

Round shapes suggest a steak or a hamburger. A fillet shape suggests fish. A curve suggests shrimp. There are no limits to what you can create on the plate using your imagination. You can create stripes, straight or wiggly. Sausage shapes piped next to one another are very good for proteins. Use your imagination to make an appetizing plate.

For a smear look, find a spatula in your kitchen, squeeze a dollop of the desired puree onto the plate, and using a light touch, wand the spatula over the food to create a smooth look. This is good for sauces. Dip the spoonful of puree into the sauce, and enjoy!

Try using a 2-ounce ice cream scoop or two spoons to dollop the puree into small mounds on the plate. This creates the look of mashed potato.

For more on piping (and photos), see The iddsi Guy: *www.theiddsiguy.com/*.

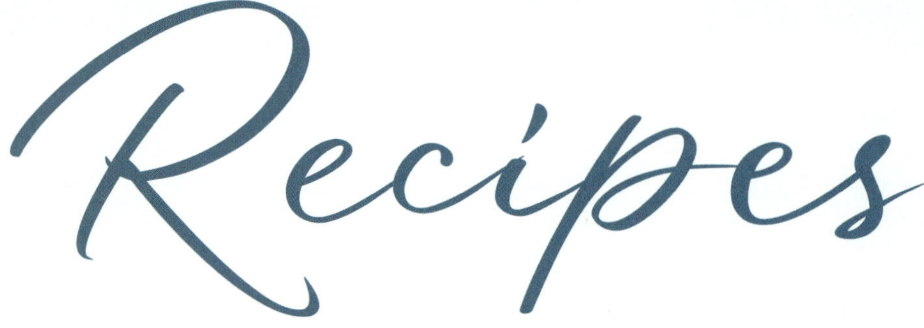

79 Soups

89 Salads

99 Poultry

110 Vegetable-Based

120 Seafood

132 Meat

154 Pasta

170 Vegetable-Side Dishes

194 Whole Grains

203 Legumes and Pulses

208 Breakfasts

215 Smoothies

221 Desserts

Serving

The dishes shown in the photos accompanying the recipes that follow are IDDSI Level 7. Please use the IDDSI instructions (pages 42-47) to modify the texture of each dish to the individual IDDSI level prescribed by your healthcare provider. Please refer to Andrew Cullum's section (pages 74-75) on piping to create a beautiful plate.

The recipes that follow allow for serving right away to yourself, to the person with dysphagia, or to family and friends. Generally, if not serving immediately, divide the extra servings (the beauty of the batch-cooking method!) between freezer- and oven-safe glass storage dishes. Allow to cool completely, cover, and refrigerate for up to 48 hours or freeze for up to 3 months (exceptions noted in individual recipes).

When you wish to serve a dish from the freezer, I recommend heating the servings by using a stovetop multi-tiered stainless steel pot or a steaming appliance.

1. For the steamer, add water to your steamer; for stovetop, put water in a pot to boil and place a colander or steamer basket in the pot.
2. Bring water to a low boil and place your covered food storage dishes in the steamer or in the pot (cover the pot) and steam for 30 minutes. Be careful about escaping steam.
3. Use gloves or a pair of tongs to remove the dishes from the steamer or pot. Let cool for five minutes, and test the internal temperature of the food (it should be 165°F [75°C].)

When serving from thawed, heat the servings using a steamer appliance or the above stovetop method, but the steaming time needed to come to the required internal temperature might be shorter.

Alternately, you can use a boil-in-bag method for storing and heating individual servings.

1. Use watertight zip bags, or vacuum-sealed bags instead of glass storage dishes to store the finished servings. (You can find inexpensive suction vacuum units at discount retailers; I suggest using a cake-decorating rack to hold the bags upright to make filling them easier.)
2. Place a bag in a stockpot filled with several quarts of water and boil until the dish reaches an internal temperature of 165°F (75°C).

Steamed Parchment Parcels

Cooking with this technique is the essence of easy meal prep. It's quick, it's simple and fuss-free, making it ideal for busy times. Follow the steps below to learn how to use this method to combine your favorite fish, or another protein, with veggies and seasonings in one delicious package. See also Cod and Vegetable Parcels, page 122.

1. Ask the person who is eating the dish to name their favorite proteins. Some suggestions: tuna, cod, or salmon; thinly sliced pieces of chicken breast; shrimp or scallops.
2. Shop the day before—get enough to make five servings (allow 4 to 6 ounces per serving, depending on the appetite).
3. Cut five 12 x 12-inch squares of parchment paper (aluminum foil can also be used).
4. If needed, cut the chosen protein into servings. Season lightly with salt and pepper.
5. Place one serving of protein on each of the parchment paper squares.
6. Add aromatics like grated ginger, garlic, or thinly sliced scallion. If desired, add veggies like carrots, zucchini, or red pepper, cut into matchsticks.
7. Make a parchment parcel by folding the paper in half to enclose the portions and crimping the edges all around to seal.
8. Place the parcels in a steamer and cook for the number of minutes required for the chosen protein.
9. Remove the parcels from the steamer using tongs, place on a plate, and allow to cool.
10. When cooled, the contents of each parcel can be pureed and thickened.
11. Store 1 or 2 servings in the fridge for serving within 48 hours. Store the rest in the freezer for serving within 1 month. (See Serving, page 77.)
12. Serve with a sauce thickened to the prescribed IDDSI level (see page 41), either on the side or added on top. Suggested sauces: lemon butter, pesto, remoulade, marinara, barbecue, curry, or Alfredo.

Soups

80 Roasted Tomato Soup

82 Matzo Ball Soup

84 Split Pea Soup

85 Minestrone

86 Wonton Soup

87 Mushroom Barley Soup

88 Chawan Mushi
(Japanese Teacup Soup)

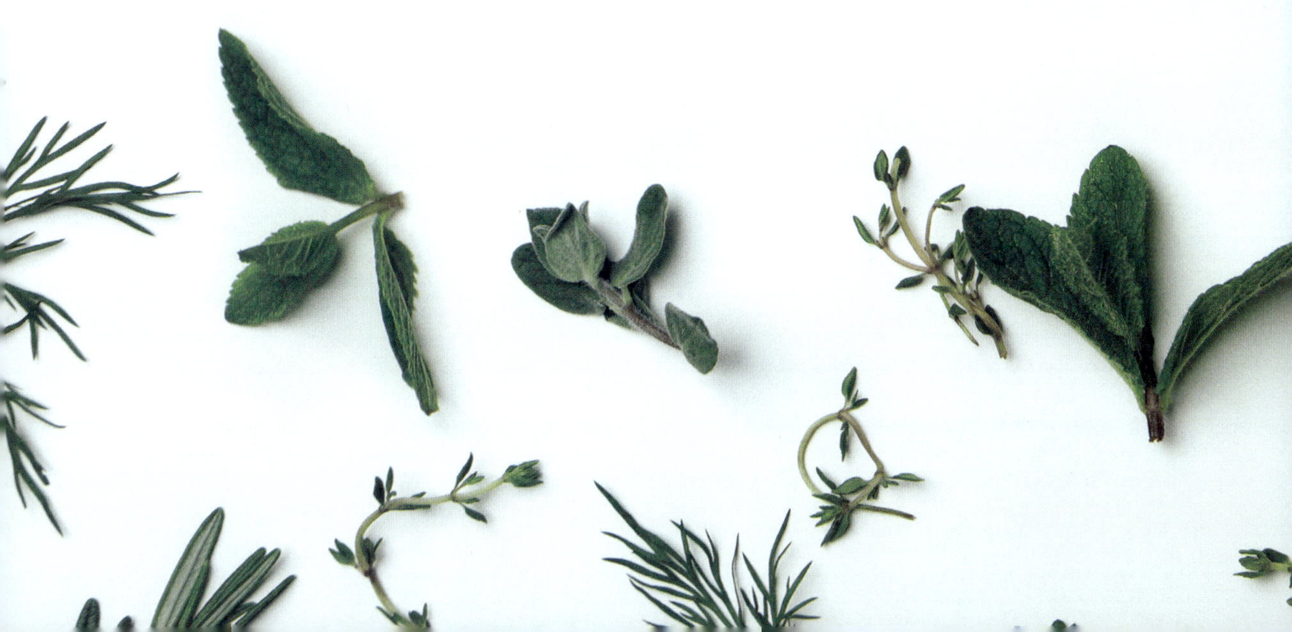

Roasted Tomato Soup

SERVINGS: 4-6 | IDDSI LEVELS 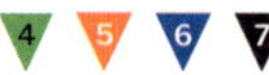

This vibrant soup is best made in summer, at the height of tomato season. Choose the ripest small to medium tomatoes available. When tomatoes are not in season, a good substitution is a 28-ounce can of roasted or whole peeled tomatoes, crushed by hand before being added to the soup. As a shortcut, or when I don't have fresh herbs on hand, I use a store-bought herb paste. It purees smoothly and adds great flavor.

- 3 pounds cherry, grape, or plum tomatoes, halved
- 3 tablespoons extra-virgin olive oil, divided
- ½ teaspoon sea salt
- ⅛ teaspoon white pepper
- 1 large onion, sliced
- 4 garlic cloves, sliced
- 2½ cups low-sodium vegetable broth
- 1 tablespoon chopped fresh basil or basil paste
- 1 tablespoon chopped fresh parsley or parsley paste

1. Place a rack in the center of the oven and preheat to 400°F (205°C). Line a baking sheet with parchment paper. Place the halved tomatoes on the baking sheet, cut side up.

2. Drizzle with 2 tablespoons olive oil and season with salt and white pepper. Transfer the sheet pan to the oven and roast until the tomatoes have collapsed and are lightly caramelized, about 30 minutes.

3. Meanwhile, heat the remaining 1 tablespoon olive oil in a large pot over medium-high heat. Add the onion and sauté until softened and just beginning to brown, about 5 minutes. Add the garlic and sauté for 1 more minute. Add the roasted tomatoes along with their juices, the vegetable broth, and the herbs, and stir to combine.

4. Remove the pot from the heat. Working in batches, transfer the soup to a blender, filling the pitcher only two-thirds full and venting the lid. Blend until smooth.

5. Run each batch of blended soup through a mesh strainer set over a large bowl to collect any skins and seeds. Discard the skins and seeds. Set aside servings for family meals, if desired.

6. Test as you go and at time of serving to see if a thickening agent, thickened sauce, or thickened stock is needed; use IDDSI Testing Methods (*iddsi.org*) to help achieve the desired IDDSI level. See pages 42-47.

7. Serve immediately or divide into servings for storage or freezing, following the directions for Serving, page 77.

NUTRITIONAL ANALYSIS PER SERVING | 1 cup
112 calories, 0.7 g fat, 0.1 g saturated fat, 172 mg sodium, 4.1 g sugar, 23.3 g carbohydrates, 2.7 g fiber, 5.2 g protein

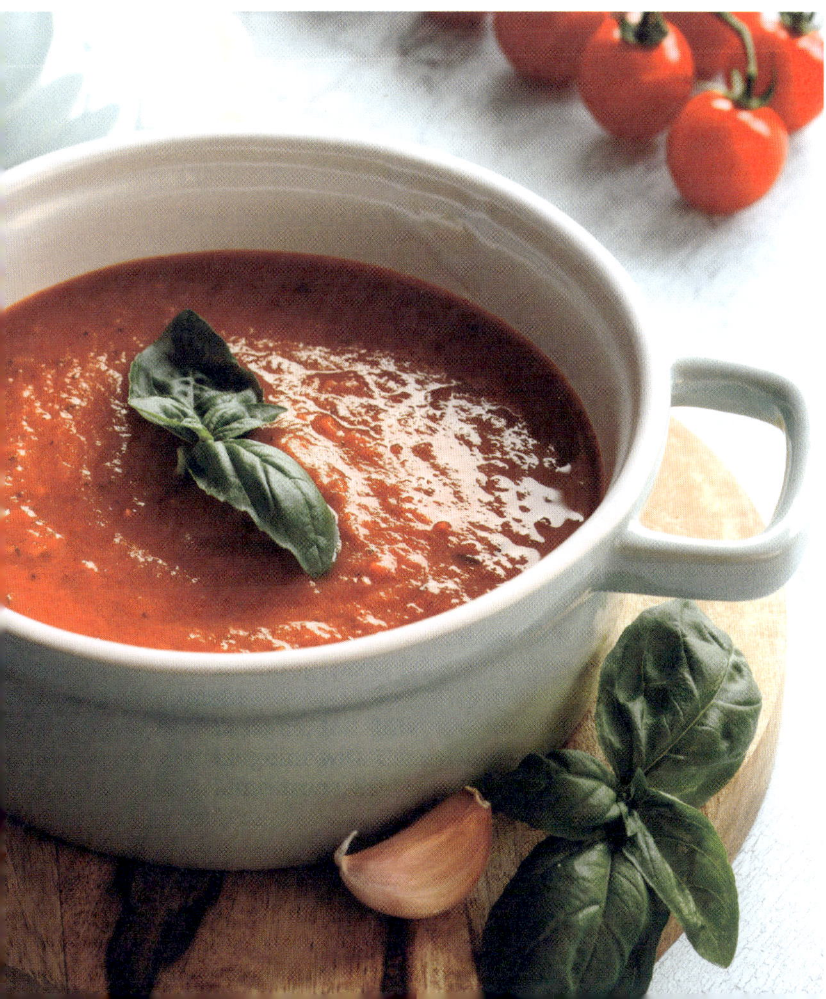

Herb paste

For 1 teaspoon chopped fresh herbs, use an equal amount of herb paste, or half the amount of dried herbs, as dried herbs have a more intense flavor. I use Gourmet Garden Herb Pastes in my recipes—they are convenient, as they can be stored in the refrigerator and are already pureed.

If using dried herbs, make sure they have softened in the cooking process. To remove pieces of herbs, run the puree through a mesh strainer lined with cheesecloth using a silicone spatula.

Matzo Ball Soup

SERVINGS: 4 | IDDSI LEVELS  

The secret to these tender matzo balls lies in the addition of beaten egg whites and room-temperature club soda. Frozen matzo balls are available in the international freezer section of the supermarket, but this homemade recipe is so much more delicious.

FOR THE MATZO BALLS

½ cup matzo meal*
1 teaspoon chopped fresh parsley or parsley paste (optional)
¼ teaspoon sea salt
⅛ teaspoon white pepper
2 tablespoons vegetable oil
2 tablespoons low-sodium chicken broth
2 tablespoons club soda, at room temperature
1 large egg white

* *If matzo meal isn't available, break up five matzo crackers, place in a mini food processor, and pulse until the crackers turn into a fine meal. This should yield ½ cup.*

To make the matzo balls

1. In a medium mixing bowl, combine the matzo meal, parsley, salt, and pepper. Add the oil, broth, and club soda, and stir to combine.

2. In a separate small bowl, whisk the egg white until frothy, about 1 minute. Add the egg white to the matzo ball mixture and mix well. Cover the bowl with plastic wrap and refrigerate for 30 minutes.

3. Once the matzo ball mix has rested, in a large pot, bring 2 quarts of water to a gentle boil. Using wet hands or a 1-inch ice cream scoop, form 1-inch matzo balls. Take care to handle the matzo balls gently and pack them loosely; this is the secret to making them tender.

4. Gently slide the matzo balls into the boiling water and cook, uncovered, for about 20 minutes. Use a slotted spoon to remove one matzo ball; cut it open to make sure it is cooked through. Once they are done cooking, transfer the remaining matzo balls to a plate.

FOR THE SOUP

- 1 quart low-sodium chicken broth
- 1 pound boneless, skinless chicken breasts
- 2 carrots, peeled and cut into rounds
- 2 parsnips, peeled and cut into rounds
- ½ yellow onion
- 1 teaspoon chopped fresh parsley or parsley paste
- 1 teaspoon chopped fresh dill or dill paste

To make the soup

1. In a soup pot, combine the broth, chicken, carrot, parsnip, onion, and herbs. Bring the broth to a boil, then lower to a simmer. Simmer until the chicken is cooked through and the vegetables are soft, about 15 minutes. Remove from the heat and allow to cool slightly.

2. Transfer the chicken breasts to a cutting board and cut into 1-inch cubes. Remove and discard the onion.

3. Set aside any family servings before pureeing, adding matzo balls, carrots, and parsnips to each serving.

4. For the puree, add 4 ounces chicken breast per serving to a blender or food processor. Pulse a few times to chop the chicken, add 2 matzo balls, ¼ cup broth, and a few pieces of carrot and parsnip, and blend until smooth, adding additional broth, 1 tablespoon at a time, as needed to achieve a smooth puree.

5. Transfer the blended portions to a bowl. Test as you go and at time of serving to see if a thickening agent, thickened sauce, or thickened stock is needed; use IDDSI Testing Methods (*iddsi.org*) to help achieve the desired IDDSI level. See pages 42-47.

6. Serve immediately or divide into servings for storage or freezing, following the directions for Serving, page 77.

NUTRITIONAL ANALYSIS PER SERVING | 1 cup
202 calories, 9 g fat, 2 g saturated fat, 352 mg sodium, 4 g sugar, 17 g carbohydrates, 0.5 g fiber, 8 g protein

Split Pea Soup

SERVINGS: 4 | IDDSI LEVELS 

This vegetarian version of split pea soup omits the traditional ham hock. In its place is cumin, which imparts a smoky depth of flavor, and soy sauce for savoriness. I buy organic French lentils and split peas at a health food store because they are fresher in bulk.

¾ cup split peas
¼ cup French lentils
1 tablespoon extra-virgin olive oil
1 medium yellow onion, diced
2 carrots, halved lengthwise and sliced into half moons
1 garlic clove, sliced
1 tablespoon low-sodium soy sauce
½ teaspoon cumin
¼ teaspoon dried thyme
⅛ teaspoon white pepper
4 cups low-sodium vegetable broth
⅛ teaspoon sea salt

1. Place the split peas and lentils in a medium bowl, cover with cold water, and let sit for at least 1 hour. Drain the peas and lentils and rinse them in a mesh strainer, picking through to remove any stones. Set aside.

2. In a large pot, warm the olive oil over medium-high heat. Add the onion and sauté until translucent, about 3 minutes. Add carrots and sauté for 3 minutes. Add garlic and sauté, stirring, for 1 more minute. Add the soy sauce, cumin, thyme, and white pepper, and cook for another 30 seconds.

3. Add the peas, lentils, and broth, and bring to a boil. Lower the heat and simmer, skimming and discarding foam, until the peas and lentils are very soft, about 1 hour. If the soup thickens too much, add a splash of water. Season with salt, stir, and remove from the heat.

4. Working in batches, transfer the soup to a blender, filling the pitcher only two-thirds full and venting the lid. Blend until smooth, transferring each batch to a large bowl. Set aside any servings for family meals.

5. Test as you go and at time of serving to see if thickening is needed; use IDDSI Testing Methods (*iddsi.org*) to help achieve the desired IDDSI level. See pages 42-47.

6. Serve immediately or divide into servings for storage or freezing, following the directions for Serving, page 77.

NUTRITIONAL ANALYSIS PER SERVING | 1 cup
190 calories, 4 g fat, 4 g saturated fat, 676 mg sodium, 5 g sugar, 27 g carbohydrates, 9 g fiber, 13 g protein

Minestrone

SERVINGS: 4 | IDDSI LEVELS 

This version of the classic Italian vegetable soup is packed with nutrition and fiber, with heartiness from beans and pasta. This soup also presents a good opportunity to clean out the fridge—you can add whatever vegetables you have on hand, like string beans and spinach.

- 1 tablespoon extra-virgin olive oil
- 1 medium yellow onion, sliced
- 1 carrot, halved lengthwise and sliced into half moons
- 1 zucchini, halved lengthwise and sliced into half moons
- 1 garlic clove, sliced
- 1 quart low-sodium vegetable broth
- 1 (15-ounce) can diced tomatoes, or 1½ cups fresh plum tomatoes, seeded and chopped
- 1 cup small shell pasta
- 1 can light red kidney or cannellini beans, drained and rinsed
- 1 teaspoon chopped fresh parsley or parsley paste
- 1 teaspoon chopped fresh basil or basil paste

1. In a soup pot, warm the olive oil over medium heat. Add the onion and sauté until translucent, about 3 minutes. Add the carrot and zucchini and sauté until just softened, about 3 minutes. Add the garlic and sauté for 1 more minute.

2. Add the broth, tomato, and pasta, and bring to a boil. Lower to a simmer and cook until the pasta and vegetables are tender, about 15 minutes. Add the beans and herbs and simmer for another 5 minutes.

3. Set aside any servings for family meals. Working in batches, transfer the remaining soup to a blender. Only fill the blender pitcher two-thirds full and vent the lid to allow steam to escape.

4. Blend until smooth, transferring each blended batch to a large bowl. Test as you go and at time of serving to see if a thickening agent, thickened sauce, or thickened stock is needed; use IDDSI Testing Methods (*iddsi.org*) to help achieve the desired IDDSI level. See pages 42-47.

5. Serve immediately or divide into servings for storage or freezing, following the directions for Serving, page 77.

NUTRITIONAL ANALYSIS PER SERVING | 1 cup
199 calories, 1 g fat, 0 g saturated fat, 153 mg sodium, 1 g sugar, 34 g carbohydrates, 11 g fiber, 16 g protein

Wonton Soup

SERVINGS: 4 | IDDSI LEVELS 

This homemade version of a classic takeout favorite contains protein, green veggies, and carbs, with far less sodium than takeout. You can also add extra cooked vegetables to the puree for a nutritional boost.

- 1 quart low-sodium chicken broth
- 1 (½-inch) piece ginger, or 1 teaspoon ginger paste
- 2 scallions, sliced thinly on the bias
- ½ teaspoon low-sodium soy sauce
- 2 cups fresh spinach
- 2 packages gluten-free chicken or vegetable potstickers*
- 8 ounces roast pork loin (see page 140), sliced into matchsticks

* *Different brands of potstickers have different numbers per package. To make sure you have enough, buy two packages. Hint: Try to buy the brand with the thinnest pastry wrapping. Too much dough makes for a gummy puree.*

1. In a soup pot, bring the broth to a boil. Lower to a simmer and add the ginger, scallions, and soy sauce. Simmer for 2 minutes. Add the spinach and simmer for another 2 minutes, just until the spinach is wilted and bright green.
2. Remove the soup from the heat. Allow it to cool slightly. If using fresh ginger, remove and discard it.
3. Prepare the potstickers according to the package instructions.
4. Set aside any family servings of soup before pureeing, and serve with the potstickers and sliced pork.
5. For the puree, place 2 ounces of pork in a food processor or blender. Pulse 5 times to chop up the pork. Add 2 tablespoons broth and process until smooth. Add 3 potstickers per serving, and pulse to puree until smooth. Add the scallions, spinach, and 1 cup broth, and blend until completely smooth.
6. Return the puree to the pot with the remaining broth. Test as you go and at time of serving to see if a thickening agent, thickened sauce, or thickened stock is needed; use IDDSI Testing Methods (*iddsi.org*) to help achieve the desired IDDSI level. See pages 42-47.
7. Serve immediately or divide into servings for storage or freezing, following the directions for Serving, page 77.

NUTRITIONAL ANALYSIS PER SERVING | 1 cup
279 calories, 12.4 g fat, 1.3 g saturated fat, 499 mg sodium, 4.4 g sugar, 27.2 g carbohydrates, 3.2 g fiber, 4.5 g protein

Mushroom Barley Soup

SERVINGS: 4 | IDDSI LEVELS 

I made mushroom barley soup for my mother with chicken or vegetable stock, but you can use beef stock if you prefer. Served with a salad, this makes a lovely lunch. I like the flavor of baby Bella mushrooms, also known as cremini, but you can use any variety of mushrooms you prefer.

1 tablespoon extra-virgin olive oil
4 scallions, or ½ yellow onion, sliced
2 carrots, halved lengthwise and sliced into ¼-inch half moons
1 pound baby Bella or cremini mushrooms, quartered
1 cup pearl barley, rinsed
6 cups low-sodium chicken broth

1. In a large sauté pan, warm the olive oil over medium-high heat. Add the scallions and sauté until softened, about 2 minutes. Add the carrots and sauté 3 more minutes. Add the mushrooms and cook, stirring occasionally, until they soften, release their liquid, and turn a light golden brown, about 10 minutes. If they begin to brown too quickly, lower the heat to medium. Add the barley and stir to coat the grains in the oil.

2. Add the broth, bring the soup to a boil, and lower to a simmer. Cook, skimming any light foam that rises to the surface of the pot, until the barley is tender, about 30 minutes. Remove from the heat. Set aside any family servings before pureeing.

3. For the puree, working in batches, transfer the soup to a blender, filling the pitcher only two-thirds full and venting the lid. Blend until smooth, transferring each blended batch to a large bowl.

4. Test as you go and at time of serving to see if a thickening agent, thickened sauce, or thickened stock is needed; use IDDSI Testing Methods (*iddsi.org*) to help achieve the desired IDDSI level. See pages 42-47.

5. Serve immediately or divide into servings for storage or freezing, following the directions for Serving, page 77.

NUTRITIONAL ANALYSIS PER SERVING | 1 cup
261 calories, 6 g fat, 1 g saturated fat, 181 mg sodium, 3 g sugar, 46 g carbohydrates, 9 g fiber, 9 g protein

Chawan Mushi (Japanese Teacup Soup)

SERVINGS: 1 | IDDSI LEVELS 

Chawan means "teacup" in Japanese—this Japanese egg custard soup is traditionally steamed and served in a small teacup. The custard has a soft and delicate texture and is comforting and tasty. The vegetables and proteins are pureed before they are added to the custard, so once the soup has been steamed and cooled, it is ready to eat. These instructions call for a steamer basket, but you can also use an electric pressure cooker with a steam setting. For the broth, you can also use Japanese broths such as dashi or miso.

1 teaspoon vegetable oil
4 ounces cooked chicken breast, cut into cubes
4 cooked shrimp, tails removed
¼ cup sliced button mushrooms, wiped with a damp paper towel
2 tablespoons grated or julienned carrots
2 scallions, thinly sliced
1 cup low-sodium chicken broth, vegetable broth, or dashi
2 large eggs
1 teaspoon low-sodium soy sauce

1. Add the oil to a small sauté pan over medium heat. Add the chicken, shrimp, mushrooms, carrots, and scallions and sauté, stirring occasionally, until the vegetables are softened, about 3 minutes. Add the proteins and vegetables to a food processor or high-speed blender, along with 2 tablespoons broth. Puree until smooth.

2. In a medium bowl, beat the eggs. Add the remaining broth, the puree, and the soy sauce, and whisk to combine. Pour the mixture into a ramekin.

3. Add 2 inches of water to the bottom of a stockpot fitted with a steamer basket. Bring the water to a boil over high heat. Lower the heat so the water is at a simmer.

4. Place the filled ramekin in the steamer basket, cover the pot, and steam undisturbed until the eggs are set and a toothpick inserted into the custard comes out clean, about 12 minutes. Allow to cool before serving.

5. Serve immediately. (I do not suggest freezing this.)

NUTRITIONAL ANALYSIS PER SERVING | 1 cup
86 calories, 5 g fat, 1 g saturated fat, 238 mg sodium, 0 g sugar, 1 g carbohydrates, 0 g fiber, 10 g protein

Salads

90 Tomato Cucumber Salad with Red Onion *(Vinaigrette Dressing)*

92 Tuna Avocado Salad *(Ranch Dressing)*

94 Celery Root Remoulade *(Pink Remoulade)*

96 Red Beet Salad with Ranch Dressing

97 Summer Slaw

98 Chunk Chicken Salad

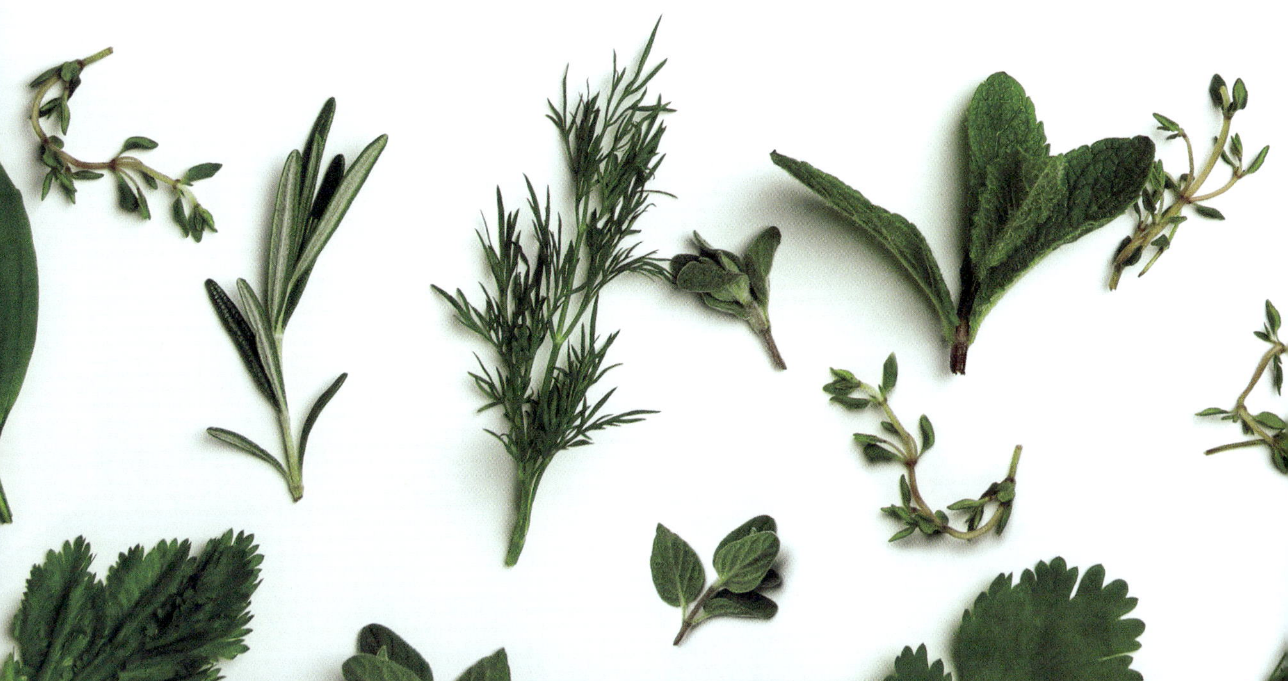

Tomato Cucumber Salad with Red Onion

SERVINGS: 2 | IDDSI LEVELS  

An easy-to-make fresh salad that purees and thickens beautifully.

1 medium tomato, quartered and seeded
½ cucumber, peeled, seeded, and sliced
¼ small red onion, diced
3 tablespoons Vinaigrette Dressing (see page 91)

1. Add the tomato, cucumber, red onion, and Vinaigrette Dressing to a medium bowl and stir to combine. If reserving a portion for family meals, set aside, cover, and refrigerate until ready to serve.

2. For the puree, add the remaining salad to a blender or nutrition extractor. Blend until completely smooth. Using a silicone spatula, rub the puree through a strainer set over a medium bowl to remove any fibers, discarding the fibers in the strainer.

3. Test as you go and at time of serving to see if a thickening agent, thickened sauce, or thickened stock is needed; use IDDSI Testing Methods (*iddsi.org*) to help achieve the desired IDDSI level. See pages 42-47.

4. Serve, or store covered in the refrigerator for up to 24 hours. (I do not suggest freezing this.)

NUTRITIONAL ANALYSIS PER SERVING | ½ cup
Salad without dressing
143 calories, 14 g fat, 2 g saturated fat, 26 mg sodium, 2 g sugar, 5 g carbohydrates, 1 g fiber, 1 g protein

Vinaigrette Dressing

SERVINGS: 2-4 | IDDSI LEVEL 

I use a ratio of 2 parts oil to 1 part vinegar. This is a low-acid vinaigrette. I like to use a mild vinegar, such as rice vinegar.

¼ cup extra-virgin olive oil
2 tablespoons rice vinegar or lemon juice
½ teaspoon Dijon mustard
Sea salt and white pepper

Place all the ingredients in a small jar with a screw-on lid and shake until well combined. Alternatively, place all the ingredients in a small bowl and mix with a fork or a whisk until well combined.

NUTRITIONAL ANALYSIS PER SERVING | 1 tablespoon
126 calories, 14.1 g fat, 2 g saturated fat, 39 mg sodium, 2.3 g sugar, 1.8 g carbohydrates, 0.1 g fiber, 0.1 g protein

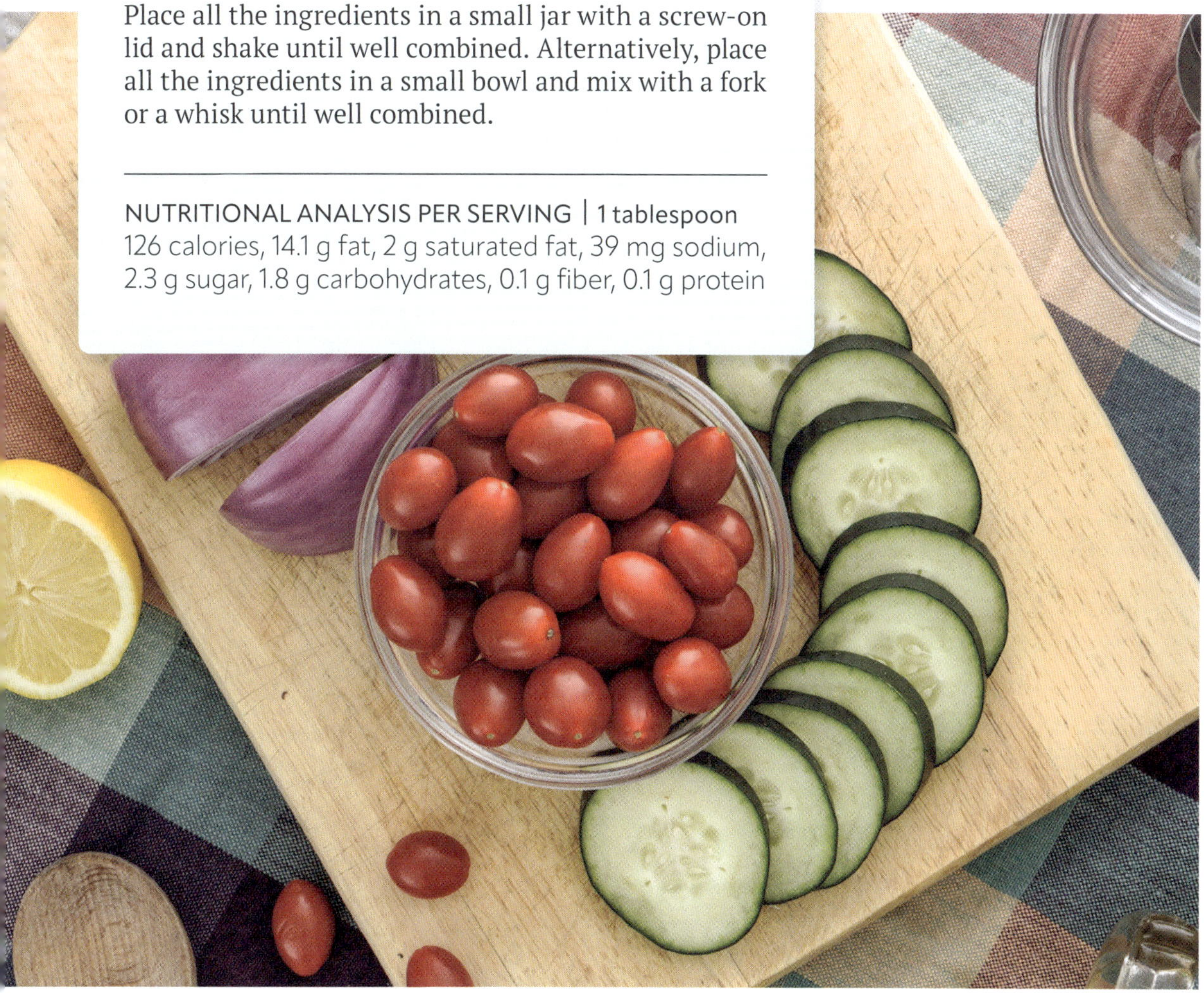

Tuna Avocado Salad

SERVINGS: 2 | IDDSI LEVELS 

A smooth, creamy salad with plenty of protein and healthy fats from the avocado. I like to serve this tasty tuna salad with a bowl of soup for a light dinner or for lunch.

1 (4.5-ounce) can low-sodium tuna, drained
1 avocado, diced
2 tablespoons Vinaigrette Dressing (see page 91)
1 tablespoon Ranch Dressing (see page 93)
1 tablespoon fresh lemon juice
Sea salt and white pepper

1. In a small bowl, combine the tuna, avocado, Vinaigrette Dressing, Ranch Dressing, lemon juice, salt, and white pepper, and stir to combine. If reserving a portion for family meals, set aside, cover, and refrigerate until ready to serve.

2. For the puree, put the salad in a food processor, pulse to incorporate, and process until you achieve the desired texture. Transfer the puree to a serving bowl, cover, and refrigerate. Test as you go and at time of serving to see if a thickening agent, thickened sauce, or thickened stock is needed; use IDDSI Testing Methods (*iddsi.org*) to help achieve the desired IDDSI level. See pages 42-47.

3. If not serving immediately, cover and store in the refrigerator for up to 24 hours. (I do not suggest freezing this.)

NUTRITIONAL ANALYSIS PER SERVING | 3 oz
Salad with dressing
396 calories, 30 g fat, 5 g saturated fat, 120 mg sodium, 0 g sugar, 6 g carbohydrates, 5 g fiber, 26 g protein

PRO TIP

You can also serve as a sandwich or a wrap, or puree the bread according to IDDSI directions (also see Resources, page 237).

Ranch Dressing

SERVINGS: 2-4 | IDDSI LEVEL 

With much better flavor than any store-bought dressing, it really takes only a few minutes to make.

2 scallions, white and light green parts, roughly chopped
1 cup buttermilk
1 cup plain Greek yogurt
½ cup mayonnaise
2 tablespoons chopped parsley or parsley paste
2 tablespoons chopped basil or basil paste
Sea salt and white pepper

1. Place the first six ingredients in a food processor or blender; process until smooth.
2. Taste and season with salt and white pepper.

NUTRITIONAL ANALYSIS PER SERVING | 2 tablespoons
102 calories, 0.6 g fat, 1.5 g saturated fat, 101 mg sodium, 1.6 g sugar, 4.2 g carbohydrates, 1.5 g fiber, 2.9 g protein

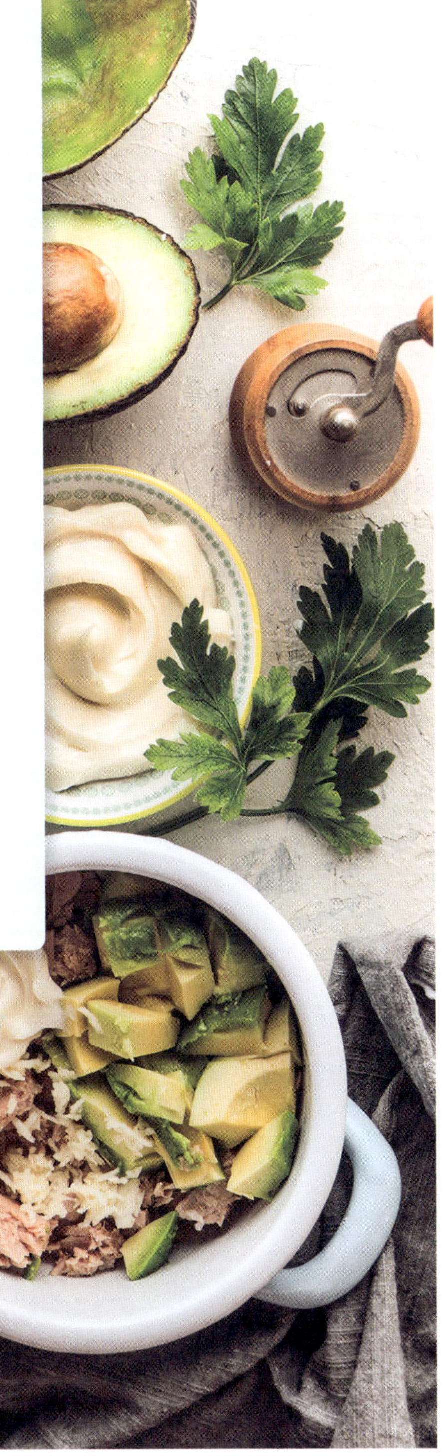

Celery Root Remoulade

SERVINGS: 4 | IDDSI LEVELS 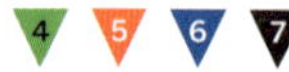

Celery root, or celeriac, may look gnarly and bumpy in the produce section, but ignore its appearance. When julienned, or sliced into thin matchsticks, and dressed with Pink Remoulade, you get a vibrant take on the classic French salad.

1 small celery root (about 1 pound), peeled and trimmed
¼ cup Pink Remoulade (see page 95)

1. Using a knife, a mandoline, a handheld julienning tool, or a food processor fitted with a julienne disc, slice the celery root into thin matchsticks.
2. Add the matchsticks to a bowl and toss with the Pink Remoulade. Set aside any servings for family meals that are not to be pureed, cover, and refrigerate until ready to serve.
3. For the puree, transfer the remaining mixture to a blender and process until you achieve the desired texture. Add water, 1 tablespoon at a time as needed (you want to avoid adding too much water and diluting the flavor of the salad).
4. Test as you go and at time of serving to see if a thickening agent, thickened sauce, or thickened stock is needed; use IDDSI Testing Methods (*iddsi.org*) to help achieve the desired IDDSI level. See pages 42-47.
5. Serve, or cover and store in the refrigerator for no more than 48 hours. (I do not suggest freezing this.)

NUTRITIONAL ANALYSIS PER SERVING | ½ cup (½ cup celeriac and 1 tablespoon remoulade)
167 calories, 6 g fat, 1 g saturated fat, 410 mg sodium, 7.5 g sugar, 27.2 g carbohydrates, 7 g fiber, 4.7 g protein

Pink Remoulade

SERVINGS: 2-4 | IDDSI LEVEL 

This sauce comes from regional Texas cuisine. A daring pink, the remoulade is perfect for summer dishes of all kinds. I like to use a healthier mayonnaise called Lemonaise, from a California company called the Ojai Cook, but new products are coming out all the time. Read the labels. Alternatively, your favorite mayo is just fine. Thicken to IDDSI Moderately Thick, Level 3, for sauces and gravies.

1 cup mayonnaise
2 tablespoons fresh lemon juice
1 teaspoon smooth brown mustard
1 garlic clove, grated, or 1 teaspoon garlic paste
1 teaspoon paprika
¼ teaspoon Worcestershire sauce
¼ teaspoon ketchup

Combine all the ingredients in a bowl and whisk until smooth. Add 1 to 3 tablespoons water, if needed, to reach the desired consistency. Taste and adjust the seasoning as needed.

NUTRITIONAL ANALYSIS PER SERVING | 2 tablespoons
120 calories, 6 g fat, 1 g saturated fat, 394 mg sodium, 5.5 g sugar, 17.7 g carbohydrates, 5 g fiber, 3 g protein

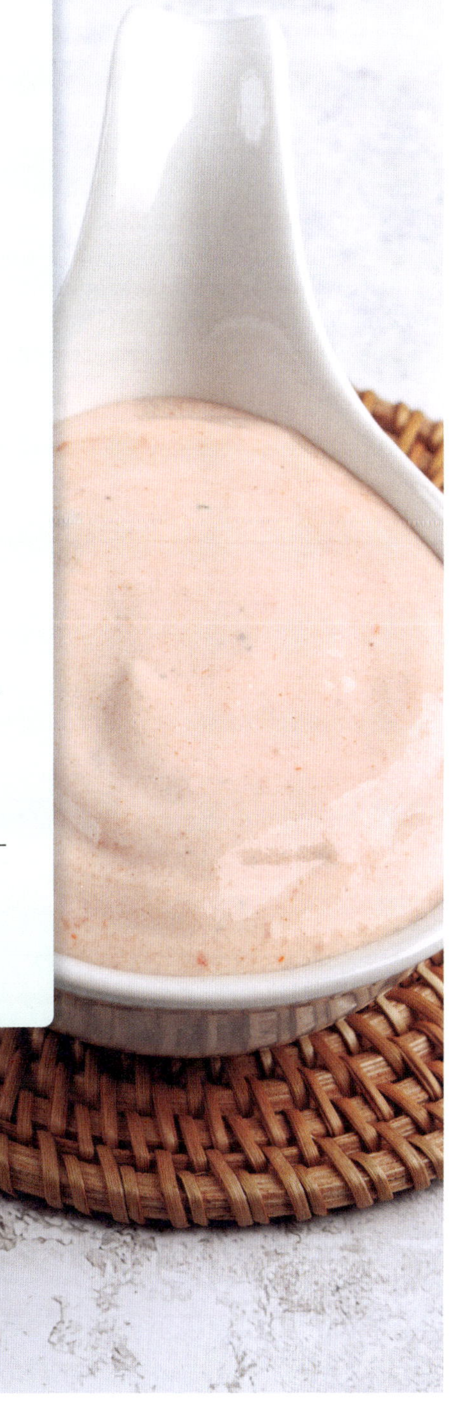

Red Beet Salad with Ranch Dressing

SERVINGS: 2 | IDDSI LEVELS 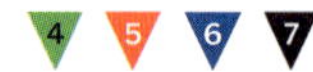

Beets are a nutritional powerhouse, and fermented foods are good for the human gut. This tangy salad has wonderful flavor and a beautiful pink color. Remember, we eat with our eyes, so adding this vibrant pink salad to the menu is a sure way to avoid boredom. **The Ranch Dressing tames the acid in the pickling juice, but check with your healthcare provider for clearance on pickled items to ensure they are safe for the swallow.** You do not want the person with dysphagia to aspirate due to a sudden intake of breath because of the vinegar.

1 (16-ounce) jar sliced pickled beets, such as Aunt Nellie's, drained, with pickling liquid reserved
½ cup red onion, thinly sliced (optional)
2 tablespoons pickling liquid from the jar of beets
6 tablespoons Ranch Dressing (see page 93), or store-bought
Sea salt and white pepper

For the person with dysphagia:

1. Add the beets, onion, and pickling liquid to a food processor and pulse until coarsely chopped. Process until you achieve the desired texture.

2. Using a silicone spatula, run the puree through a strainer set over a bowl to remove any fibers.

3. Stir the Ranch Dressing, salt, and white pepper into the beet puree. Test as you go and at time of serving to see if a thickening agent, thickened sauce, or thickened stock is needed; use IDDSI Testing Methods (*iddsi.org*) to help achieve the desired IDDSI level. See pages 42-47.

4. Serve, or cover and store in the refrigerator for no more than 48 hours. (I do not suggest freezing this.)

For non-pureed servings for family members:

Mix the beets and onion in a medium bowl. (Do not add the pickling liquid.) Add the Ranch Dressing, salt, and pepper, and mix to combine. Cover and refrigerate until ready to serve.

NUTRITIONAL ANALYSIS PER SERVING | ½ cup
90 calories, 6 g fat, 1 g saturated fat, 257 mg sodium, 0 g sugar, 10 g carbohydrates, 1 g fiber, 1 g protein

Summer Slaw

SERVINGS: 4-6 | IDDSI LEVELS   

You can make this crunchy summer slaw for a gathering of family and friends and simply separate the serving for the person with swallowing difficulties to puree it. To julienne the vegetables, you can use a knife, a mandoline, a handheld julienning tool, or a food processor fitted with a julienne disc. The Pink Remoulade is excellent as a substitute for store-bought coleslaw dressing.

1 small jicama, peeled and cut into thin matchsticks
1 small Granny Smith or Gala apple, peeled, cored, and cut into thin matchsticks
1 small Asian pear, peeled, cored, and cut into thin matchsticks
1 small carrot, peeled and cut into thin matchsticks
1 cup thinly sliced red cabbage
2 tablespoons Pink Remoulade (see page 95)

1. Add the first five ingredients and the dressing to a large mixing bowl and toss thoroughly to combine. Set aside any servings for family meals that are not to be pureed, cover, and refrigerate until ready to serve.

2. For the puree, transfer 1 cup slaw to a food processor or high-speed blender and pulse until the slaw breaks down into a smooth puree.

3. Test as you go and at time of serving to see if a thickening agent, thickened sauce, or thickened stock is needed; use IDDSI Testing Methods (*iddsi.org*) to help achieve the desired IDDSI level. See pages 42-47.

4. Serve, or cover and store in the refrigerator for up to 48 hours. (I do not suggest freezing this.)

NUTRITIONAL ANALYSIS PER SERVING | 3 oz
106 calories, 6 g fat, 1 g saturated fat, 197 mg sodium, 9.5 g sugar, 13.3 g carbohydrates, 2.1 g fiber, 1 g protein

Chunk Chicken Salad

SERVINGS: 2 | IDDSI LEVELS 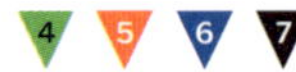

A delicious and creamy chicken salad that can be made with leftovers from a rotisserie chicken or Cornish Game Hens (page 102), or from scratch with poached chicken breasts.

1 cup cubed cooked chicken (from a rotisserie chicken*)
1 stalk celery, peeled and finely diced
2 tablespoons mayonnaise
2 tablespoons low-fat sour cream
2 tablespoons chopped fresh parsley or parsley paste
Sea salt and white pepper

* *If you are not using a rotisserie chicken, use the following method to poach chicken: Place 1 pound boneless, skinless chicken breasts or thighs in a large saucepan and cover with water or broth. Bring to a boil, lower the heat to a simmer, and cook until the chicken reaches an internal temperature of 165°F (75°C), 10 to 15 minutes. If you poach chicken for this recipe, you can use the poaching liquid in place of water in the puree.*

1. In a medium bowl, combine the chicken, celery, mayonnaise, sour cream, parsley, salt, and white pepper. If reserving a portion for family meals, set aside, cover, and refrigerate until ready to serve.

2. For the puree, transfer the remaining salad to a blender and add 2 tablespoons water. Pulse until the chicken is broken down. Then process until you achieve the desired texture, adding more water if needed for blending.
   › **Tip:** I recommend peeling the celery to remove the strings before pureeing. It's an extra step, but it makes for a smoother puree. A high-speed blender or nutrition extractor will eliminate most of the celery fibers, but to eliminate any possibility of strings, push the puree through a mesh strainer to remove them.

3. Test as you go and at time of serving to see if a thickening agent, thickened sauce, or thickened stock is needed; use IDDSI Testing Methods (*iddsi.org*) to help achieve the desired IDDSI level. See pages 42-47.

4. If not serving immediately, cover and store in the refrigerator for no more than 48 hours. (I do not suggest freezing this.)

NUTRITIONAL ANALYSIS PER SERVING | ½ cup
180 calories, 15 g fat, 2 g saturated fat, 70 mg sodium, 0 g sugar, 1 g carbohydrates, 1 g fiber, 12 g protein

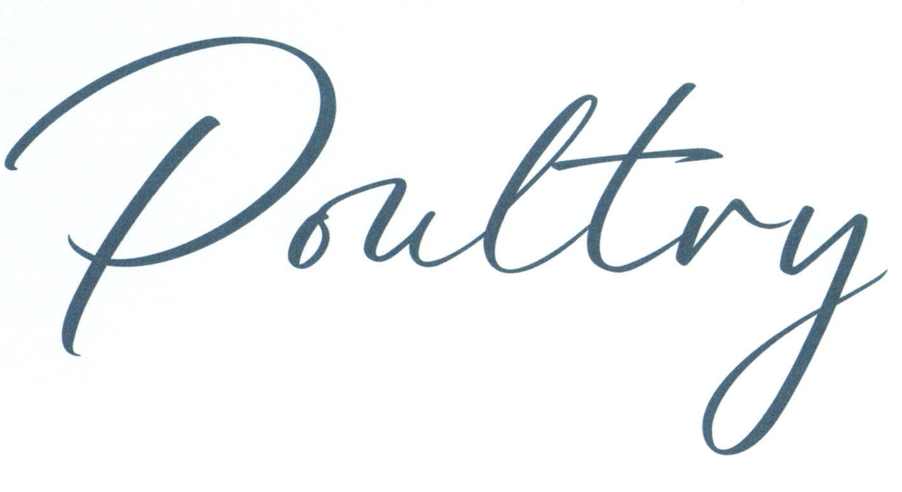

Poultry

100 Chicken Pot Pie
(*Pot Pie Crust*)

102 Cornish Game Hens
with Pan Gravy

104 Chicken Marsala

106 Roast Turkey Breast
with Lemon and Herbs
(*Herb Gravy*)

108 Mom's Turkey Meatloaf

Chicken Pot Pie

SERVINGS: 4 | IDDSI LEVELS 

Chicken pot pie is a favorite American comfort food. This recipe is simple to prepare because it uses store-bought cream of chicken soup and store-bought pie crust, and it is delicious.

1 tablespoon extra-virgin olive oil
1 medium carrot, cut into ¼-inch rounds
½ cup pearl onions, or ½ yellow onion, diced
1 packet instant cream of chicken soup mix
1 pound cooked chicken meat, torn or chopped into bite-size pieces (from a rotisserie chicken*)
½ cup to 1 cup frozen peas
1 Pot Pie Crust (see page 101)

* *If you are not using a rotisserie chicken, use the following method to poach chicken. Place 1 pound boneless, skinless chicken breasts or thighs in a large saucepan and cover with water or broth. Bring to a boil, lower to a simmer, and cook until the chicken reaches an internal temperature of 165°F (75°C), 10 to 15 minutes.*

1. Heat the olive oil in a medium saucepan over medium heat. Add the carrot and onions and cook, stirring occasionally, until softened, about 5 minutes.

2. Add the soup mix to the saucepan along with ½ cup water and stir to combine. Bring to a simmer and cook for 2 minutes. Add the chicken and peas, stir to combine, and simmer for another 2 minutes. Remove from the heat.

3. After setting aside any servings for family meals that are not to be pureed, add one serving to the food processor. Pulse to break up the chicken, then process until you achieve the desired texture.

4. Test as you go and at time of serving to see if a thickening agent, thickened sauce, or thickened stock is needed; use IDDSI Testing Methods (*iddsi.org*) to help achieve the desired IDDSI level. See pages 42-47.

5. Divide the servings between the dishes or storage containers and using a squeeze bottle or piping bag with a wide nozzle, pipe Pot Pie Crust puree onto the filling, in the shape of dots, slices, or swirls. You can also simply dollop the crust puree onto the filling with a spoon. For family servings, add a reserved baked crust round.

6. Serve immediately, or allow to cool completely, cover, and refrigerate for up to 48 hours or freeze for up to 3 months.

NUTRITIONAL ANALYSIS PER SERVING | 4 oz
Without pie crust
261 calories, 6 g fat, 1 g saturated fat, 181 mg sodium, 3 g sugar, 46 g carbohydrates, 9 g fiber, 9 g protein

Pot Pie Crust

SERVINGS: 4 | IDDSI LEVEL 

Unbleached all-purpose flour, for dusting
1 pie crust, preferably unbleached flour
1 large egg
2 tablespoons warm broth or water

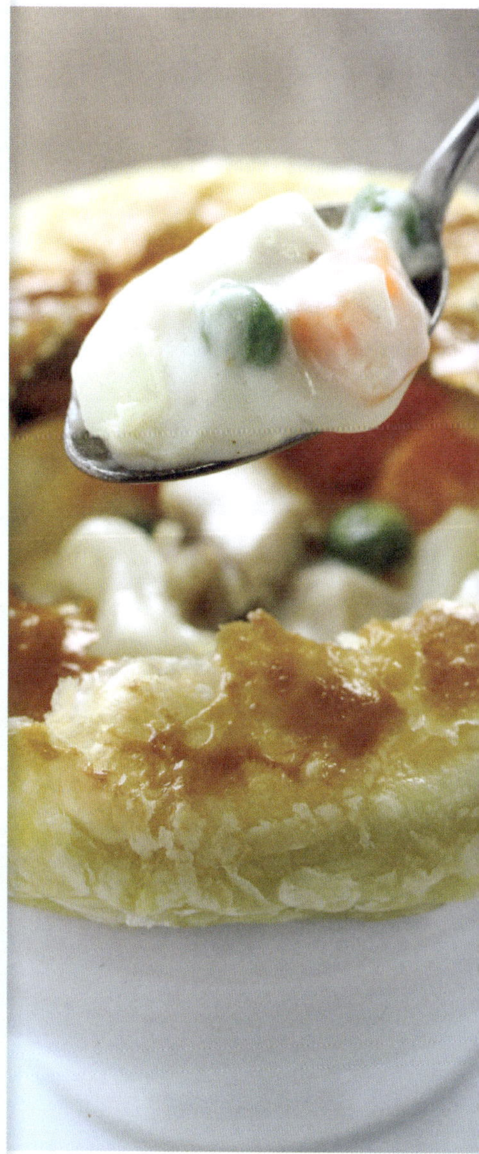

1. Place a rack in the center of the oven and preheat to 400°F (205°C). Line a baking sheet with parchment paper and set aside.

2. Dust a clean work surface with flour. Roll the pie crust to ¼ inch thick. Using a biscuit cutter, cut four 4-inch rounds of pie crust and transfer them to the prepared baking sheet.

3. Beat the egg with 1 tablespoon water. Using a pastry brush, brush the surface of the crust with the egg wash. Transfer to the oven and bake until golden brown, about 8 minutes. Set aside to cool.

4. Reserve baked crust rounds for any servings that are being frozen for family meals.

5. Break the remaining cooled crusts into a food processor. Add 1½ teaspoons warm broth or water per crust round and pulse to combine.

6. Process until smooth. Add thickener to IDDSI Pureed, Level 4 (see page 44), and pulse to combine. Transfer the crust mixture to a chef's squeeze bottle with a large opening or a piping bag. Let stand until thickened, about 3 minutes, before topping your pot pie.

NUTRITIONAL ANALYSIS PER SERVING | ⅛ crust (25 g)
120 calories, 7 g fat, 3.5 g saturated fat, 85 mg sodium, 0 g sugar, 12 g carbohydrates, 0 g fiber, 1 g protein

Cornish Game Hens with Pan Gravy

SERVINGS: 4 | IDDSI LEVELS 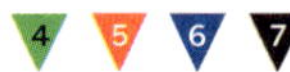

These little hens have plenty of flavor and present a change from takeout rotisserie roast chicken that may be high in sodium. Buy hens that have never been frozen, if they are available. Otherwise, thaw the frozen hen in the fridge overnight. You can puree the carrots and onion and serve them as a side dish with the hens.

- 2 Cornish game hens
- 1 yellow onion, cut into wedges
- 2 carrots, peeled and cut into 1-inch sections
- 1 celery stalk, cut into 1-inch sections
- 1 bay leaf
- 1 cup low-sodium chicken broth
- ¼ cup white wine (optional)
- 1 small lemon, halved
- 2 sprigs rosemary
- 2 garlic cloves
- 1 tablespoon extra-virgin olive oil
- Sea salt and white pepper
- 2 tablespoons Wondra flour

1. Place a rack in the center of the oven and preheat to 400°F (205°C). Remove and reserve any giblets from inside the hens. In the bottom of a roasting pan with a rack, arrange the onion, carrots, celery, bay leaf, and giblets. Add the broth and wine, if using, and top with the rack. This will be the base of your gravy.

2. Into the cavity of each bird, place ½ lemon, a sprig of rosemary, and a garlic clove. Rub the outside of the hens with the olive oil, then season with salt and white pepper.

3. Place the birds on top of the roasting rack, with some room between them to allow air to circulate. Roast for 20 minutes per pound, until the juices run clear when a knife is inserted into the joint between the breast and the thigh, or until a thermometer inserted into the thickest part of the thigh registers 165°F (75°C).

4. Remove from the oven and transfer the birds to a cutting board or platter to cool.

5. To make the gravy, remove the rack from the roasting pan. Remove the vegetables, giblets, and bay leaf from the drippings in the pan. In a small bowl, combine the Wondra flour with 2 tablespoons water to make a slurry, and whisk until the mixture is smooth.

6. Place the roasting pan on the stovetop over medium heat and bring the pan drippings to a simmer. Add the slurry to the pan drippings and cook, whisking constantly, until the mixture comes to a boil and thickens. Lower the heat to low and simmer for 5 minutes. Remove from the heat.
   › **Tip:** If you like liver, you can add the liver to the gravy puree. You can discard the bay leaf and then puree the carrot and onions—I find the celery can become a bit stringy; thicken them to the prescribed IDDSI level [see page 41], and serve them as a side dish with the hens.

7. Once the birds have cooled, carve off the breasts and remove the meat from the legs and wings. Divide the meat into servings of 4 to 6 ounces and reserve any servings for family meals, if desired.

8. Place the remaining portions to be pureed in a food processor or blender. Add ½ cup gravy per serving, and process until you achieve the desired texture. Test as you go and at time of serving to see if a thickening agent, thickened sauce, or thickened stock is needed; use IDDSI Testing Methods (*iddsi.org*) to help achieve the desired IDDSI level. See pages 42-47.

9. Serve, or divide into servings for storage or freezing, following the directions for Serving, page 77.

NUTRITIONAL ANALYSIS PER SERVING | 6 oz
173 calories, 4 g fat, 1 g saturated fat, 243 mg sodium, 3 g sugar, 8 g carbohydrates, 2 g fiber, 26 g protein

Chicken Marsala

SERVINGS: 2 | IDDSI LEVELS 

This flavorful recipe uses Marsala wine to make a pan sauce that purees beautifully. **Check with your healthcare provider to make sure there is no conflict between the Marsala wine and your medications.**

1 boneless, skinless chicken breast (8 ounces)
Salt and white pepper
2 tablespoons extra-virgin olive oil
8 ounces mushrooms, sliced
¼ cup Marsala wine
¼ cup low-sodium chicken broth
1 tablespoon finely chopped fresh parsley, or ¼ teaspoon dried parsley
2 teaspoons Wondra flour

1. Cut the chicken breast in half horizontally to create two thinner portions. If the chicken breasts are not of even thickness, place them between two sheets of plastic wrap and gently pound them with a kitchen mallet. Season the breasts with a pinch of salt and white pepper.

2. Heat 1 tablespoon olive oil in a large sauté pan over medium-high heat. Add the chicken breasts and sear until lightly golden brown, about 2 minutes per side. Transfer to a plate and set aside.

3. Warm the remaining 1 tablespoon oil, add the mushrooms, and sauté until softened and lightly golden in spots, about 3 minutes. Add the Marsala and the chicken broth and bring the mixture to a simmer.

4. Return the chicken to the pan and simmer, turning the breasts once, until they are cooked through, about 5 minutes. Add the parsley, stir to combine, and simmer for 1 more minute.

5. Remove the chicken and mushrooms from the pan, leaving behind the liquid.

6. In a small bowl, whisk 2 teaspoons Wondra flour with 4 teaspoons water. Whisk the mixture into the liquid in the pan. Bring to a simmer and cook, stirring occasionally, until the sauce is thickened, about 4 minutes.

7. Remove the pan from the heat. If reserving a portion for family meals, set aside one of the chicken breast portions, half the mushrooms, and half the sauce.

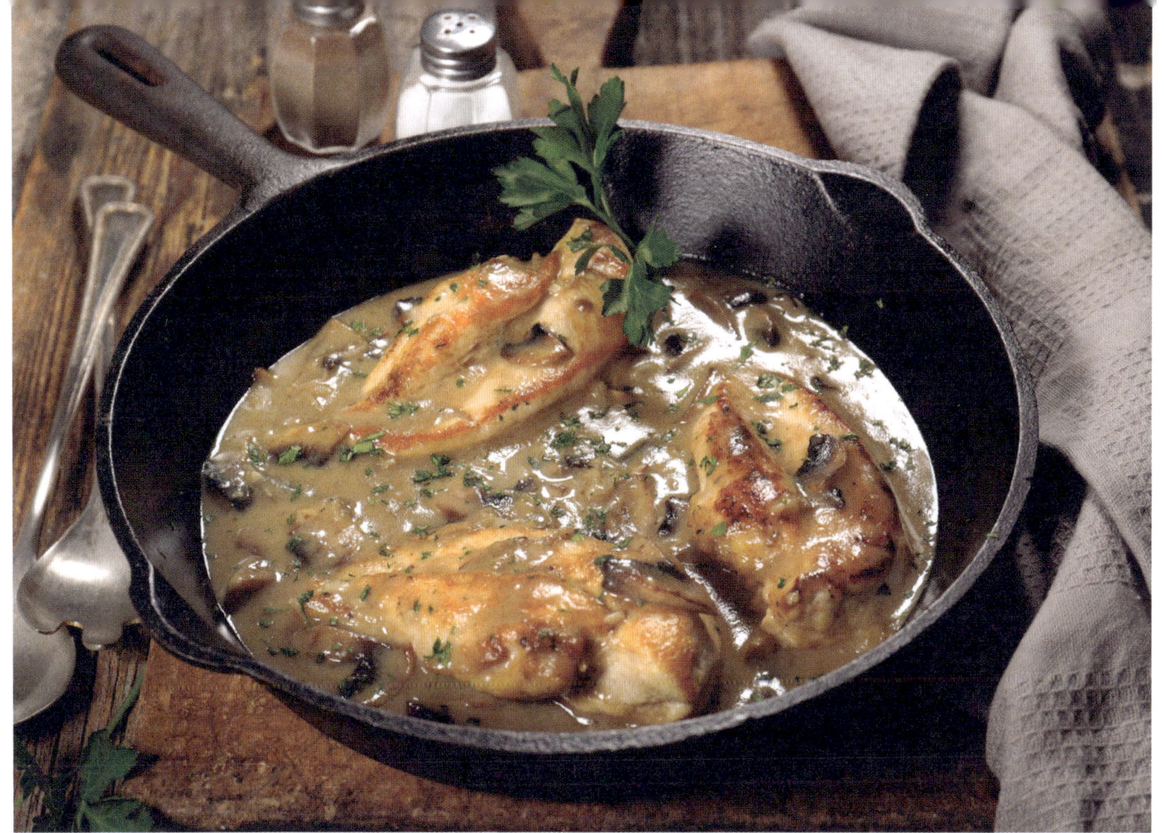

8. For the puree, chop the chicken breast into ½-inch pieces. Per serving, add 1 chicken breast portion, half the mushrooms, and ¼ cup Marsala sauce to a food processor or blender, and pulse to break up the chicken and the mushrooms. Process until you achieve the desired texture.

9. Test as you go and at time of serving to see if a thickening agent, thickened sauce, or thickened stock is needed; use IDDSI Testing Methods (*iddsi.org*) to help achieve the desired IDDSI level. See pages 42-47.

10. Serve immediately or divide into servings for storage or freezing, following the directions for Serving, page 77.

NUTRITIONAL ANALYSIS PER SERVING | 6 oz
167 calories, 4 g fat, 1 g saturated fat, 348 mg sodium, 2 g sugar, 6 g carbohydrates, 1 g fiber, 27 g protein

Roast Turkey Breast with Lemon and Herbs

SERVINGS: 8 | IDDSI LEVELS 

A turkey breast is more manageable than a whole bird. If you like dark meat, use the same herbs, but buy a package of legs. This is a festive centerpiece for a holiday meal. If you would like to serve the turkey with cranberry sauce, puree the cranberry sauce to a smooth texture and bind it with instant thickener (IDDSI Pureed, Level 4 works best for dipping sauces). I recommend serving this turkey breast with Mashed Potatoes (see page 176), as well as other pureed side vegetables—the more colorful, the better. As long as all the components of the holiday meal are the same thickness, the meal is safe for the swallow.

- 1 (6-pound) turkey breast
- 3 tablespoons extra-virgin olive oil
- 2 tablespoons chopped fresh rosemary or rosemary paste
- 2 tablespoons chopped fresh parsley or parsley paste
- 3 tablespoons chopped fresh sage or sage paste
- 2 tablespoons chopped fresh thyme leaves or thyme paste
- Zest of half a lemon
- Sea salt and white pepper
- 1 cup low-sodium turkey or chicken broth, plus more as needed
- ½ cup white wine (optional)
- Herb Gravy (see page 107)

1. Place a rack in the center of the oven and preheat to 325°F (165°C). Loosen the skin from the breast to prepare it for the herb paste. In a food processor, combine 2 tablespoons oil, the herbs, and the lemon zest. Process into a paste. Use your hands to apply the herb paste under the skin. Drizzle 1 tablespoon olive oil onto the breast and massage it into the skin. Season the breast liberally with salt and white pepper.

2. Place the breast on a rack in a roasting pan. Add the broth and wine to the roasting pan. Place the pan on the center rack and roast for 2 hours (20 minutes per pound), until the skin is golden brown, and a thermometer inserted into thickest part of the breast reads 160°F (70°C). If the skin becomes too brown during roasting, cover it loosely with aluminum foil.

3. Transfer the breast to a cutting board to rest for 15 minutes.

4. For any family meal servings, slice the turkey breast against the grain and serve with the gravy. For the puree, cut up the turkey meat (4 ounces per serving) and add it to a food processor or blender. Pulse to break up the turkey. Add ½ cup gravy per serving and process until you achieve the desired texture.

5. Test as you go and at time of serving to see if a thickening agent, thickened sauce, or thickened stock is needed; use IDDSI Testing Methods (*iddsi.org*) to help achieve the desired IDDSI level. See pages 42-47.

6. Serve immediately or divide into servings for storage or freezing, following the directions for Serving, page 77.

NUTRITIONAL ANALYSIS PER SERVING | 4 oz
Without gravy
212 calories, 14 g fat, 3 g saturated fat, 85 mg sodium, 0 g sugar, 0 g carbohydrates, 0 g fiber, 20 g protein

Herb Gravy

YIELD: 8 (¼-CUP) SERVINGS | IDDSI LEVEL 

This recipe uses the pan drippings from the Roast Turkey Breast with Lemon and Herbs (see page 106), for added flavor. If you do not have any pan drippings, you can use 2 full cups of broth. Store leftover gravy in a glass storage container in the freezer.

2 cups pan drippings, plus turkey or chicken broth, as needed
2 tablespoons extra-virgin olive oil
2 tablespoons unbleached all-purpose flour
1 teaspoon finely chopped fresh parsley or parsley paste
1 teaspoon finely chopped fresh thyme leaves or thyme paste
1 teaspoon finely chopped sage or sage paste
Sea salt and white pepper

1. Transfer the juices from the turkey breast roasting pan to a measuring cup. Add broth, as needed, to reach 2 cups liquid.

2. In a small saucepan, warm the olive oil over medium heat. Add the flour and cook, stirring constantly, until the flour is lightly golden brown, 2 to 3 minutes. Add the pan drippings and broth, a little at a time, whisking constantly to prevent lumps. Add the parsley, sage, thyme, salt, and pepper, stir to combine, and bring to a simmer. Simmer, stirring, until the gravy is thickened, about 3 minutes.

3. Remove from the heat, allow to cool for five minutes, then run the gravy through a mesh strainer set over a bowl or measuring cup. Stir in thickener to IDDSI Moderately Thick, Level 3, for gravy and sauces.

NUTRITIONAL ANALYSIS PER SERVING | ¼ cup
331 calories, 24.7 g fat, 3.7 g saturated fat, 93 mg sodium, 0.5 g sugar, 27.9 g carbohydrates, 5.7 g fiber, 4.2 g protein

Mom's Turkey Meatloaf

SERVINGS: 4 | IDDSI LEVELS 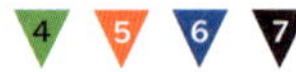

Meatloaf is the ultimate American comfort food. It's a diner classic, served with a side of Mashed Potatoes (see page 176) and Garlic Green Beans (see page 191). This recipe is for ground turkey, but it can also be made with ground chicken, ground beef, or a combination of ground beef and pork.

- 1 tablespoon extra-virgin olive oil
- ½ onion, finely diced
- 1 garlic clove, finely chopped, or 1 teaspoon garlic paste
- 1 pound ground turkey
- ¼ cup breadcrumbs*
- 2 tablespoons finely chopped fresh flat-leaf parsley or parsley paste
- 2 tablespoons parmesan cheese
- 1 large egg, lightly beaten
- 1 teaspoon Worcestershire sauce or low-sodium soy sauce
- ½ teaspoon sea salt
- ¼ teaspoon white pepper
- ½ cup ketchup (optional)
- Herb Gravy (see page 107)
- Mashed Potatoes (see page 176)

* *For those on gluten-free diets, use ½ cup old-fashioned oats in place of the breadcrumbs. Run the oats through a blender or food processor.*

1. Place a rack in the center of the oven and preheat to 375°F (190°C). Warm the olive oil in a medium sauté pan over medium heat. Add the onion and sauté until translucent, 3 minutes. Add the garlic and sauté 1 minute. Remove from the heat and set aside to cool.

2. Line a baking sheet with parchment paper. In a large bowl, combine the cooled onion and garlic with the ground turkey, breadcrumbs, parsley, parmesan, egg, Worcestershire, salt, and white pepper. Use clean hands to thoroughly incorporate the mixture, taking care not to overmix or compact the meat.

3. Transfer the mixture to the prepared baking sheet and gently form into a loaf. Spread the ketchup over the surface. (This is optional, but it prevents the meatloaf from drying out.)

4. Place the meatloaf in the oven. Cook to an internal temperature of 160°F (70°C). Depending on the heat of your oven and the shape of your baking pan or loaf pan, begin testing for temperature at 35 minutes. My oven cook time is 50 minutes.

5. Allow to rest for at least 10 minutes. Slice, and set aside any servings for family meals.
   - **Tip:** For pureeing, **use only the glaze on top of the meatloaf, not the glaze that adheres to the pan, to ensure the safe swallow.**

6. For the puree, add two slices (¼ of the loaf) per serving to a food processor or blender and pulse to break up. Add 2 tablespoons gravy and ½ cup mashed potatoes per serving and process until you achieve the desired texture, adding more gravy as needed.

7. Test as you go and at time of serving to see if a thickening agent, thickened sauce, or thickened stock is needed; use IDDSI Testing Methods (*iddsi.org*) to help achieve the desired IDDSI level. See pages 42-47.

8. Serve immediately or divide into servings for storage or freezing, following the directions for Serving, page 77.

NUTRITIONAL ANALYSIS PER SERVING | 4 oz
199 calories, 10 g fat, 3 g saturated fat, 186 mg sodium, 1 g sugar, 4 g carbohydrates, 1 g fiber, 22 g protein

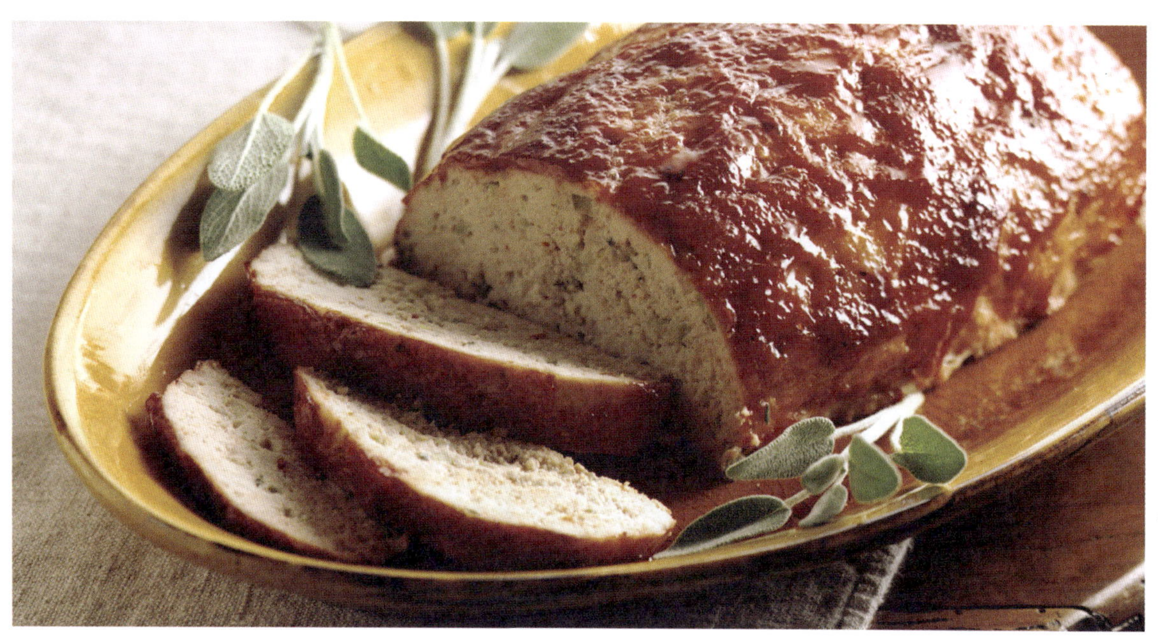

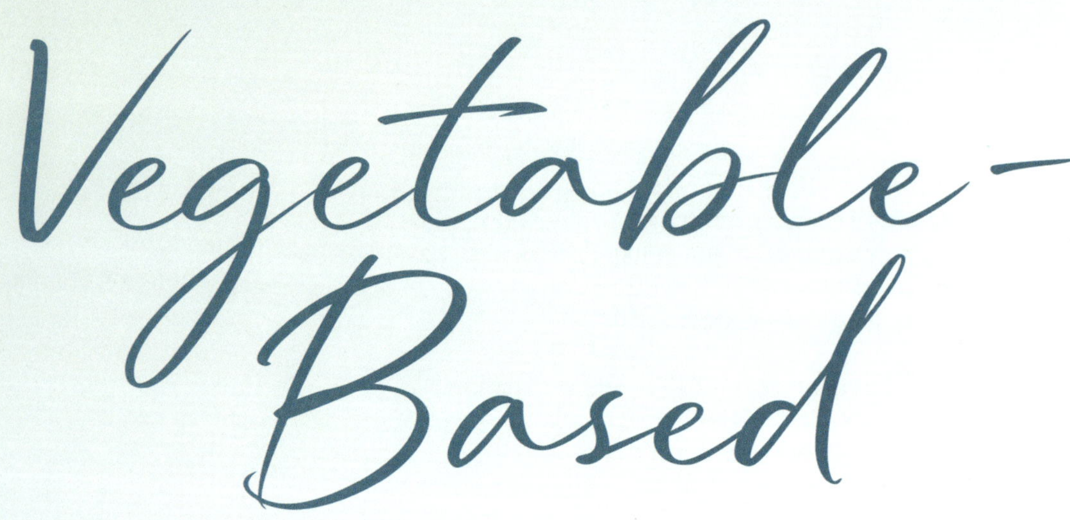

Vegetable-Based

111 Tempeh, Black Bean, and Veggie Chili

112 Asparagus and Mushroom Pot Pie

114 Eggplant Parmesan with Ricotta Topping

116 Vegetarian Almond Lentil Loaf

118 Vegetable Curry

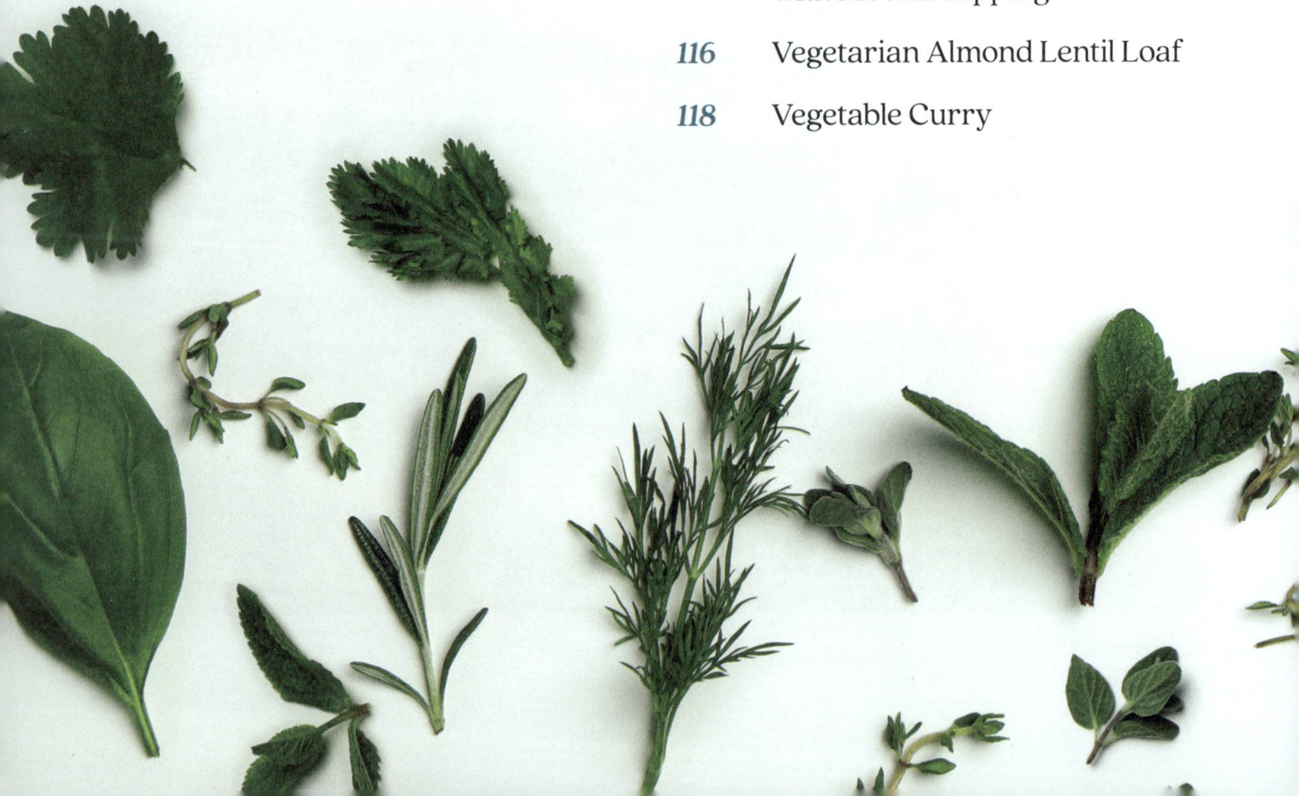

Tempeh, Black Bean, and Veggie Chili

SERVINGS: 6 | IDDSI LEVELS 

7

This vegetarian chili is so satiating and flavorful, you won't miss the meat. Tempeh, a protein source made from organic soybeans with millet, brown rice, and barley, is a traditional ingredient in Indonesian and Japanese cuisine. I prefer one from LightLife. To serve this dish as a family meal, top with cheddar cheese, sour cream, and sliced scallions.

2 tablespoons extra-virgin olive oil
6 ounces tempeh, cut into ½-inch cubes
2 teaspoons low-sodium soy sauce
1 red onion, finely diced
1 garlic clove, sliced
½ jalapeño pepper, stemmed, seeded, and finely diced
1 red bell pepper, diced
2 cups kabocha squash, cut into 2-inch pieces
3 large portobello mushrooms, cut into 2-inch pieces
2 leeks, white parts only, cleaned and sliced
1 (15-ounce) can diced tomatoes
1 (8-ounce) can tomato sauce
¼ cup tomato paste
1 (15-ounce) can black beans, drained
1 teaspoon Worcestershire sauce
2 tablespoons red wine (optional)
1 teaspoon chili powder (optional)

1. Warm the oil in a pot over medium heat or in a slow cooker with a sauté function. Add the tempeh and sauté, stirring occasionally, until lightly golden. Season with the soy sauce and stir to coat. Transfer the tempeh to a plate.

2. Add the onion, garlic, jalapeño, bell pepper, kabocha, portobellos, and leeks to the pot. Sauté, stirring occasionally, until softened and lightly caramelized, about 10 minutes. Add the diced tomatoes, tomato sauce, tomato paste, beans, Worcestershire, red wine, and chili powder, if using.

3. Return the tempeh to the pot and stir. If using a stove, bring to a boil, lower to a simmer, and cook, covered, with the lid ajar, about 1 hour. If using a slow cooker, cook on high for 1 hour. Set aside any servings for family meals.

4. For the puree, blend chili in batches, filling the pitcher only two-thirds full and venting the lid. Blend until you achieve the desired texture, transferring each batch to a large bowl.

5. Test as you go and at time of serving to see if a thickening agent, thickened sauce, or thickened stock is needed; use IDDSI Testing Methods (*iddsi.org*) to help achieve the desired IDDSI level. See pages 42-47.

6. Serve immediately or divide into servings for storage or freezing, following the directions for Serving, page 77.

NUTRITIONAL ANALYSIS PER SERVING | 1 cup
165 calories, 4 g fat, 1 g saturated fat, 214 mg sodium, 6 g sugar, 27 g carbohydrates, 6 g fiber, 10 g protein

Asparagus and Mushroom Pot Pie

SERVINGS: 4-6 | IDDSI LEVELS   

This vegetarian pot pie is delicious, and it presents an opportunity to get creative and use up leftover vegetables. Vary the vegetables in this pot pie according to the tastes of your household—in place of the asparagus, use leftovers of grilled, steamed, or roasted vegetables like broccoli, cauliflower, zucchini, string beans, Brussels sprouts, or squash. You can use another variety of soup as the base, add a can of cannellini beans for creaminess and protein, and get creative with the added cheese, using parmesan, cheddar, or goat cheese. These variations on vegetarian pot pie are easy, quick, and infinitely better than anything commercially packaged.

- 1 pound asparagus, woody ends trimmed, peeled if skins are tough, and cut into bite-sized pieces
- 1 (12-ounce) can mushroom bisque or cream of mushroom soup, such as Amy's
- ¼ cup grated Monterey Jack cheese
- 1 Pot Pie Crust (see page 101)

1. Fill a large pot fitted with a steamer basket with 2 inches of water. Bring the water to a boil, then reduce the heat to a simmer. Add the asparagus, cover the pot, and steam until tender, about 4 minutes.

2. Meanwhile, in a small saucepan, warm the mushroom bisque. Add only half the amount of water indicated on the can, so the liquid is thick. Add the cheese and stir until melted and thoroughly combined. Add the asparagus and stir to combine. Set aside any family servings before pureeing, adding a reserved baked crust round.

3. For the puree, add the cooled mixture to a food processor or blender. Pulse to break up the asparagus, then process until you achieve the desired texture.

4. Test as you go and at time of serving to see if a thickening agent, thickened sauce, or thickened stock is needed; use IDDSI Testing Methods (*iddsi.org*) to help achieve the desired IDDSI level. See pages 42-47.

5. Prepare the Pot Pie Crust puree according to directions (page 101).

6. Divide the servings between the dishes or storage containers, and using a squeeze bottle or piping bag with a wide nozzle, pipe Pot Pie Crust puree onto the filling, in the shape of dots, slices, or swirls. You can also simply dollop the puree crust onto the filling with a spoon.

7. Serve immediately, or allow to cool completely, cover, and refrigerate for up to 48 hours or freeze for up to 3 months.

NUTRITIONAL ANALYSIS PER SERVING | 4 oz
155 calories, 6.5 g fat, 0.9 g saturated fat, 426 mg sodium, 2.1 g sugar, 18.5 g carbohydrates, 7.6 g fiber, 8.6 g protein

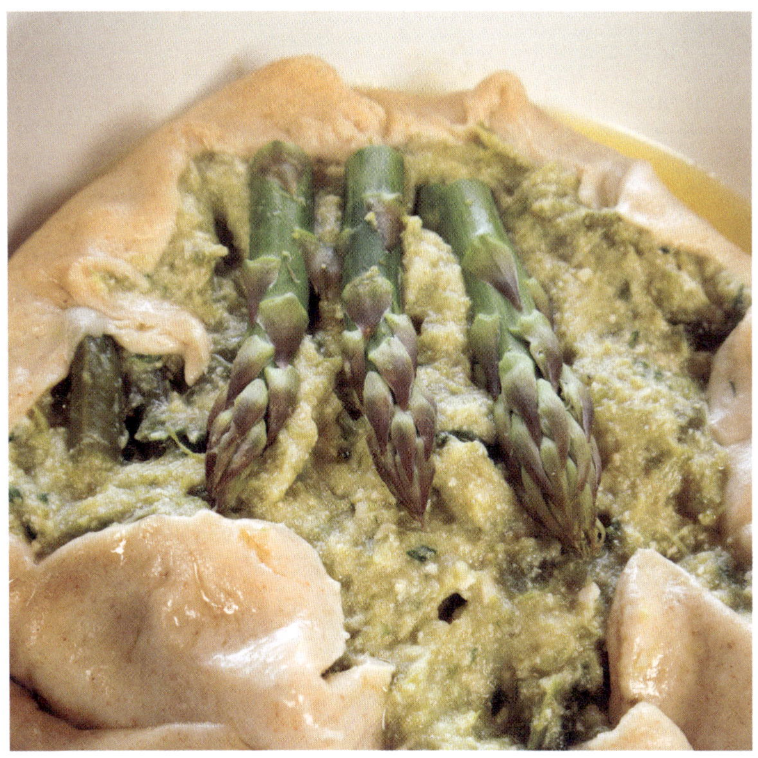

PRO TIP

To serve a whole pot pie for a family event, such as Game Day, add all the filling to an 8- or 9-inch baking dish and top with a store-bought pie crust. Paint the pie crust with an egg wash (a beaten egg and a tablespoon of water) and bake according to package instructions, usually forty minutes. Family and friends cut their own slices. For the loved one, puree the crust according to the directions for Pot Pie Crust puree given in the recipe on page 101 and puree and thicken the filling. In the serving dish, add the filling and top with the crust according to the directions.

Eggplant Parmesan with Ricotta Topping

SERVINGS: 6 | IDDSI LEVELS 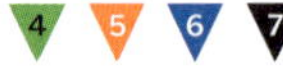

This version of the dish does not require breading and deep-frying. You can add sautéed ground beef or sliced, sautéed mushrooms to the tomato sauce for heartier variations of this recipe.

1 medium eggplant, peeled and sliced ⅜ inch thick
2 tablespoons extra-virgin olive oil
Sea salt and white pepper
2 cups part-skim ricotta*
¼ cup grated parmesan cheese, divided
2 large eggs
1 tablespoon freshly chopped parsley or parsley paste
1 tablespoon freshly chopped basil or basil paste
1 (16-ounce) jar pasta sauce, or 2 cups homemade tomato sauce (see Spaghetti with Tomato Sauce, page 156)

* *Ricotta expands when pureed, so one serving will puree to a larger volume than unpureed.*

1. Place a rack in the center of the oven and preheat the oven to 400°F (205°C). Line a baking sheet with parchment paper. Using a pastry brush, paint the slices of eggplant on both sides with oil and place on the baking sheet in a single layer. Season the slices with salt and white pepper.

2. Roast until soft and lightly golden, flipping once halfway through cooking, about 25 minutes. This eliminates the step of frying the eggplant. It is much less messy and saves time.

3. Meanwhile, in a medium mixing bowl, combine the ricotta, 2 tablespoons parmesan, the eggs, herbs, ¼ teaspoon salt, and ⅛ teaspoon white pepper. Stir until thoroughly combined and smooth.

4. Lower the oven temperature to 375°F (190°C). Spread 1 cup sauce into the base of a 9 x 13-inch baking dish. Place the cooked eggplant over the sauce in a single layer, overlapping as needed. Spread another 1 cup sauce over the top of the eggplant to cover, then top with the ricotta filling and spread evenly to cover. Sprinkle the surface with the remaining 2 tablespoons parmesan.

5. Place in the oven and bake for 35 minutes, until browned and bubbling. Allow to cool, and set aside any family servings before pureeing.

6. For the puree, add the desired number of servings (one-sixth of the baking dish per serving) to a food processor or blender. Process until you achieve the desired texture.

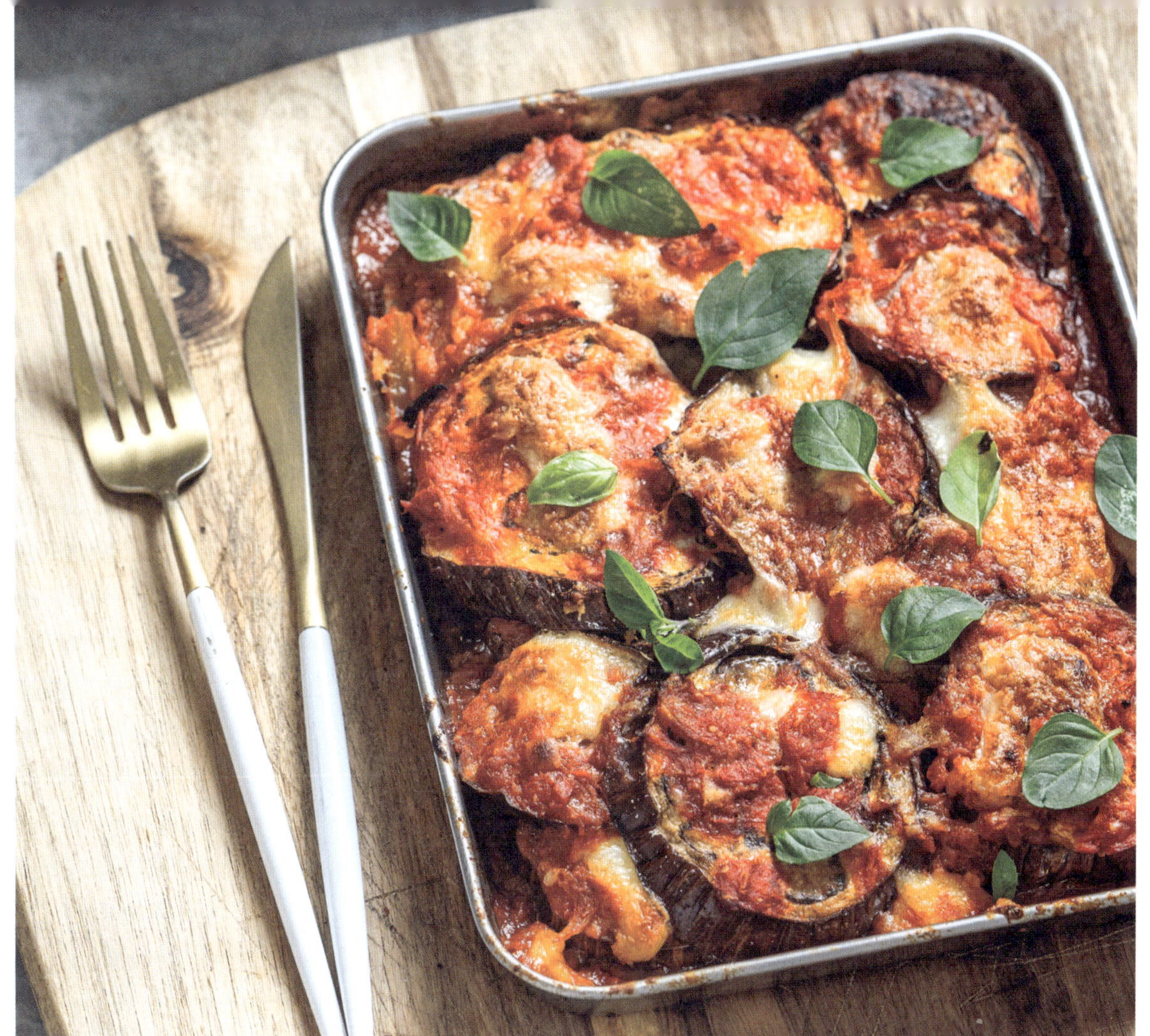

7. Test as you go and at time of serving to see if a thickening agent, thickened sauce, or thickened stock is needed; use IDDSI Testing Methods (*iddsi.org*) to help achieve the desired IDDSI level. See pages 42-47.

8. Serve immediately or divide into servings for storage or freezing, following the directions for Serving, page 77.

NUTRITIONAL ANALYSIS PER SERVING | 1 cup
245 calories, 11 g fat, 5 g saturated fat, 201 mg sodium, 7 g sugar, 25 g carbohydrates, 10 g fiber, 16 g protein

Vegetarian Almond Lentil Loaf

SERVINGS: 4 | IDDSI LEVELS   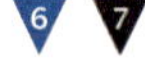

I created this vegetable loaf as a light version of meatloaf.

1 tablespoon extra-virgin olive oil
3 large shallots, diced
1 carrot, peeled and diced
2 garlic cloves, sliced
1 cup red lentils, rinsed
3 cups low-sodium vegetable broth or water
⅔ cup almond butter loosened with 2 tablespoons warm water and whisked
½ cup minced fresh flat-leaf parsley, or 3 tablespoons parsley paste
1 large egg, lightly beaten
¼ teaspoon sea salt
⅛ teaspoon white pepper
Nonstick cooking spray
Mushroom Gravy (see page 141)

1. Place a rack in the center of the oven and preheat to 350°F (175°C).

2. In a soup pot, warm the oil over medium heat. Add the shallots and sauté until softened, about 3 minutes. Add the carrot and sauté 3 more minutes. Add the garlic and sauté 1 more minute.

3. Add the lentils and the broth or water, bring to a boil, and reduce to a simmer. Place a lid on the pot slightly ajar, and cook until the lentils are tender, stirring occasionally and skimming any foam that rises to the surface, about 20 minutes. Transfer the lentil mixture to a large mixing bowl and allow to cool.
   › **Tip:** To get a good texture for the loaf, use an immersion blender to puree the lentils before adding the rest of the ingredients.

4. Add the almond butter, parsley, and egg. Season with salt and white pepper, and stir thoroughly to combine.

5. Grease a loaf pan or silicone muffin pan with nonstick cooking spray. Transfer the mixture to the loaf pan and use a spatula to smooth the surface, or scoop ¼-cup portions into the muffin pan.

6. Bake until firm and lightly golden, 30 minutes for the loaf, 20 minutes for the muffins. Allow to cool, and set aside any family servings before pureeing.

7. For the puree, place 1 loaf slice or 1 muffin per serving, torn, in a food processor with ½ cup Mushroom Gravy per portion. Pulse to combine and process until you achieve the desired texture.

8. Test as you go and at time of serving to see if a thickening agent, thickened sauce, or thickened stock is needed; use IDDSI Testing Methods (*iddsi.org*) to help achieve the desired IDDSI level. See pages 42-47.

9. Serve immediately or divide into servings for storage or freezing, following the directions for Serving, page 77.

PRO TIP

For a vegan version of this recipe, buy vegan "eggs"; make according to package directions, and substitute for the egg.

NUTRITIONAL ANALYSIS PER SERVING | 1 cup
Without gravy (for gravy see page 141)
233 calories, 16.5 g fat, 2.3 g saturated fat, 335 mg sodium, 1.9 g sugar, 14 g carbohydrates, 3.7 g fiber, 9.5 g protein

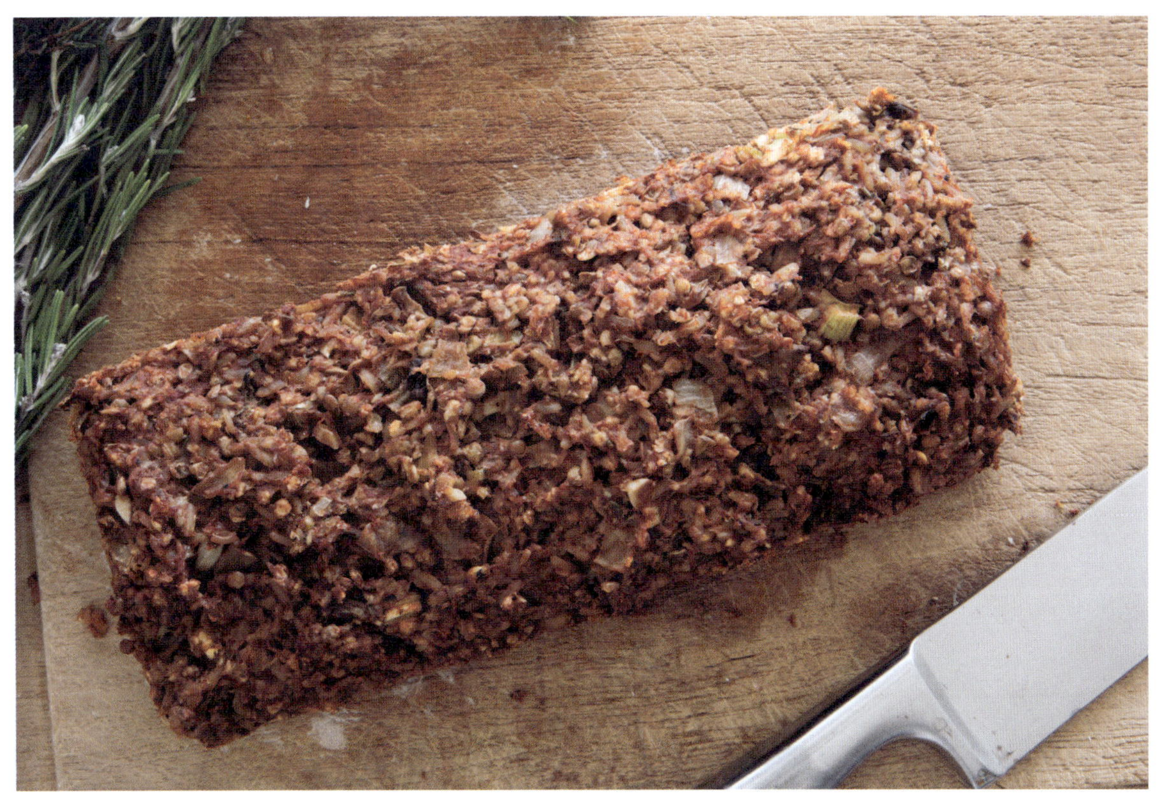

Vegetable Curry

SERVINGS: 4 | IDDSI LEVELS 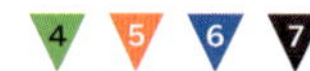

Vegetables may be mixed and matched according to your preference. Each combination is unique. I suggest serving with Rice Congee (see page 196) on the side.

- 1 tablespoon grapeseed oil
- ½ yellow onion, thinly sliced (about ½ cup)
- 1 garlic clove, finely chopped, or ½ teaspoon garlic paste
- 1 small carrot, peeled and thinly sliced (about ½ cup)
- ½ sweet potato, peeled and cut into ½-inch dice (about ½ cup)
- 1 small Yukon Gold potato, peeled and cut into ½-inch dice (about ½ cup)
- ½ cup low-sodium vegetable broth
- ½ red bell pepper, finely diced (about ½ cup)
- ½ cup cauliflower florets
- ½ cup frozen peas
- ½ small zucchini, cut into matchsticks (about ½ cup)
- 1 block firm tofu, cut into ½-inch cubes
- 1 (12- to 16-ounce jar) Panang curry sauce
- Coconut milk, as needed

1. In a large skillet with a lid or a Dutch oven, warm the oil over medium heat. Add the onion and cook until translucent, about 2 minutes. Add the garlic and cook for 1 minute. Add the carrot and both potatoes.

2. Stir to combine, cover the pan, and cook for 5 minutes. If the vegetables begin to stick or the pan looks dry, add ¼ cup vegetable broth.

3. Add the red pepper and cauliflower and the remaining ¼ cup vegetable broth. Cover and cook for 5 more minutes. Check to see if the potatoes and cauliflower are fork tender. If not, cover and cook for a few more minutes.

4. Add the peas, zucchini, and tofu. Stir to combine and simmer, uncovered, for 2 minutes. Add the curry sauce, lower the heat to medium-low, and cook for 2 minutes, until warmed through. If the curry sauce is too spicy or strong in flavor, add coconut milk, a few tablespoons at a time, to make the dish milder.

5. Remove from the heat and allow to cool, and set aside any family servings before pureeing.

6. For the puree, transfer as many portions as desired to a food processor or blender. Pulse the dish to incorporate all the elements, venting the lid to allow heat to escape. Process until you achieve the desired texture.

7. Use thickener as needed to modify texture (for IDDSI Level 5) or thicken (for IDDSI Level 4). See pages 42-47.

8. Serve immediately or divide into servings for storage or freezing, following the directions for Serving, page 77.

NUTRITIONAL ANALYSIS PER SERVING | 1 cup
409 calories, 32 g fat, 7.9 g saturated fat, 149 mg sodium, 6.7 g sugar, 0 g carbohydrates, 4.7 g fiber, 7.1 g protein

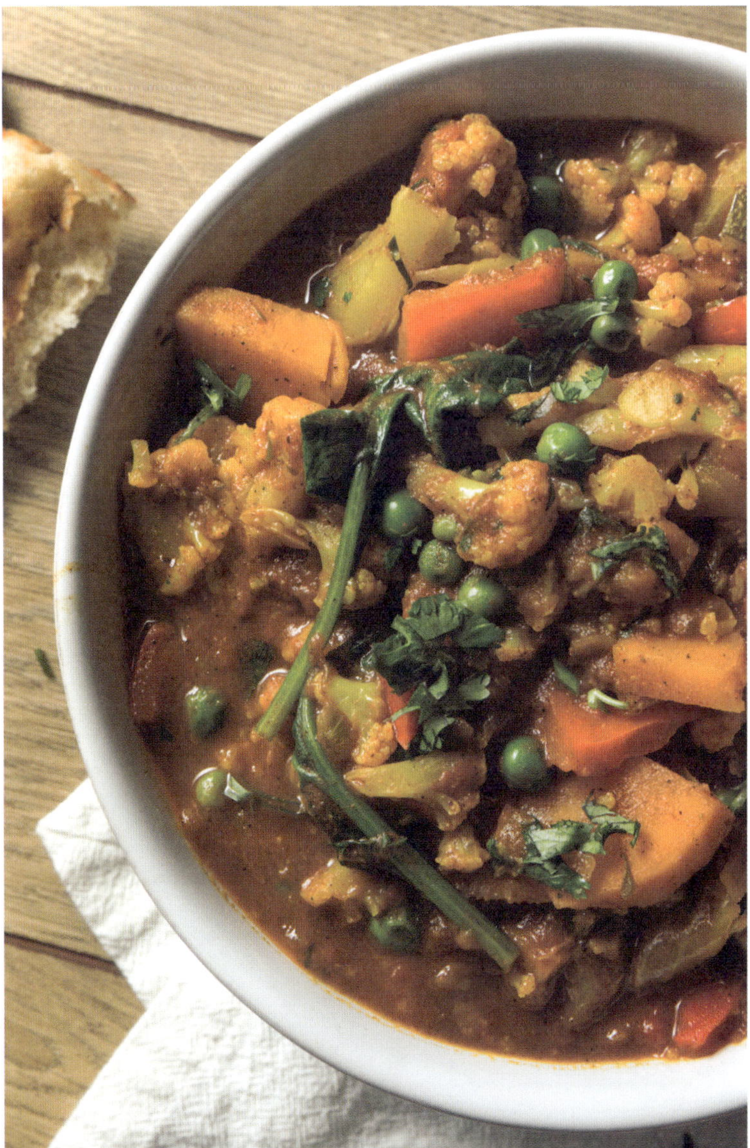

PRO TIP

For added flavor, serve the curry with traditional accompaniments: yogurt and chutney. Serve 1 tablespoon yogurt and 1 tablespoon sweet chutney in small dishes for flavoring the curry. If the chutney has particles of fruit, puree it in a food processor with yogurt and run it through a mesh strainer to remove any solids. Add a pump of thickener to bind the puree to IDDSI Moderately Thick, Level 3, for sauces and gravies. The way to eat this is to dip a spoonful of curry into the dipping sauce.

Seafood

121 Baked Cod with Lemon and Mashed Potatoes

122 Cod and Vegetable Parcels

124 Salmon in Puff Pastry

126 New England Crab Cakes

128 Shrimp, Cheese, and Spinach–Stuffed Portobellos

130 Shrimp and Vegetable Stir-Fry

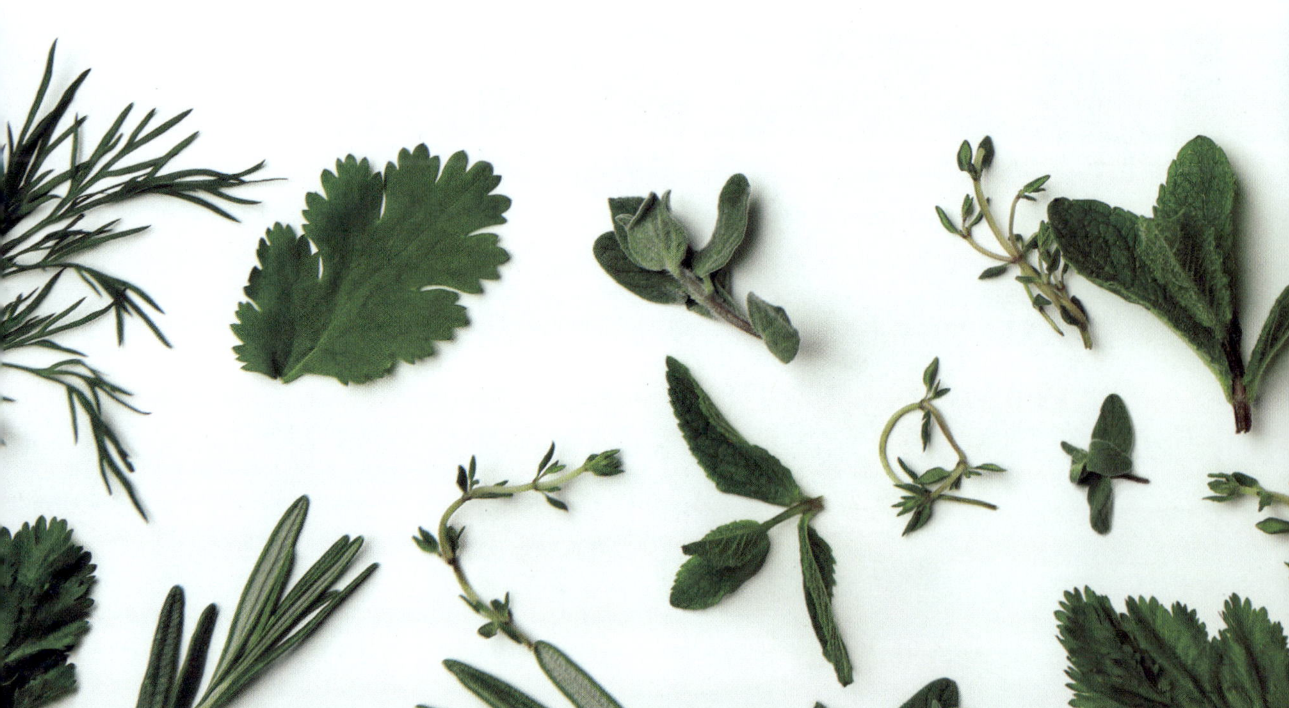

Baked Cod with Lemon and Mashed Potatoes

SERVINGS: 2 | IDDSI LEVELS 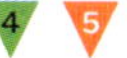

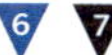

7

This recipe may be made with any white fish: tilapia, halibut, snapper, mahi-mahi, perch, or grouper. Fish may be fresh or frozen (thawed in water in a bowl in the refrigerator). Serve this dish with Garlic Green Beans (see page 191) or Spinach and Parmesan Sauté (see page 185).

8 ounces fresh or frozen cod or any other white fish
2 tablespoons extra-virgin olive oil
Sea salt and white pepper
¼ lemon, thinly sliced
Mashed Potatoes (see page 176)

1. Place a rack in the center of the oven and preheat to 350°F (175°C). Place the fish in a baking dish. Drizzle with the olive oil, turn to coat evenly, and season with salt and pepper on both sides. Lay 2 or 3 lemon slices on top of the fish. Bake until the fish is firm to the touch and flakes easily when pressed, 15 to 20 minutes.

2. Set aside any family serving before pureeing.

3. For the puree, once the fish has cooled slightly, remove and discard the lemon slices. Break up the fish into a food processor or blender. Add 1 to 2 tablespoons pan juice and ½ cup mashed potatoes per serving and process until you achieve the desired texture, adding more pan juice or water as needed. Process gently so the potatoes do not become gummy. Transfer the mixture to a bowl.

4. Test as you go and at time of serving to see if a thickening agent, thickened sauce, or thickened stock is needed; use IDDSI Testing Methods (*iddsi.org*) to help achieve the desired IDDSI level. See pages 42-47.

5. Serve immediately or divide into servings for storage or freezing, following the directions for Serving, page 77.

NUTRITIONAL ANALYSIS PER SERVING | 4 oz
Fish only (for potatoes, see page 176)
121 calories, 1 g fat, 0 g saturated fat, 63 mg sodium, 0 g sugar, 7 g carbohydrates, 1 g fiber, 21 g protein

Cod and Vegetable Parcels

SERVINGS: 2 | IDDSI LEVELS 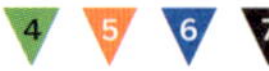

In the culinary world, this technique is called *en papillote*, but I call it the parcel method. Steaming food in parchment paper is a quick and easy way to prepare individual servings of fish. See page 78 for more ideas about how to make best use of the parcel cooking method.

½ cup shaved vegetables, such as carrots, zucchini, scallions, parsnips, or asparagus*
8 ounces fresh or frozen cod or any other white fish, halved
2 tablespoons extra-virgin olive oil
Sea salt and white pepper
¼ lemon, thinly sliced

* *You can use any vegetable you like; just make sure they are cut or shaved with a vegetable peeler thinly enough to be tender after a 10-minute steaming.*

1. Place a rack in the center of the oven and preheat to 350°F (175°C), or fill a large pot fitted with a steamer basket with 2 inches of water and bring to a boil over medium-high heat.

2. Cut 2 pieces of parchment paper into 12 x 12-inch squares. Place ¼ cup shaved vegetables on the parchment and lay a 4-ounce fillet of cod over top. Drizzle each piece of cod with 1 tablespoon olive oil, and season with salt and white pepper. Top the fish with the lemon slices.

3. Fold and crimp the edges to seal the parchment. (Aluminum foil can be used as a substitute for parchment paper.)

4. Place the parcels on a baking sheet and place in the oven, or add the parcels to the steamer basket, cover, and lower the heat to medium-low. Steam until the fish is cooked through, about 10 minutes.

5. Open the packets carefully and allow the fish to cool slightly. If reserving a portion for family or friends, serve directly from the parcel.

6. For the puree, remove and discard the lemon. Break up the fish and add to a food processor or blender, along with the vegetables and the juices that have accumulated in the parchment packet. Pulse to combine and process until you achieve the desired texture.

7. Test as you go and at time of serving to see if a thickening agent, thickened sauce, or thickened stock is needed; use IDDSI Testing Methods (*iddsi.org*) to help achieve the desired IDDSI level. See pages 42-47.

8. Serve immediately or divide into servings for storage or freezing, following the directions for Serving, page 77.

PRO TIP

Serve with a side of whole grain such as rice, quinoa, or farro, or with mashed potatoes.

NUTRITIONAL ANALYSIS PER SERVING | 4 oz

326 calories, 1.5 g fat, 0.3 g saturated fat, 1,985 mg sodium, 0 g sugar, 13.1 g carbohydrates, 4.4 g fiber, 62 g protein

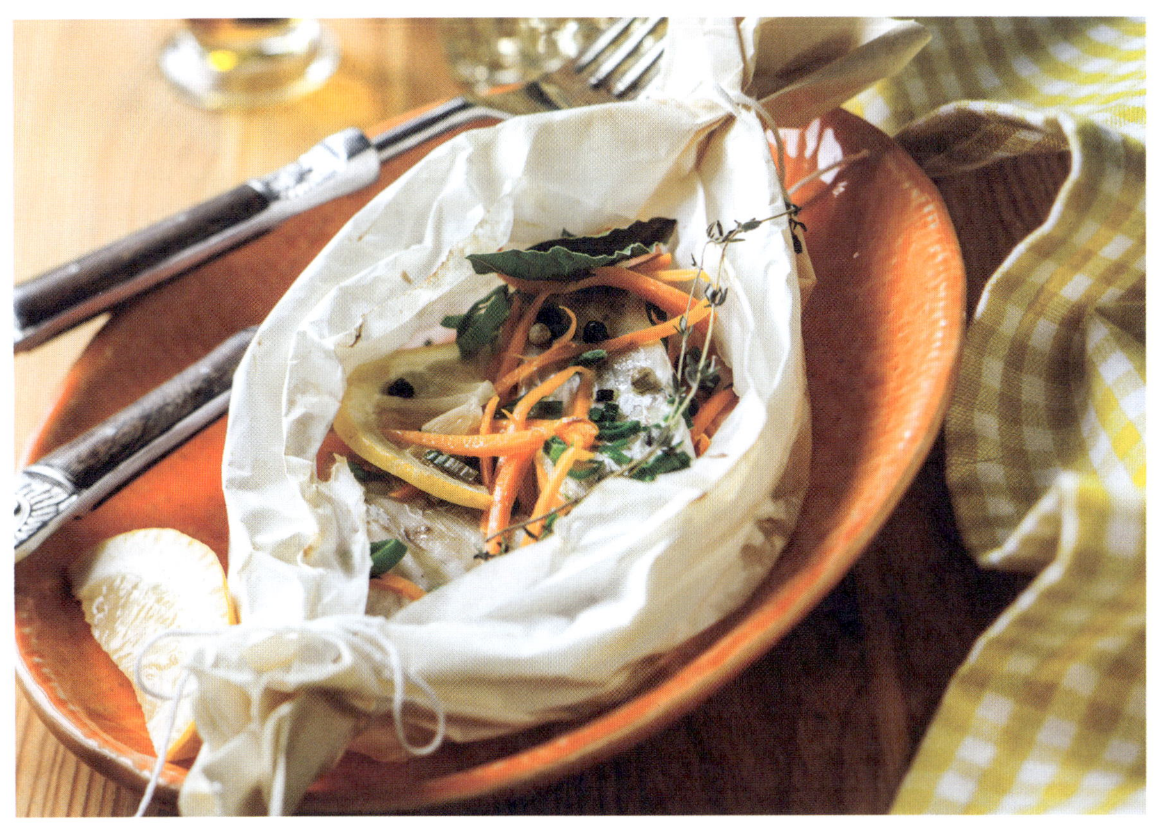

Salmon in Puff Pastry

SERVINGS: 4 | IDDSI LEVELS 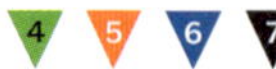

This recipe offers a protein, a carb, and a green in one dish—and it comes together quickly, thanks to store-bought puff pastry and jarred Alfredo sauce doctored with lemon juice and a shot of Tabasco. It freezes beautifully. The sauce makes for an excellent puree. This is a festive dish and may be served at a holiday or special occasion.

2 tablespoons low-sodium soy sauce
¼ cup freshly squeezed lemon juice, divided
Sea salt and white pepper
2 (8-ounce) salmon fillets
1 tablespoon extra-virgin olive oil
1 shallot, thinly sliced
1 garlic clove, thinly sliced
1 bunch spinach, washed and drained, or ½ bag frozen spinach
1 sheet store-bought frozen puff pastry, thawed
2 cups Rice Congee (see page 196)
1 large egg, beaten with 1 teaspoon water (for egg wash)
1 (15-ounce) jar Alfredo sauce
1–2 dashes hot sauce (optional)

1. To a zip-top plastic bag, add the soy sauce, 2 tablespoons lemon juice, and a pinch of salt and pepper. Add the salmon fillets and turn the bag several times to coat the fish. Marinate in the refrigerator for 1 hour.

2. Place a rack in the center of the oven and preheat to 375°F (190°C).

3. Meanwhile, in a medium skillet, heat the oil over medium heat. Add the shallot and sauté just until softened, about 3 minutes. Add the garlic and sauté for 1 minute. Add the spinach and cook, stirring, until the spinach wilts and begins to give off liquid, about 1 more minute. Season lightly with salt and white pepper and stir to combine. Remove the spinach mixture from the pan, draining off any liquid.

4. Line a sheet pan with parchment paper. Lay out the sheet of puff pastry on the paper. Arrange the Rice Congee down the center, leaving enough pastry on either side to fold up and enclose the filling.
   - **Tip:** If you're using previously frozen Rice Congee and the rice needs hydrating after being defrosted, add it to a pan with several tablespoons of broth or water. Simmer, stirring, until the rice absorbs the liquid.

5. Place the drained spinach mixture on top of the Rice Congee. Remove the salmon from the marinade and arrange the salmon fillets on top of the spinach. Fold the edges of the puff pastry to enclose the filling. Squeeze the edges together firmly to seal.

6. Using a sharp knife, make 2 slices in the pastry top to allow steam to escape. Brush the pastry with the egg wash.

7. Place in the oven and bake until the pastry is golden brown, approximately 30 minutes. If pastry is browning too quickly after 20 minutes, cover loosely with aluminum foil. To check for doneness, you can insert a knife into the salmon for a few seconds. The flesh should feel firm, and the knife should feel warm to the touch. Set aside to cool.

8. Place the Alfredo sauce in a small saucepan over low heat. Add the remaining 2 tablespoons lemon juice and the hot sauce, if using.

9. Remove the pastry from the oven, and divide into 4 servings. Set aside any portions being served for family meals and serve with the warm Alfredo sauce.

10. For the puree, break up the pastry and the salmon and add to a food processor or blender. Add ½ cup sauce per serving. Pulse to break up the components and process until you achieve the desired texture.

11. Test as you go and at time of serving to see if a thickening agent, thickened sauce, or thickened stock is needed; use IDDSI Testing Methods (*iddsi.org*) to help achieve the desired IDDSI level. See pages 42-47.

12. Serve immediately, or allow to cool completely before wrapping tightly in plastic wrap and then aluminum foil. Packages can be placed in a zip-top bag for storage. Refrigerate for up to 48 hours or freeze for up to 1 month. To reheat, follow the directions for Serving, page 77.

NUTRITIONAL ANALYSIS PER SERVING | 4 oz
483 calories, 1.5 g fat, 3 g saturated fat, 141 mg sodium, 0 g sugar, 32 g carbohydrates, 2 g fiber, 28 g protein

New England Crab Cakes

SERVINGS: 4 | IDDSI LEVELS   

Crab cakes are a huge favorite and can be made easily in the puree kitchen. The dipping sauce is a favorite in my family.

CRAB CAKES

8 ounces jumbo lump crabmeat
¾ cup breadcrumbs (store-bought, or see sidebar)
½ cup mayonnaise
1 teaspoon fresh lemon juice
¼ teaspoon Dijon mustard
1 scallion, finely chopped
½ teaspoon finely chopped fresh chives, or ¼ teaspoon dried chives
Sea salt and white pepper

TANGY DIPPING SAUCE

2 tablespoons mayonnaise
1 tablespoon plain Greek yogurt
1 teaspoon lemon juice
½ teaspoon Dijon mustard

1. Place a rack in the center of the oven and preheat to 425°F (220°C). Line a baking sheet with parchment paper.

2. In a medium bowl, combine the crabmeat, breadcrumbs, mayonnaise, lemon juice, dijon, scallion, and chives, and season with salt and white pepper.

3. Scoop ¼ cup of the crab mixture and form a patty with your hands, taking care not to pack the mixture too tightly. Repeat with the remaining mixture, placing each formed patty on the lined baking sheet. Let chill in the refrigerator for 10 minutes.

4. Place the baking sheet in the oven and bake until the crab cakes lift easily off the baking sheet and are lightly browned on the bottoms, about 10 minutes. Carefully flip and continue to bake until the second side lifts easily off the pan and is lightly browned, 5 to 8 minutes more.

5. Meanwhile, make the dipping sauce. In a small bowl, stir together the mayonnaise, yogurt, lemon juice, and Dijon. Thicken to Moderately Thick, Level 3, for sauces and gravies. This sauce may be served on the side for dipping or added to the puree.

6. Set aside any servings for family meals, and serve with the dipping sauce alongside.

7. For the puree, break 1 crab cake per serving into a food processor or blender. Add 3 tablespoons water or broth and 2 teaspoons dipping sauce per serving. Pulse to break up the crab cake and then process until you achieve the desired texture.

8. Test as you go and at time of serving to see if a thickening agent, thickened sauce, or thickened stock is needed; use IDDSI Testing Methods (*iddsi.org*) to help achieve the desired IDDSI level. See pages 42-47.

9. Serve immediately or divide into servings for storage or freezing, following the directions for Serving, page 77. (I freeze this for up to 1 month, not 3 months.)

NUTRITIONAL ANALYSIS PER SERVING | 2 oz
226 calories, 17 g fat, 2 g saturated fat, 692 mg sodium, 1 g sugar, 8 g carbohydrates, 1 g fiber, 10 g protein

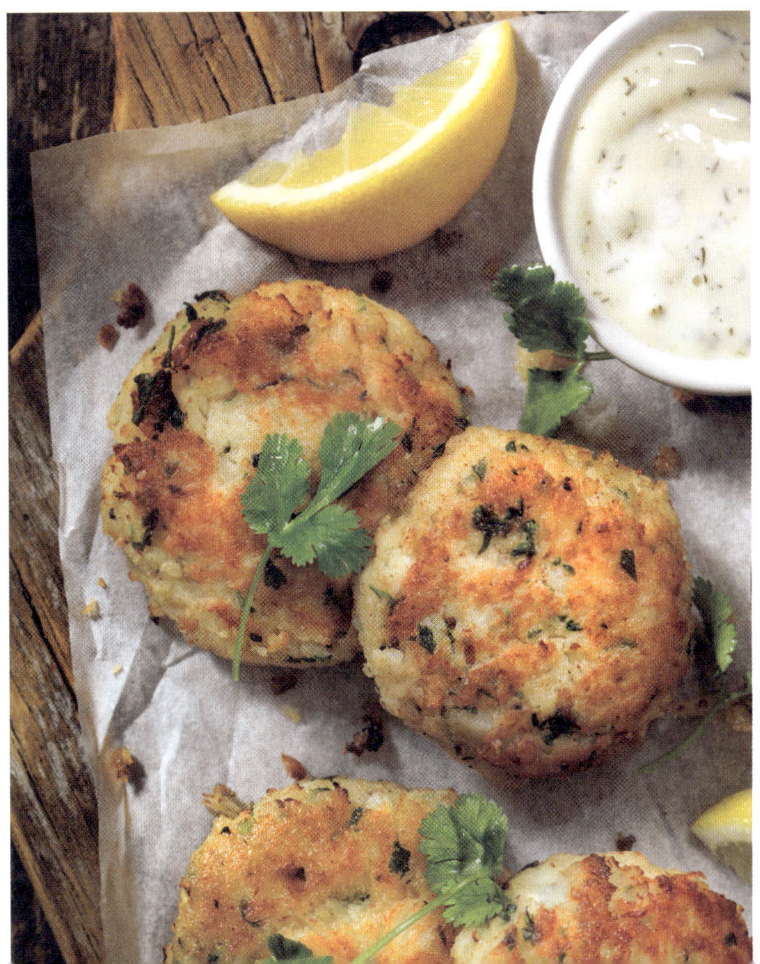

Fresh Breadcrumbs

To make fresh breadcrumbs, which are far more moist than packaged breadcrumbs, cut or tear slices of bread into ½-inch pieces and put them in a food processor. Pulse until the bread reaches the desired crumb texture. I learned this method from Jacques Pépin.

Shrimp, Cheese, and Spinach–Stuffed Portobellos

SERVINGS: 4 | IDDSI LEVELS 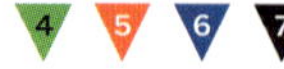

Because of the inclusion of shellfish, this is a festive dish and is great for a holiday or a special occasion. You can use scallops, sautéed in a pan with olive oil, or warmed lump crabmeat in place of the shrimp.

4 portobello mushroom caps (each about 3 inches in diameter)
2 tablespoons extra-virgin olive oil, divided
1 tablespoon low-sodium soy sauce
White pepper
2 shallots, or ½ yellow onion, thinly sliced
1½ cups spinach leaves, coarsely chopped
½ cup ricotta or mascarpone cheese
¼ cup grated parmesan
1 large egg
Sea salt
16 cooked medium shrimp (about 8 ounces), peeled, deveined, tails removed
Dried parsley, for serving

1. Place a rack in the center of the oven and preheat to 400°F (205°C). Line a baking sheet with parchment paper.

2. In a small bowl, combine 1 tablespoon of the olive oil, the soy sauce, and a pinch of white pepper. Transfer the mushrooms to the baking sheet and, using a pastry brush, paint the caps on both sides with the marinade. Set aside.

3. Warm the remaining 1 tablespoon olive oil in a skillet over medium heat. Add the shallots and sauté until translucent, about 3 minutes. Add the spinach and stir just until it wilts.

4. Transfer the shallots and spinach to a large mixing bowl to cool slightly. Add the ricotta, parmesan, egg, and a pinch of salt and pepper. Stir until thoroughly combined.

5. Add about 2 tablespoons filling to each of the prepared mushroom caps. Transfer to the oven and bake until the mushrooms are fork tender and the filling is lightly golden, 12 to 15 minutes.

6. Meanwhile, warm the cooked shrimp in the oven or a skillet over low heat. For family meal portions, top each mushroom cap with 4 shrimp and sprinkle with dried parsley, and set aside.

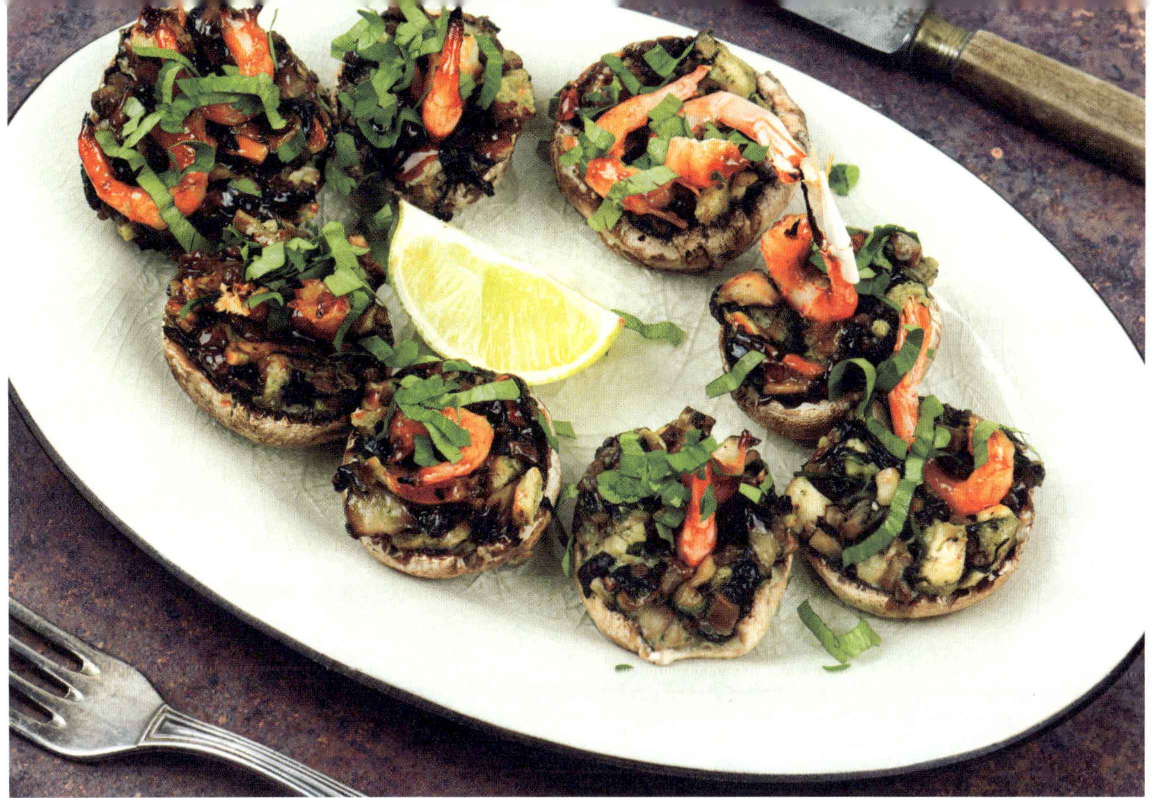

7. For the puree, cut a baked mushroom cap into quarters and transfer to a food processor or blender, along with 4 shrimp per serving and any juices that have accumulated on the sheet pan. Pulse to break up the shrimp and mushrooms and process until you achieve the desired texture.

8. Test as you go and at time of serving to see if a thickening agent, thickened sauce, or thickened stock is needed; use IDDSI Testing Methods (*iddsi.org*) to help achieve the desired IDDSI level. See pages 42-47.

9. Serve immediately or divide into servings for storage or freezing, following the directions for Serving, page 77. (I freeze this for up to 1 month, not 3 months.)

NUTRITIONAL ANALYSIS PER SERVING | 2 oz
196 calories, 15 g fat, 8 g saturated fat, 160 mg sodium, 0 g sugar, 5 g carbohydrates, 1 g fiber, 16.2 g protein

Shrimp and Vegetable Stir-Fry

SERVINGS: 2 | IDDSI LEVELS 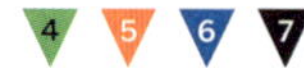

You can prepare this recipe with cooked frozen shrimp. Just thaw the shrimp in a bowl of water in the refrigerator, drain, and pat dry. For other variations, you can use leftover cooked chicken or frozen scallops. This stir-fry can also be made vegetarian or vegan with 4 ounces of diced silken tofu and a selection of vegetables such as onions, mushrooms, broccoli, and cabbage. Serve with a side dish of 4 ounces of Rice Congee, page 196.

- 1 pound shrimp, peeled, with tails left on, and deveined
- 2 tablespoons grapeseed oil, divided
- 1 garlic clove, finely chopped or grated, or 1 teaspoon garlic paste
- 1-inch piece ginger, peeled and finely chopped or grated, or 1 tablespoon ginger paste
- 2 scallions, thinly sliced
- 1 medium zucchini, thinly sliced
- 2 tablespoons teriyaki sauce (I like Soy Vay brand because it is readily available in supermarkets and is made without stabilizers, gums, or artificial ingredients)

1. I like to cook the shrimp with tails on for flavor and remove the tails for the puree. Heat 1 tablespoon oil in a wok or a large skillet over medium heat. Add the garlic, ginger, and scallions. Stir-fry, stirring frequently, until fragrant, 2 minutes.

2. Add the shrimp and cook until the shrimp all turn pink, 2 to 3 minutes. Remove the shrimp mixture from the pan, cover with aluminum foil to keep warm, and set aside.

3. Add the zucchini to the skillet and stir-fry for 2 minutes, until they start to turn lightly golden. Add 3 tablespoons water to the skillet, cover the pan, and steam the zucchini until soft, about 4 minutes. Add more water if needed to keep things from sticking or burning.

4. Return the shrimp to the pan along with 2 tablespoons teriyaki sauce and stir until well combined. Remove the pan from the heat and allow the contents to cool. Set aside a 1-cup family serving before pureeing.

5. For the puree, add the stir-fry (remember to remove the tails from the shrimp) to a food processor or blender. Pulse several times to break up the veggies and the shrimp, and then process until you achieve the desired texture, adding 1 tablespoon water and scraping down the sides of the bowl as needed.

6. Test as you go and at time of serving to see if a thickening agent, thickened sauce, or thickened stock is needed; use IDDSI Testing Methods (*iddsi.org*) to help achieve the desired IDDSI level. See pages 42-47.

7. Serve immediately or divide into servings for storage or freezing, following the directions for Serving, page 77. (I freeze this for up to 1 month, not 3 months.)

NUTRITIONAL ANALYSIS PER SERVING | 1 cup
370 calories, 18 g fat, 3 g saturated fat, 691 mg sodium, 3 g sugar, 7 g carbohydrates, 1 g fiber, 45 g protein

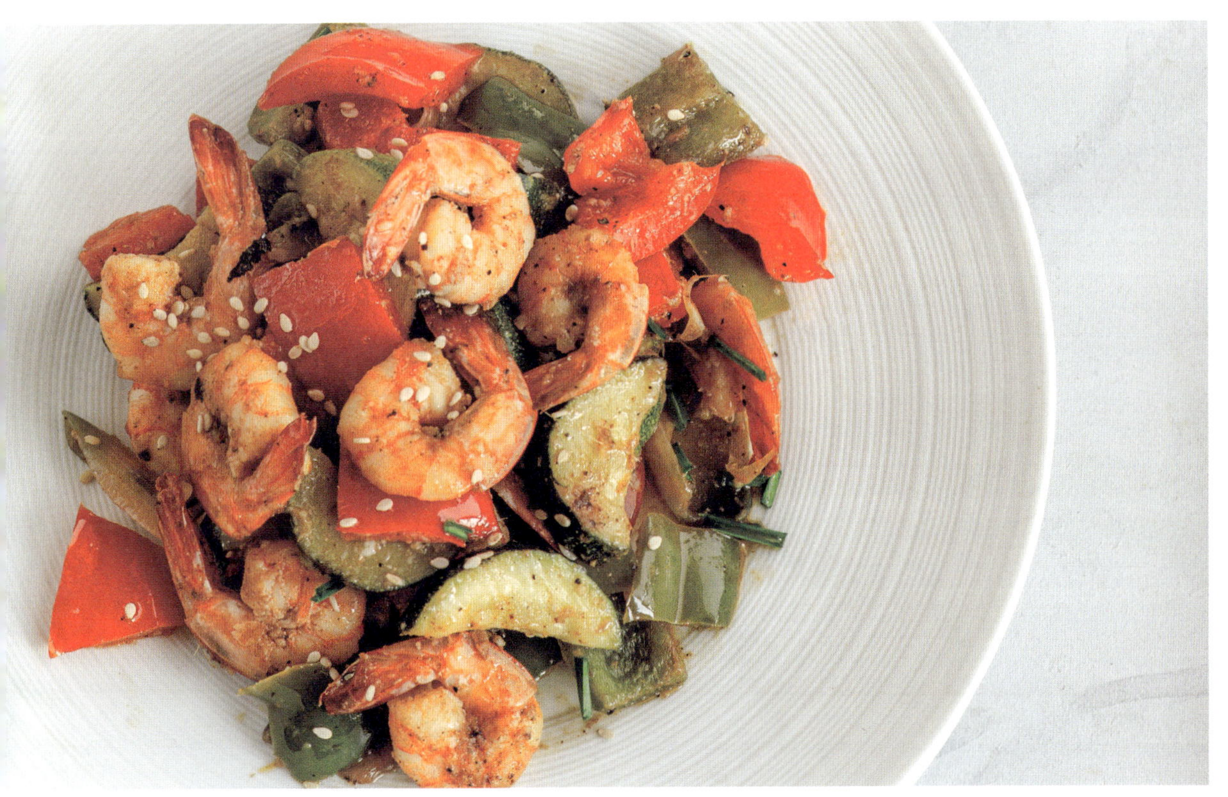

Meat

133 Shepherd's Pie

134 Beef Stew

136 Pot Roast

138 Mild Steak Chili

140 Classic Roast Loin of Pork
(Mushroom Gravy)

142 Barbecued Pork Loin
(Barbecue Sauce)

144 Pork Fried Rice

145 Garlic and Rosemary Lamb Chops

146 Holiday Ham
(Pineapple Honey Mustard Glaze)

148 Stuffed Cabbage

150 Sausage and Rice–Stuffed Peppers

152 Sausage and Peppers
(Onion and Pepper Smother Gravy)

Shepherd's Pie

SERVINGS: 2 | IDDSI LEVELS 

The great chef Jacques Pépin is forever praising the use of leftovers to make a second dish. This recipe follows the principle of using everything in the kitchen and wasting nothing. If you have leftover lamb or beef stew, use it to make this quick and simple Shepherd's Pie.

1 cup Beef Stew (or Lamb and Sweet Potato variation) (see page 135)
1 cup Mashed Potatoes (see page 176)
1 tablespoon butter or non-trans-fat margarine (often called a tub spread)

1. Place a rack in the center of the oven and preheat to 350°F (175°C). Place the stew in a small baking dish. Top with the mashed potatoes and spread to cover the stew. Dot the mashed potatoes with butter or margarine. Bake until the potatoes are lightly browned on top, about 15 minutes. Set aside any servings for family meals that are not to be pureed.

2. For the puree, once the pie has cooled, put the desired number of portions into a food processor or blender. Pulse a few times to break up the meat and vegetables. Process until you achieve the desired texture. If the dish is too thick, add a splash of gravy, broth, or water.

3. Test as you go and at time of serving to see if a thickening agent, thickened sauce, or thickened stock is needed; use IDDSI Testing Methods (*iddsi.org*) to help achieve the desired IDDSI level. See pages 42-47.

4. Serve immediately or divide into servings for storage or freezing, following the directions for Serving, page 77.

PRO TIP

For an even easier shepherd's pie for the busy cook, I highly recommend using Bob's Red Mill Instant Mashed Potatoes. It tastes like the real thing. Make the mashed potatoes according to directions on the package for two cups of mashed potatoes. My mother's secret ingredient was two teaspoons of good mayonnaise for two cups of mashed potatoes.

NUTRITIONAL ANALYSIS PER SERVING | 1 cup
Shepherd's pie without mashed potatoes
353 calories, 13 g fat, 5 g saturated fat, 473 mg sodium, 4 g sugar, 22 g carbohydrates, 4 g fiber, 36 g protein

---

NUTRITIONAL ANALYSIS PER SERVING | ½ cup
Mashed potatoes, see page 176
65 calories, 0 g fat, 0 g saturated fat, 11 mg sodium, 0 g sugar, 14 g carbohydrates, 1 g fiber, 3 g protein

Beef Stew

SERVINGS: 6 | IDDSI LEVELS 

Keep in mind when browning the meat in this and the following recipes to sear the meat lightly, as **a heavy sear is not safe for the swallow**. This can also be made in a slow cooker set on low for 4 hours. About potatoes: you may add 1 pound of cubed Yukon Gold potatoes to the stew. If you plan to use this dish as the basis for the Shepherd's Pie, page 133, leave out the potatoes.

- 2 tablespoons vegetable oil
- 2 pounds beef chuck, trimmed of excess fat and membrane, cut into 1½-inch cubes
- 1 teaspoon sea salt
- ½ teaspoon white pepper
- 1 medium yellow onion, chopped
- 2 medium carrots, halved lengthwise and cut into ½-inch half moons
- 1 garlic clove, finely chopped, or 1 teaspoon garlic paste
- 1 tablespoon tomato paste
- 1 tablespoon low-sodium soy sauce
- 2 medium Yukon Gold potatoes, cubed (optional)
- 1 quart low-sodium beef or chicken stock
- ¼ cup unbleached all-purpose flour
- 1 cup frozen peas

1. Heat the oil in a Dutch oven or large saucepan over medium-high heat. Season the beef with salt and pepper. In batches, add the beef to the pot and cook, turning occasionally, until lightly browned on all sides, about 6 minutes. Transfer to a plate.

2. Reduce the heat to medium. Add the onion and cook, stirring occasionally, until softened, about 3 minutes. Stir in the carrots and cook for 2 minutes. Stir in the garlic and cook just until fragrant, about 1 minute.

3. Move the vegetables off to one side, and add the tomato paste to the empty side of the pot and let cook without stirring until the edges brown, about 2 minutes. Add 3 tablespoons water and the soy sauce and stir to dissolve the tomato paste, then mix with the vegetables.

4. Return the beef and any juices to the pot. Add the stock (and potatoes if desired) and stir to combine. Bring to a boil over medium-high heat. Reduce the heat to medium-low and cover tightly. Simmer until the beef is tender, about 2 hours.

5. Whisk the flour and ¼ cup water in a small bowl to make a smooth slurry. Whisk in enough of the slurry into the simmering stew to get the gravy consistency of IDDSI Moderately Thick, Level 3, sauces and gravies.

6. Stir in the peas and simmer for 5 minutes. Season with additional salt and pepper. Let cool completely. Reserve portions for family meals (or to make Shepherd's Pie, see page 133).

7. For the puree, transfer portions of the stew to a food processor or blender (filling the pitcher only two-thirds full and venting the lid). Pulse to break up the stew, then process until you achieve the desired texture. Transfer to a bowl and repeat until all the stew is pureed.

8. Test as you go and at time of serving to see if a thickening agent, thickened sauce, or thickened stock is needed; use IDDSI Testing Methods (*iddsi.org*) to help achieve the desired IDDSI level. See pages 42-47.

9. Serve immediately or divide into servings for storage or freezing, following the directions for Serving, page 77.

NUTRITIONAL ANALYSIS PER SERVING | 1 cup
353 calories, 13 g fat, 5 g saturated fat, 473 mg sodium, 4 g sugar, 22 g carbohydrates, 4 g fiber, 36 g protein

Cooking Garlic

Be careful when cooking garlic. If it burns, the entire dish will taste bitter. I always add it at the end of sautéing the onions and other vegetables, and then only cook it for a minute, just enough for it to soften and smell fragrant. When it reaches that point, stir in some liquid to stop it from browning further.

VARIATIONS

- For **Lamb and Sweet Potato Stew**, substitute boneless lamb shoulder for the beef. Substitute sweet potatoes for the Yukon Gold potatoes.
- For **Veal and Rosemary Stew**, substitute boneless veal shoulder for the beef. Add 1 large sprig of rosemary with the stock. After cooking, remove the rosemary stem, then serve.

Pot Roast

SERVINGS: 6 | IDDSI LEVELS 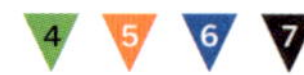

This can be made in a Dutch oven or any heavy pot with a cover, or a slow cooker set on low for 4 hours. It is delicious served with Mashed Potatoes (see page 176) or a side of whole grains (see pages 194 to 202).

2½-pound beef chuck roast, trimmed of excess fat and membrane, tied with kitchen twine
Sea salt and white pepper
1 tablespoon extra-virgin olive oil
2 medium yellow onions, chopped
2 large carrots, cut into ½-inch pieces
2 garlic cloves, finely chopped
1 (15-ounce) can tomato puree
½ teaspoon dried thyme or thyme paste
1 bay leaf
⅛ teaspoon low-sodium soy sauce
1 quart low-sodium beef or chicken stock
1 tablespoon unbleached all-purpose flour

1. Place an oven rack low enough to fit the Dutch oven with a lid and preheat to 350°F (175°C).

2. Liberally season the beef on all sides with salt and white pepper. In a large pot or Dutch oven, warm the oil over medium-high heat. Sear the beef lightly on all sides. **(A heavy sear is not safe for the swallow.)** Transfer the seared beef to a plate.

3. Add the onions to the pot and sauté until translucent, 3 minutes. Add the carrots and sauté for 2 minutes. Add the garlic and sauté for 1 minute. Add the tomato puree, thyme, bay leaf, and soy sauce. Stir to combine, and bring the mixture to a simmer for 1 minute.

4. If using a slow cooker, transfer the ingredients in the pot to the slow cooker, add the stock and the beef, and cook on low for 4 hours.

5. If using a Dutch oven, add the stock and return the beef to the pot. Cover the pot and transfer to the oven. Cook for 1 hour. Reduce the oven temperature to 325°F (165°C) and simmer for 1½ more hours.

6. When done, uncover the pot roast and allow to cool. Transfer the beef to a cutting board. Remove the twine.

7. Remove and discard the bay leaf. Transfer the braising liquid and vegetables to a blender, vent the lid to allow steam to escape, and puree until smooth. Return the puree to the pot, or transfer to a saucepan.

8. In a small bowl, whisk together 1 tablespoon flour with 2 tablespoons of the puree to make a slurry. Add the slurry to the puree in the pot, whisk to combine, and set over medium heat. Bring to a boil, lower to a simmer, and cook for 3 minutes, until the puree thickens into a sauce.

9. Set aside servings for family meals, with slices of pot roast topped with a ladleful of sauce and vegetables.

10. For the puree, cut the pot roast into 1-inch pieces and transfer to a food processor or blender. Add ½ cup sauce per serving. Pulse a few times to break down the meat. Process until you achieve the desired texture.

11. Test as you go and at time of serving to see if a thickening agent, thickened sauce, or thickened stock is needed; use IDDSI Testing Methods (*iddsi.org*) to help achieve the desired IDDSI level. See pages 42-47.

12. Serve immediately or divide into servings for storage or freezing, following the directions for Serving, page 77.

NUTRITIONAL ANALYSIS PER SERVING | 1 cup
392 calories, 17 g fat, 6 g saturated fat, 496 mg sodium, 3 g sugar, 15 g carbohydrates, 3 g fiber, 43 g protein

Mild Steak Chili

SERVINGS: 6 | IDDSI LEVELS   

The heat in this chili is very mild but **remember to get clearance from a healthcare provider before eating or serving spicy foods.** For a heat-free version, simply eliminate the chili powder, Tabasco, and cayenne.

1 pound ribeye or sirloin steak, trimmed of excess fat, cut into 1-inch cubes
Sea salt and white pepper
2 tablespoons grapeseed oil
1 medium yellow onion, diced
2 garlic cloves, thinly sliced
2 tablespoons tomato paste
1 teaspoon chili powder (optional)
½ teaspoon cumin
½ teaspoon cayenne powder (optional)
2 dashes Tabasco (optional)
1 (28-ounce) can crushed tomatoes
1 (8-ounce) can tomato sauce
1 (15-ounce) can low-sodium kidney beans, rinsed and drained
Optional toppings: cheddar cheese, sour cream, thinly sliced scallion

1. Season the steak cubes with salt and white pepper. In a large pot or Dutch oven, warm the oil over medium-high heat. Working in batches if needed, lightly brown the steak on all sides. Transfer the meat to a plate and set aside.

2. Lower the heat to medium. Add the onion and sauté until translucent, 3 minutes. Add the garlic and sauté for 1 minute. Add the tomato paste, chili powder, cumin, cayenne, and Tabasco. Stir to coat the aromatics in the tomato paste and sauté to toast the spices, 2 minutes.

3. Return the meat to the pot, along with any juices that have accumulated on the plate. Add the crushed tomatoes, tomato sauce, and beans. Stir to combine, and bring the mixture to a boil.

4. Lower the heat to a simmer and cook for 1 hour, adding a splash of water if the chili becomes too thick. Remove from the heat and allow to cool. Set aside any servings for family meals.

5. For the puree, transfer portions of the chili to a food processor or blender (only fill it two-thirds full and vent the lid). Add optional toppings to the blender, if desired. Pulse to break up the meat, then process until you achieve the desired texture. Transfer to a bowl and repeat until all the chili is pureed.

6. Test as you go and at time of serving to see if a thickening agent, thickened sauce, or thickened stock is needed; use IDDSI Testing Methods (*iddsi.org*) to help achieve the desired IDDSI level. See pages 42-47.

PRO TIP

You can also make this chili with ground beef or ground turkey.

7. Serve immediately or divide into servings for storage or freezing, following the directions for Serving, page 77.

NUTRITIONAL ANALYSIS PER SERVING | 1 cup
273 calories, 12 g fat, 3 g saturated fat, 283 mg sodium, 6 g sugar, 23 g carbohydrates, 6 g fiber, 21 g protein

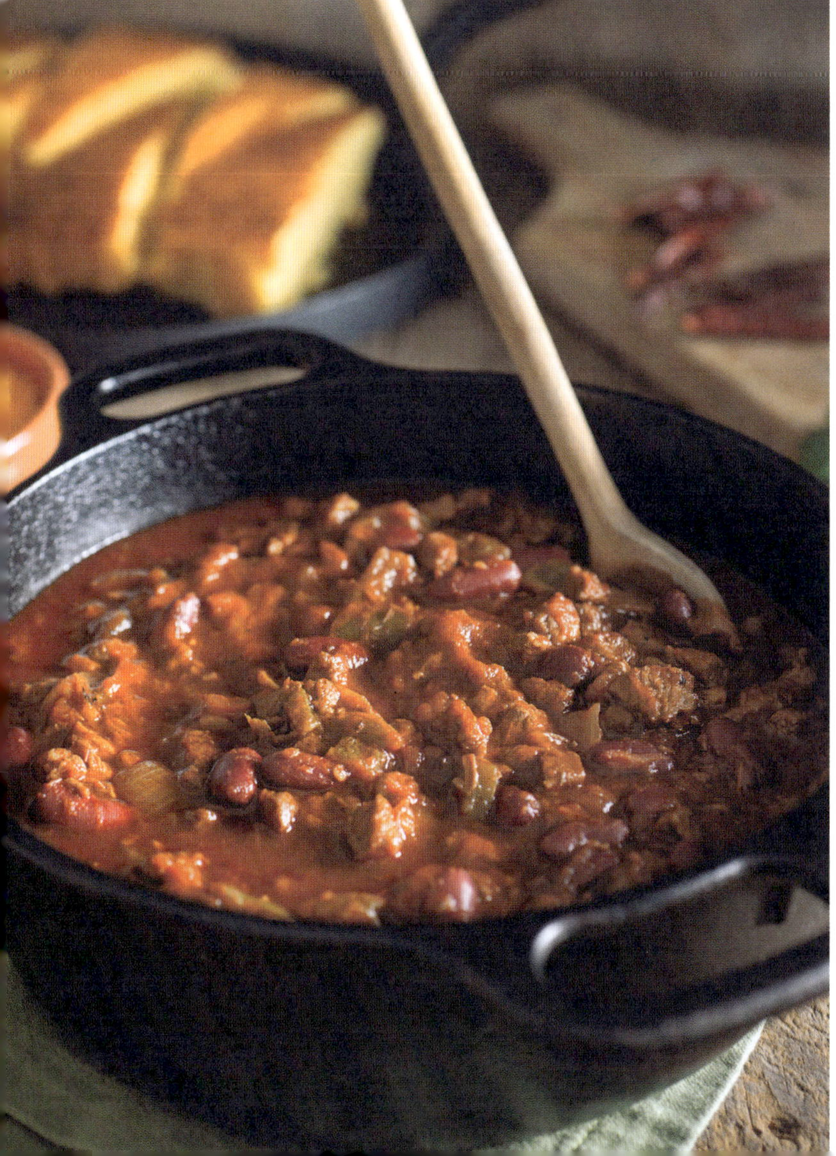

Cornbread

Cornbread makes a great side for this chili. For the puree, blend a four-ounce piece of homemade or store-bought cornbread with 3 tablespoons very hot water. Test as you go and at time of serving to see if a thickening agent, thickened sauce, or thickened stock is needed; use IDDSI Testing Methods (*iddsi.org*) to help achieve the desired IDDSI level (see pages 42-47). Pipe cornbread into a desired shape. Serve alongside the chili. Store leftover cornbread, wrapped tightly in plastic wrap and then aluminum foil, in the freezer for up to 3 months.

Classic Roast Loin of Pork

SERVINGS: UP TO 8 | IDDSI LEVELS 

This simple method for roasting pork will yield several other delicious dishes. Here it is served with a rich and flavorful Mushroom Gravy. The gravy is important because it is what flavors the puree.

2 pounds pork loin
2 garlic cloves, thinly sliced
2 tablespoons grapeseed oil, divided
1 tablespoon low-sodium soy sauce
Sea salt and white pepper
Mushroom Gravy (see page 141)

1. Place a rack in the center of the oven and preheat to 350°F (175°C). Make small slits in the surface of the pork and insert the slices of garlic. Coat the bottom of a shallow baking dish with 1 tablespoon oil. Add the pork to the pan. Rub the pork with the remaining oil and the soy sauce, and season with salt and white pepper.
2. Roast until a thermometer inserted into the center of the loin reads 145°F (65°C), about 1 hour. Transfer the meat to a cutting board and allow to rest for at least 10 minutes.
3. Divide the pork into 4-ounce portions and set aside any pork that will be used to make other dishes. Set aside any servings for family meals. To serve, slice the pork and serve with warm Mushroom Gravy spooned over the top.
4. For the puree, cut the pork into 1-inch pieces and place in a food processor or blender. Pulse a few times to break up the pork. Add ½ cup Mushroom Gravy and process until you achieve the desired texture. If needed, add a few tablespoons of broth or water to create a good consistency.
5. Test as you go and at time of serving to see if a thickener is needed; use IDDSI Testing Methods (*iddsi.org*) to help achieve the desired IDDSI level. See pages 42-47.
6. Serve immediately or divide into servings for storage or freezing, following the directions for Serving, page 77.

NUTRITIONAL ANALYSIS PER SERVING | 1 cup
Without gravy
273 calories, 24.3 g fat, 3.7 g saturated fat, 77 mg sodium, 0.3 g sugar, 8.3 g carbohydrates, 0.5 g fiber, 8.1 g protein

PRO TIP

The Classic Roast Loin of Pork (see page 140) is perfect for the Batch Cooking Method (see page 60). Once you cook it, you can make several meals out of it. In addition to serving it with Mushroom Gravy (see page 141), you can use it to make Barbecued Pork Loin (see page 142), Pork Fried Rice (see page 144), and Wonton Soup (see page 86).

This is the beauty of batch cooking—a quick meal is always on hand. Depending on your schedule, you can freeze the cooked pork until you are ready to make the variations.

Mushroom Gravy

YIELD: 1½ CUPS | IDDSI LEVEL 

This beats anything you can buy packaged off the shelf or in the freezer section. Most store-bought gravies are high in sodium and contain preservatives and fillers. This homemade gravy is fresher, of higher quality, and cheaper—not to mention it tastes delicious. The baby Bella mushrooms, also called cremini, have more flavor than white button mushrooms, but you can use whatever mushrooms are in season. I use Wondra flour for thickening because it is light and has less tendency to form lumps. Double the recipe if you want to have extra gravy on hand for a social gathering or in the freezer.

¼ cup extra-virgin olive oil, divided
1 pound baby Bella or cremini mushrooms, sliced
1 cup low-sodium vegetable broth
2 tablespoons Wondra flour
1 teaspoon fresh thyme, or ½ teaspoon dried thyme
1 teaspoon low-sodium soy sauce
Sea salt and white pepper

1. Warm 2 tablespoons oil in a large sauté pan over medium-high heat. Add the mushrooms and sauté, stirring occasionally and adding a little more oil if needed, until the mushrooms have softened and are golden brown, about 10 minutes. Transfer the mushrooms to a bowl and set aside.

2. Meanwhile, bring the broth to a simmer in a small saucepan. Add the remaining oil to the sauté pan. Add the Wondra flour to the oil and cook, stirring constantly, until just starting to turn lightly golden brown, 1 to 2 minutes. Slowly add the simmering broth, whisking constantly to avoid lumps.

3. Add the mushrooms, thyme, and soy sauce along with any juices that have accumulated in the bowl, and stir to combine. Simmer for 6 minutes, until thickened. Remove from the heat. Set aside some gravy for family meals, if desired.

4. Test as you go and at time of serving to see if a thickening agent, thickened sauce, or thickened stock is needed; use IDDSI Testing Methods (*iddsi.org*) to help achieve the desired IDDSI level. See pages 42-47.

5. Serve immediately or divide into ½ cup servings for storage or freezing, following the directions for Serving, page 77.

NUTRITIONAL ANALYSIS PER SERVING | ½ cup
214 calories, 10.8 g fat, 6.4 g saturated fat, 197 mg sodium, 4.2 g sugar, 25.4 g carbohydrates, 2.7 g fiber, 6.7 g protein

Barbecued Pork Loin

SERVINGS: 1 | IDDSI LEVELS   

This dish combines 4 ounces of Classic Roast Loin of Pork with store-bought or homemade barbecue sauce. While I prefer my homemade sauce, I think it is better to have a modified version of the dish than not to have the dish at all. When purchasing barbecue sauce, it is important to read labels for sugar content and degree of mildness. **Check with your healthcare provider about eating or serving spicy food.**

4 ounces Classic Roast Loin of Pork (see page 140), cut into 1-inch cubes, warmed
¼ cup low-sodium chicken broth, warmed
¼ cup Barbecue Sauce, homemade (see page 143) or store-bought

1. Add the pork, broth, and Barbecue Sauce to a food processor or blender. Pulse to break up the pork, and then process until you achieve the desired texture. Adjust the puree with sauce or broth as needed for a good consistency.

2. Test as you go and at time of serving to see if a thickening agent, thickened sauce, or thickened broth is needed; use IDDSI Testing Methods (*iddsi.org*) to help achieve the desired IDDSI level. See pages 42-47.
   - **Tip:** For the puree, I use broth along with the barbecue sauce to get a dish that tastes good but does not contain too much sugar, sodium, or heat. For a family meal serving, warm a thinly sliced 4-ounce portion of the pork loin with the barbecue sauce.

3. Serve immediately or divide into servings for storage or freezing, following the directions for Serving, page 77.

NUTRITIONAL ANALYSIS PER SERVING | 1 cup
Without barbecue sauce
273 calories, 24.3 g fat, 3.7 g saturated fat, 77 mg sodium, 0.3 g sugar, 8.3 g carbohydrates, 0.5 g fiber, 8.1 g protein

Barbecue Sauce

YIELD: 1½ CUPS | IDDSI LEVEL 

This quickie homemade barbecue sauce was inspired by chef Bobby Flay. I've adapted it for the puree kitchen. It's easy to prepare, it's made from pantry items, and hoisin sauce is its secret ingredient. Hoisin sauce can be found in most supermarkets and in Asian markets. It is made from plums and imparts a rich, deep flavor to the sauce. This sauce is customizable and can be adjusted according to individual taste.

1 cup ketchup
½ cup molasses
2 tablespoons Dijon mustard
2 tablespoons hoisin sauce
1 tablespoon honey
1 teaspoon low-sodium soy sauce

1. In a small saucepan, combine the ketchup, molasses, Dijon, hoisin sauce, honey, and soy sauce. Stir to combine, set over medium-low heat, and simmer for 5 minutes. Allow to cool. Set aside a portion for family servings before pureeing.

2. Test as you go and at time of serving to see if a thickening agent, thickened sauce, or thickened stock is needed; use IDDSI Testing Methods (*iddsi.org*) to help achieve the desired IDDSI level. See pages 42-47.

3. Use immediately, or store in an airtight container in the refrigerator for up to 2 weeks, or the freezer for up to 3 months.

NUTRITIONAL ANALYSIS PER SERVING | 2 tablespoons
94 calories, 1.3 g fat, 0.1 g saturated fat, 562 mg sodium, 15.8 g sugar, 20.3 g carbohydrates, 1.1 g fiber, 1.5 g protein

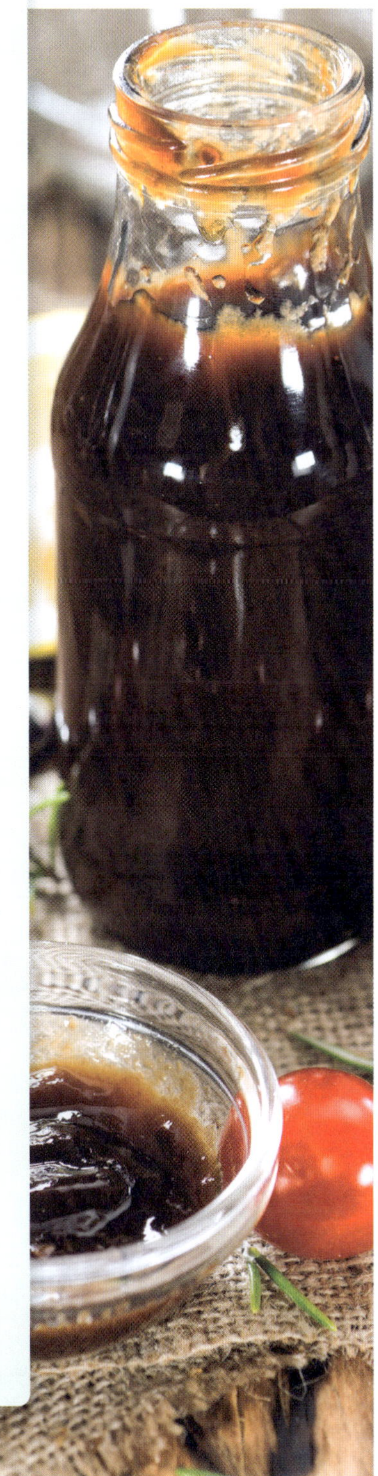

Pork Fried Rice

SERVINGS: 4 | IDDSI LEVELS 

For a Chinese takeout meal at home, you can enjoy this fried rice with a bowl of Wonton Soup (see page 86) and Shrimp and Vegetable Stir-Fry (see page 130). You can vary the fried rice by using chicken, shrimp, scallops, or any other leftover protein in place of the pork.

1 tablespoon grapeseed oil
3 scallions, white and green parts, thinly sliced
1 medium carrot, halved lengthwise and sliced into thin half moons
1 garlic clove, finely chopped, or 1 teaspoon garlic paste
4 ounces Classic Roast Loin of Pork (see page 140), cut into ½-inch dice
2 cups cooked rice (see page 196)
¼ cup low-sodium broth
2 tablespoons low-sodium soy sauce
½ cup frozen peas
1 large egg

1. In a large skillet or a wok, warm the oil over medium heat. Add the scallions and sauté until translucent, 1 minute. Add the carrot slices and 2 tablespoons water and cook until the carrot slices are softened, 2 minutes. Add the garlic and sauté for 1 minute.

2. Stir in the cubed pork and the cooked rice, and stir-fry with the vegetables, giving the rice a chance to pick up flavor and be coated with oil, 2 minutes. Add the broth, soy sauce, and peas, and continue to cook, stirring, until the flavors have melded, about 2 more minutes.

3. In a separate pan, scramble an egg. Stir the scrambled egg into the rice. Remove from the heat and allow to cool. Set aside any servings for family meals.

4. For the puree, add as many servings as you need to puree to a food processor. Pulse to break down the elements of the dish. Process until you achieve the desired texture, adding a tablespoon or so of broth as needed.

5. Test as you go and at time of serving to see if a thickening agent, thickened sauce, or thickened stock is needed; use IDDSI Testing Methods (*iddsi.org*) to help achieve the desired IDDSI level. See pages 42-47.

6. Serve immediately or divide into servings for storage or freezing, following the directions for Serving, page 77.

NUTRITIONAL ANALYSIS PER SERVING | 1 cup
179 calories, 4 g fat, 1 g saturated fat, 338 mg sodium, 0.5 g sugar, 27.9 g carbohydrates, 0.9 g fiber, 7.7 g protein

Garlic and Rosemary Lamb Chops

SERVINGS: 2 | IDDSI LEVELS   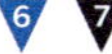

This is a surprisingly easy and delicious puree. Use an indoor grill on medium heat, or pan-sauté on low, to cook the chops to the desired degree of doneness, low and slow, without charring. Test by using an instant-read thermometer or making a cut and taking a look. Serve with Mashed Potatoes (see page 176) or Minty Pureed Peas (see page 193).

2 garlic cloves, finely chopped or grated, or 2 teaspoons garlic paste
1 sprig rosemary, chopped
1 tablespoon extra-virgin olive oil
Sea salt and white pepper
4 lamb rib chops, approximately 1½ pounds
Low-sodium stock or leftover Mushroom Gravy (see page 141), as needed

1. In a small bowl, combine the garlic, rosemary, olive oil, salt, and pepper. Rub onto the lamb chops and allow to marinate at room temperature for 15 minutes.

2. Preheat a grill to medium-high, or set a grill pan on the stove over medium-high heat. Grill the lamb chops to the desired doneness, 3 to 5 minutes per side. For medium-rare, an instant-read thermometer inserted into the center of a lamb chop should read 135°F (55°C). Remove from the grill and set aside to rest for 10 minutes. Set aside any family serving before pureeing.

3. For the puree, remove the meat from the bones, chop the lamb into 1-inch pieces, and transfer to a food processor or high-speed blender. Pulse to break up the meat. Add about ¼ cup stock per serving. (If you have leftover Mushroom Gravy [see page 141] in the freezer, you can also use that for the puree liquid.) Process until you achieve the desired texture, adding more liquid as needed.

4. Test as you go and at time of serving to see if thickening is needed; use IDDSI Testing Methods (*iddsi.org*) to help achieve the desired IDDSI level. See pages 42-47.

5. Serve immediately or divide into servings for storage or freezing, following the directions for Serving, page 77.

NUTRITIONAL ANALYSIS PER SERVING | 12 oz (2 chops)
212 calories, 12 g fat, 3 g saturated fat, 72 mg sodium, 0 g sugar, 1 g carbohydrates, 0 g fiber, 23 g protein

Holiday Ham

SERVINGS: 4 | IDDSI LEVELS 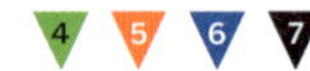

Most holiday hams come in sizes around 10 pounds, so if you only need a few servings, I have been advised by my butcher that the best smaller holiday ham, around 5 pounds, is a bone-in smoked ham. This is precooked. Heat it according to directions for the weight of the ham. This is great with a serving of Braised Greens (see page 186) or Garlic Green Beans (see page 191) as the side dish.

5-pound bone-in smoked ham
1 cup low-sodium vegetable broth
Slow-Baked Sweet Potatoes with Orange, mashed (see page 174)
Pineapple Honey Mustard Glaze (see page 147)

1. Place a rack in the center of the oven and preheat to 200°F (95°C). Place the ham on a sheet pan, cover with foil, and place in the oven until warmed through, about 1 hour.

2. Remove from the oven, transfer to a cutting board, and carve portions of the meat from the bone. Set aside any servings for family meals and tent with foil to keep warm.

3. Serve with ½ cup Slow-Baked Sweet Potatoes with Orange and 2 tablespoons Pineapple Honey Mustard Glaze per serving, for family and pureed servings.

4. For the puree, place as many 4-ounce portions of the ham as desired, cut into 1-inch pieces, into a food processor or blender. Pulse to break up the ham. Add ¼ cup broth per serving, and process until you achieve the desired texture, adding more broth as needed. Add ½ cup Slow-Baked Sweet Potatoes per serving and pulse several times to combine.

5. Test as you go and at time of serving to see if thickening is needed; use IDDSI Testing Methods (*iddsi.org*) to help achieve the desired IDDSI level. See pages 42-47.

6. Serve immediately or divide into servings for storage or freezing, following the directions for Serving, page 77.

NUTRITIONAL ANALYSIS PER SERVING | 1 cup
467 calories, 18 g fat, 4 g saturated fat, 243 mg sodium, 51 g sugar, 55 g carbohydrates, 2 g fiber, 25 g protein

Pineapple Honey Mustard Glaze

YIELD: 1½ CUPS | IDDSI LEVEL 

There are a number of store-bought glazes available, especially around the holidays. My kitchen tests revealed that the commercial brands were often too heavy on the spices for people with swallowing difficulties. They also contained preservatives and chemicals. As chef Wolfgang Puck says, "When you make it yourself, you know what's in it." Here is a simple recipe for a homemade glaze.

1 cup canned pineapple
1 tablespoon canned pineapple juice
4 tablespoons honey
2 tablespoons Dijon mustard
Pinch of ground cinnamon
Pinch of ground cloves

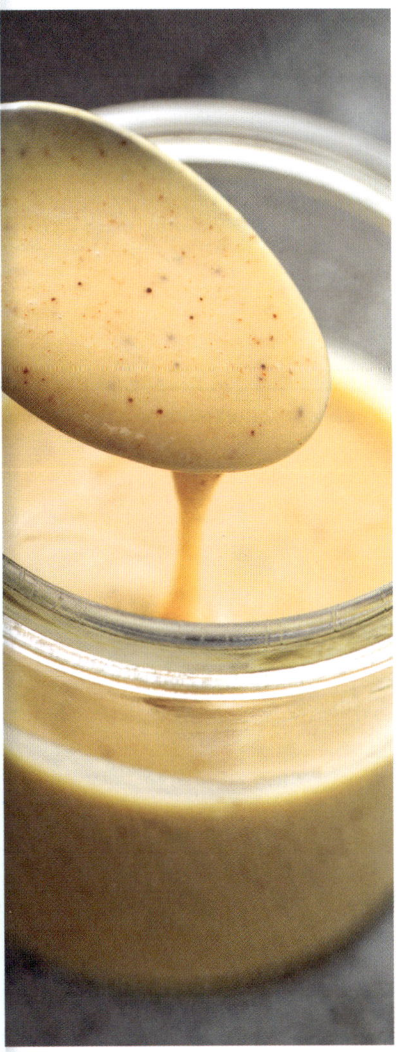

1. In a blender, combine the pineapple and its juices, honey, Dijon, and spices. Puree until smooth. Transfer to a small saucepan and warm over medium-low heat for 2 minutes. Set aside a portion for family meals, if desired.

2. Transfer the glaze to a small ramekin. Allow to cool. Test as you go and at time of serving to see if a thickening agent, thickened sauce, or thickened stock is needed; use IDDSI Testing Methods (*iddsi.org*) to help achieve the desired IDDSI level. See pages 42-47.

3. Use immediately, or store in an airtight container in the refrigerator for up to 1 week or freeze for one month.

NUTRITIONAL ANALYSIS PER SERVING | 2 tablespoons
89 calories, 0 g fat, 0 g saturated fat, 100 mg sodium, 9.7 g sugar, 10.3 g carbohydrates, 0.5 g fiber, 0.3 g protein

Stuffed Cabbage

SERVINGS: 4 | IDDSI LEVELS 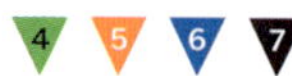

This may seem like an old-fashioned dish, but think of it as a warm wrap of vegetables, carbs, and protein baked with a sauce for puree. It is an ideal dish for the dysphagia kitchen, especially since it offers variety. The classic wrap is cabbage, but kale or chard leaves can be used as well. The protein here is ground beef, but you can use ground pork, chicken, turkey, or silken tofu. The sauce is tomato, but it could instead be gravy or a cream sauce. Any of the grains listed in the Whole Grains (see page 194) section may be used in place of the Rice Congee. This is a warm and comforting dish and offers variety.

8 leaves green or Napa cabbage, washed and dried, with hard center stalk removed
1 tablespoon extra-virgin olive oil
½ medium yellow onion, diced
1 garlic clove, finely chopped, or 1 teaspoon garlic paste
1 pound ground beef
Sea salt and white pepper
2½ cups Rice Congee (see page 196)
2 tablespoons finely chopped fresh parsley or parsley paste
1 (15-ounce) can tomato sauce
Bay leaf, optional (if using, make sure to remove after the dish is cooked)

1. Place a rack in the center of the oven and preheat to 350°F (175°C). Bring a large pot of water to a boil. Add the cabbage leaves and parboil until they are tender and pliable, 3 minutes. Drain well and set aside to cool and dry.

2. Warm the oil in a large sauté pan over medium heat. Add the onion and sauté until translucent, about 3 minutes. Add the garlic and cook for 1 more minute. Add the beef, season with salt and white pepper, and cook, stirring occasionally, until no longer pink, about 6 minutes. Add the Rice Congee and parsley and stir to combine well. Remove from the heat and allow to cool.

3. Place a cabbage leaf in the center of a clean cutting board. Place 3 to 4 tablespoons of the filling in the center. Bring the edge of the cabbage leaf that is closest to you over the filling, then tuck the two sides over the filling, and roll the leaf away from you to envelop the filling completely (You can use a sushi mat for this, to help form the roll. You can also use a toothpick to seal the roll closed.)

4. Line up the completed cabbage rolls in a 9 x 9-inch baking dish. Cover with the tomato sauce and tuck a bay leaf into the sauce. Cover the dish tightly with foil and bake for 1 hour. Remove from the oven, uncover, and

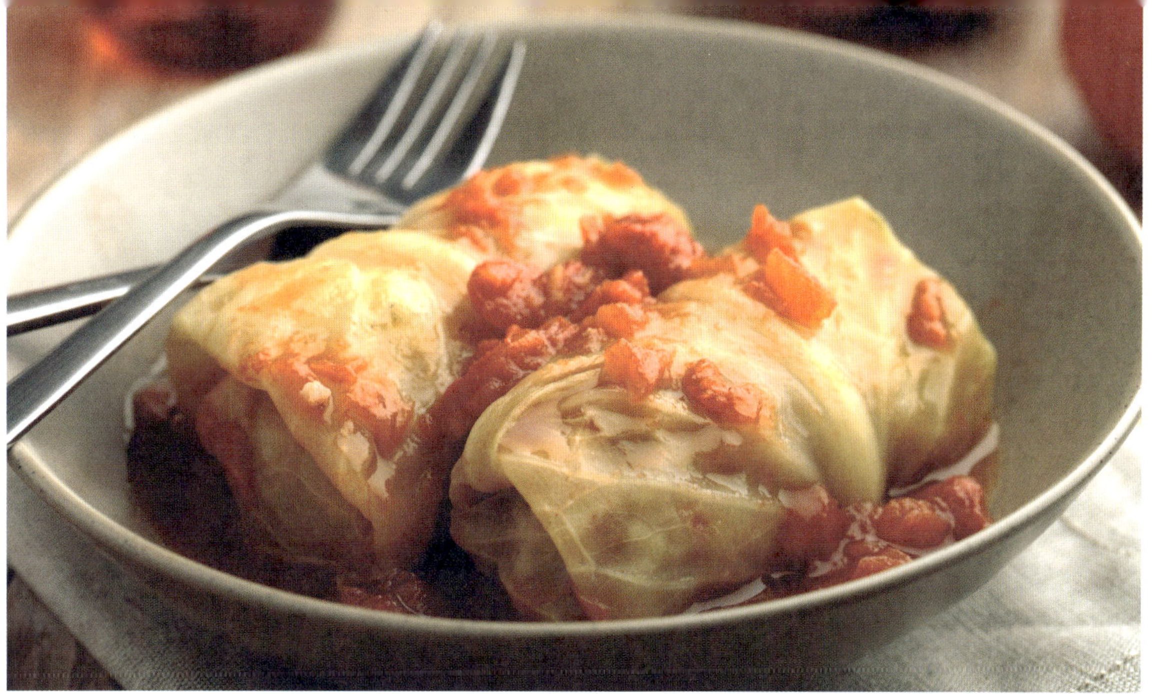

allow to cool. Remove the bay leaf and set aside any servings for family meals before pureeing.

5. For the puree, place as many cabbage rolls as you like into a food processor or blender. Pulse to break up the components. Add ½ cup of sauce and process until you achieve the desired texture. Check to make sure that the cabbage puree has no thick stems or fibers. If necessary, pass it through a mesh strainer using a silicone spatula.

6. Test as you go and at time of serving to see if a thickening agent, thickened sauce, or thickened stock is needed; use IDDSI Testing Methods (*iddsi.org*) to help achieve the desired IDDSI level. See pages 42-47.

7. Serve immediately or divide into servings for storage or freezing, following the directions for Food Storage and Labeling, page 62, and Serving, page 77.

NUTRITIONAL ANALYSIS PER SERVING | 1 cup
412 calories, 10 g fat, 3 g saturated fat, 145 mg sodium, 15 g sugar, 51 g carbohydrates, 6 g fiber, 7 g protein

Sausage and Rice–Stuffed Peppers

SERVINGS: 4 | IDDSI LEVELS   

By precooking the bell peppers, you shorten the cooking time of the whole dish, deepen the peppers' flavor, and yield a softer texture for the puree. The traditional presentation for stuffed peppers is to cut off the top and bake standing up. This is difficult for puree, so I have adopted the lengthwise cut. For variety, use different grains or vary the protein, using another ground meat or tofu in place of the sausage.

2 medium red bell peppers, sliced vertically into halves, stems and seeds removed
1 tablespoon extra-virgin olive oil, plus more for drizzling
4 ounces sweet Italian sausage, casing removed
1 shallot, thinly sliced
1 garlic clove, thinly sliced
2 cups Rice Congee (see page 196), or substitute quinoa, millet, barley, or buckwheat (see Whole Grains, page 194)
½ teaspoon dried parsley
1 (15-ounce) can diced tomatoes
1 (8-ounce) can tomato sauce

1. Place a rack in the center of the oven and preheat to 400°F (205°C). Paint the pepper halves with olive oil, place on a baking sheet cut side down, and roast until softened, about 20 minutes. Set aside to cool.

2. Meanwhile, warm 1 tablespoon olive oil in a medium skillet over medium heat. Add the sausage and cook, using a wooden spoon to break the meat into small pieces, until no longer pink and very lightly browned, about 5 minutes.

3. Use a slotted spoon to transfer the meat to a large bowl. Add the shallot to the pan and sauté, stirring occasionally, until translucent, 2 minutes. Add the garlic and cook for 1 minute.

4. Transfer the shallot and garlic to the bowl with the sausage meat. Add the Rice Congee and dried parsley to the bowl and stir to combine.

5. Lower the oven temperature to 350°F (175°C). Add the diced tomatoes and tomato sauce to a 9 x 9-inch baking dish and stir to combine.

6. Fill each pepper half with about ¾ cup of filling and carefully transfer them to the baking dish, filling side up. Cover the dish with aluminum foil and bake for 30 minutes. Allow to cool, and set aside any servings for family meals before pureeing.

7. For the puree, place as many pepper halves as you like into a food processor or blender. Pulse to break up the components. Add ½ cup of sauce and process until you achieve the desired texture. Check to make sure that the peppers have pureed smoothly. If necessary, pass through a mesh strainer using a silicone spatula.

8. Test as you go and at time of serving to see if a thickening agent, thickened sauce, or thickened stock is needed; use IDDSI Testing Methods (*iddsi.org*) to help achieve the desired IDDSI level. See pages 42-47.

9. Serve immediately or divide into servings for storage or freezing, following the directions for Serving, page 77.

NUTRITIONAL ANALYSIS PER SERVING | ½ pepper (3 oz)
253 calories, 5 g fat, 1 g saturated fat, 48 mg sodium, 6 g sugar, 38 g carbohydrates, 3 g fiber, 14 g protein

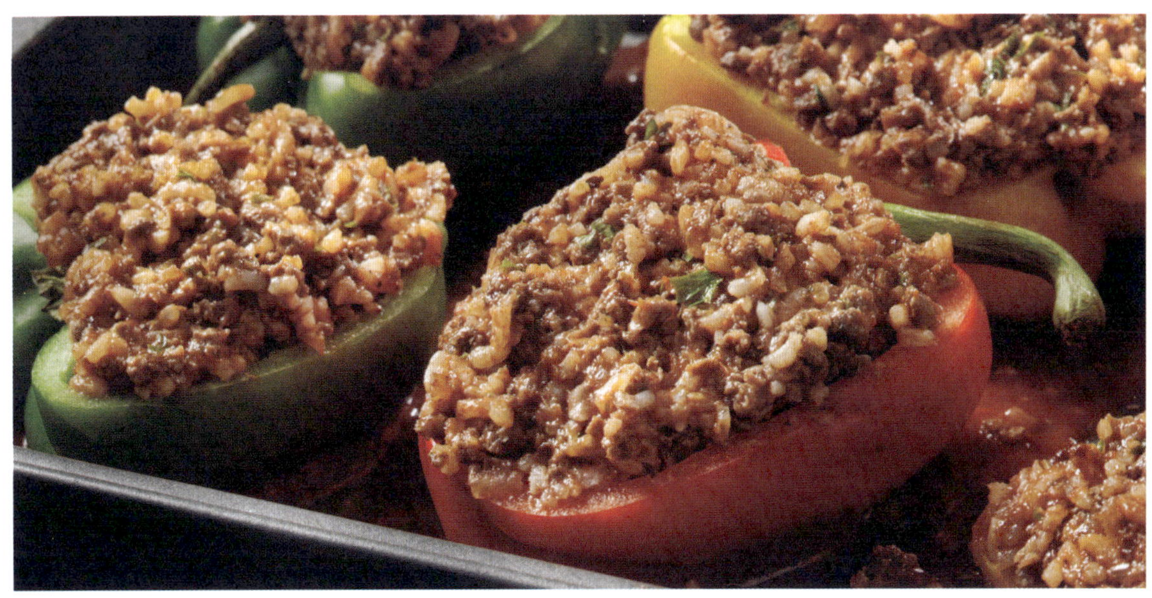

Sausage and Peppers

SERVINGS: 4 | IDDSI LEVELS 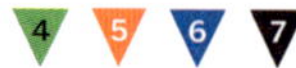

This dish is inspired by a classic flavor profile and a time-honored favorite of Italian street food. This version, adapted for home use, is also versatile, because you can use the gravy with other proteins such as a chicken breast, a small steak, a burger, or even eggs for a sausage, onion, and peppers omelet.

1 teaspoon extra-virgin olive oil
1 pound sweet Italian sausage, casings removed
Onion and Pepper Smother Gravy (see page 153)

1. Warm the olive oil in a skillet over medium heat. Add the sausage and cook, stirring occasionally, until cooked through and lightly golden, 6 to 7 minutes. Set aside to cool.

2. For family meals, set aside a portion and serve the warm sausage topped with the gravy. (For a more classic presentation for family meals, you can leave the sausage in the casing and sear it in the skillet until golden and blistered on all sides and cooked through. Serve on a plate or a roll, smothered with the gravy.)

3. For the puree, add 4 ounces sausage and ½ cup Onion and Pepper Smother Gravy per serving to a food processor or blender with the lid vented. Pulse to break up the ingredients and process until you achieve the desired texture.

4. Test as you go and at time of serving to see if a thickening agent, thickened sauce, or thickened stock is needed; use IDDSI Testing Methods (*iddsi.org*) to help achieve the desired IDDSI level. See pages 42-47.

5. Serve immediately or divide into servings for storage or freezing, following the directions for Serving, page 77.

NUTRITIONAL ANALYSIS PER SERVING | 4 oz
225 calories, 23.9 g fat, 3.5 g saturated fat, 187 mg sodium, 0 g sugar, 0.3 g carbohydrates, 0 g fiber, 4.7 g protein

Onion and Pepper Smother Gravy

YIELD: 1½ CUPS | IDDSI LEVEL 

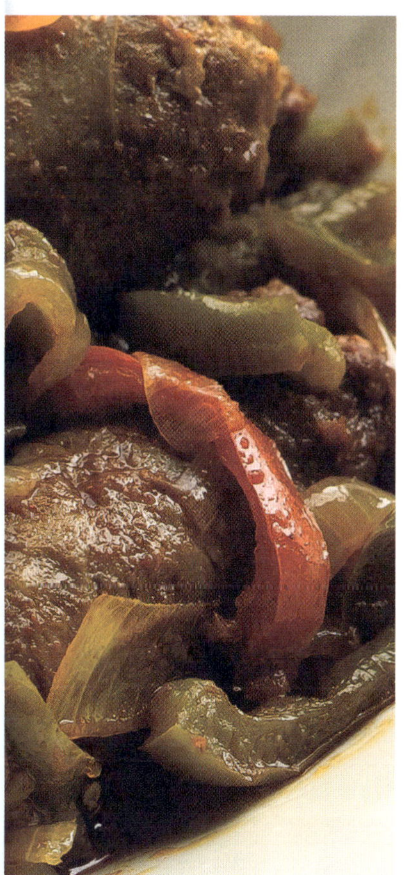

2 cups low-sodium chicken or vegetable broth
3 tablespoons extra-virgin olive oil, divided
1 large yellow onion, cut into ⅛-inch slices
1 red or green bell pepper, cut into ⅛-inch slices
2 tablespoons Wondra flour
1 teaspoon low-sodium soy sauce
⅛ teaspoon white pepper

1. Bring the broth to a simmer in a small saucepan.

2. Warm 1 tablespoon oil in a large skillet over medium-high heat. Add the onion and pepper slices and sauté, stirring often, until softened and lightly blistered, 3 minutes. Transfer to a plate.

3. Lower the heat to medium and add 2 more tablespoons oil to the skillet. Add the flour and cook, stirring constantly, until lightly golden, about 1 minute. Slowly add the simmering broth, stirring constantly to prevent lumps. Add the soy sauce and white pepper and bring the mixture to a simmer. Cook until thickened, about 2 minutes.

4. Add the vegetables back to the skillet and simmer together for 1 minute to blend the flavors. Allow to cool slightly. Puree with sausage or the protein of your choice. Process until you achieve the desired texture.

5. Serve immediately, or allow to cool completely, cover, and refrigerate for up to 48 hours or freeze for up to 3 months.

NUTRITIONAL ANALYSIS PER SERVING | ½ cup
85 calories, 6.7 g fat, 1 g saturated fat, 107 mg sodium, 1.3 g sugar, 4.9 g carbohydrates, 0.6 g fiber, 2.1 g protein

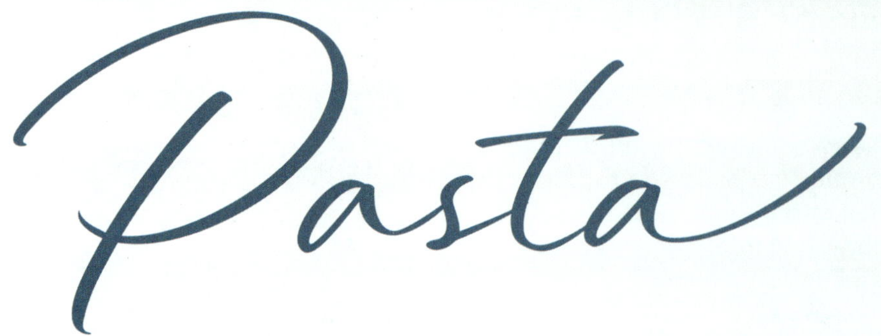

Pasta

155 Stuffed Shells

156 Spaghetti with Tomato Sauce

158 Ziti with Meat Sauce

160 Lasagna

162 Turkey Meatballs and Spaghetti

164 Linguine with Clam Sauce

166 Zucchini Noodles with Lemon, Spinach, and Asparagus

168 Penne with Pesto

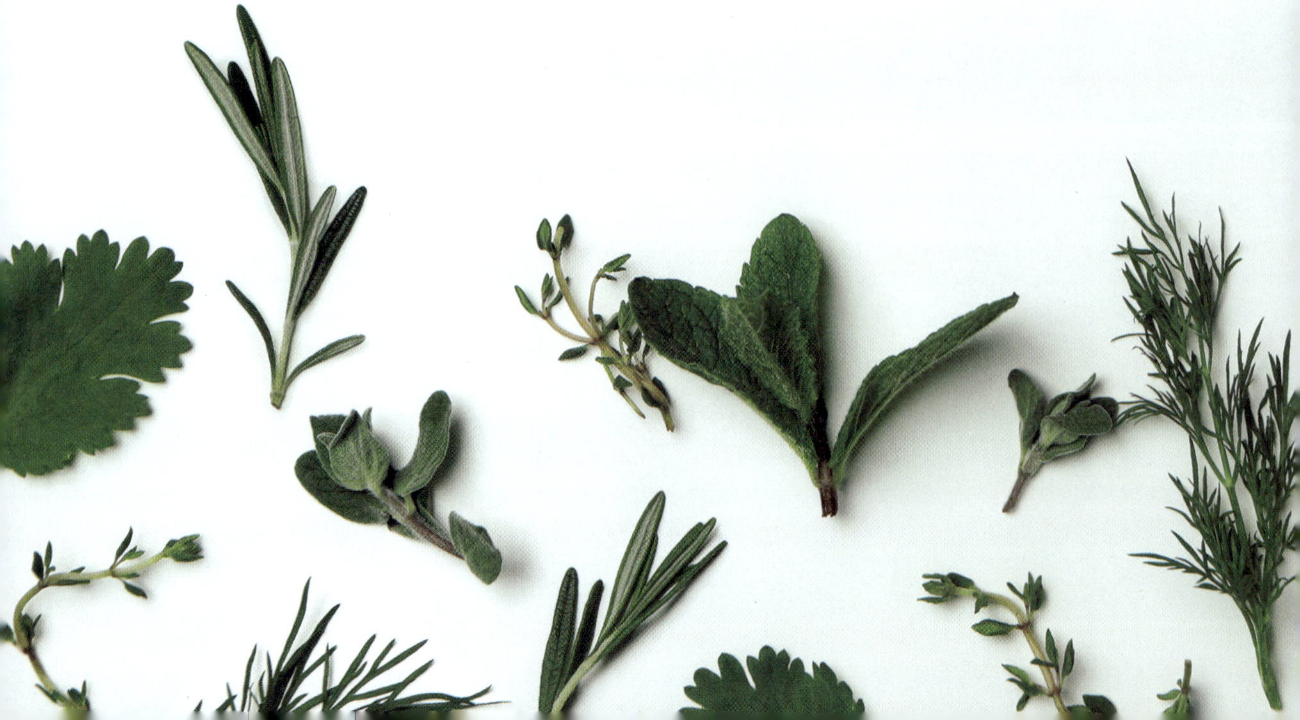

Stuffed Shells

SERVINGS: 4 | IDDSI LEVELS 

The process of pureeing adds air to the ricotta cheese mixture and increases the volume of the dish, so one serving may look like more than one serving.

Sea salt
8 jumbo shells
24 ounces of tomato sauce (from Spaghetti with Tomato Sauce, see page 156) or 1 (24-ounce) jar store-bought marinara sauce
2 cups ricotta cheese
⅓ cup grated parmesan
1 large egg
2 tablespoons finely chopped flat-leaf parsley or parsley paste
1 tablespoon finely chopped basil or basil paste
White pepper

1. Place a rack in the center of the oven and preheat to 350°F (175°C). Bring a large pot of water to a boil. Generously salt the water and cook the shells for half the time indicated in the package instructions. Drain and set aside.

2. Add the tomato sauce to the bottom of an 8 x 8-inch baking dish. Set aside.

3. In a medium bowl, combine the ricotta cheese, parmesan, egg, parsley, and basil, and season with a pinch of salt and white pepper. Stir thoroughly. Using a tablespoon, fill the parboiled shells, transferring each filled shell to the prepared baking dish.

4. Cover the dish with foil and bake until bubbling, 35 minutes. Allow to cool, and set aside any family servings.

5. For the puree, transfer the desired number of servings (2 shells per serving) to a food processor or high-speed blender. Add ⅓ cup sauce per serving. Pulse to break up the ingredients and process until you achieve the desired texture.

6. Test as you go and at time of serving to see if a thickening agent, thickened sauce, or thickened stock is needed; use IDDSI Testing Methods (*iddsi.org*) to help achieve the desired IDDSI level. See pages 42-47.

7. Serve immediately or divide into servings for storage or freezing, following the directions for Serving, page 77.

NUTRITIONAL ANALYSIS PER SERVING | 2 stuffed shells
336 calories, 13 g fat, 8 g saturated fat, 320 mg sodium, 7 g sugar, 31 g carbohydrates, 3 g fiber, 19 g protein

Spaghetti with Tomato Sauce

SERVINGS: 2 (PLUS ABOUT 2 QUARTS LEFTOVER SAUCE) | IDDSI LEVELS 4 5 6 7

In the world of Italian cooks, everyone has a favorite sauce. My mother always added a can of tomato paste, thinned out with several tablespoons of water whisked in. This adds thickness to the sauce and gives it a depth of flavor. I like to make a pot of sauce once a month; that way a good sauce is always on hand for a quick meal. This sauce freezes particularly well.

2 tablespoons extra-virgin olive oil
1 large yellow onion, diced
1 medium carrot, diced
1 medium celery stalk, diced
1 teaspoon oregano paste
1 teaspoon parsley paste
1 teaspoon basil paste
3 garlic cloves, sliced or diced
1 (4-ounce) can tomato paste
¼ cup red wine (optional)
1 (28-ounce) can crushed tomatoes
1 (28-ounce) can tomato puree
1 (28-ounce) can tomato sauce
Sea salt
8 ounces spaghetti

1. In a large stockpot, warm the oil over medium-high heat. Add the onion, carrot, celery, and the herb pastes and sauté, stirring occasionally, until softened, about 6 minutes. Add the garlic and sauté for 1 minute.

2. Add the tomato paste and cook, stirring, until the raw taste of the tomato paste cooks off and it begins to brown, about 3 minutes. Add the red wine and bring to a simmer, stirring to scrape up any tomato paste from the bottom of the pot.

3. Add the crushed tomatoes, tomato puree, and tomato sauce and stir to combine. Simmer on low heat with the lid slightly ajar until the sauce is reduced and very flavorful, about 3 hours. Season with salt. Remove from the heat and allow to cool. Reserve 1 cup of the sauce for serving with your pasta.
   › **Tip:** Transfer the rest of the sauce to storage containers. This sauce will keep in the refrigerator for up to 48 hours and in the freezer for up to 3 months.

4. Meanwhile, bring a large pot of water to a boil. Season the water generously with salt, add the spaghetti, and cook for 1 minute longer than the package instructions indicate. Drain and set aside any family servings before pureeing.

5. For the puree, add the spaghetti to a food processor or blender, along with ½ cup sauce per serving. Pulse to break down the pasta and process until you achieve the desired texture.

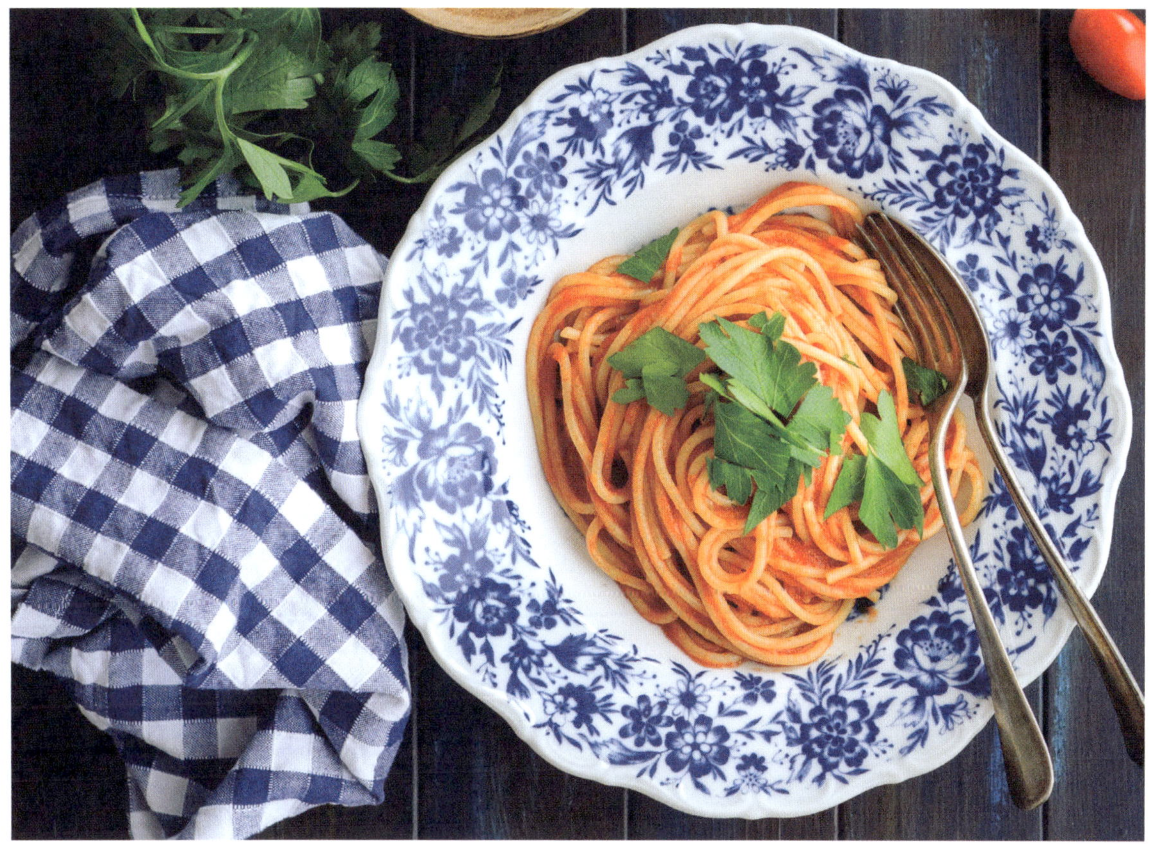

6. Test as you go and at time of serving to see if a thickening agent, thickened sauce, or thickened stock is needed; use IDDSI Testing Methods (*iddsi.org*) to help achieve the desired IDDSI level. See pages 42-47.

7. Serve immediately or divide into servings for storage or freezing, following the directions for Serving, page 77.

NUTRITIONAL ANALYSIS PER SERVING | ½ cup (20 servings)
Tomato sauce only
266 calories, 10.1 g fat, 1.4 g saturated fat, 51 mg sodium, 23.7 g sugar, 41.2 g carbohydrates, 10.7 g fiber, 11.8 g protein

(Spaghetti nutritional analysis will be on the spaghetti package; different for every brand.)

Ziti with Meat Sauce

SERVINGS: 2 (PLUS ABOUT 2 QUARTS LEFTOVER SAUCE) | IDDSI LEVELS 

7

Meat that is cooked in the sauce adds flavor and becomes very tender. You can also start the meat sauce by searing a couple of thin pork chops or browning some sweet Italian sausage. The tender pork chops and sausage will be pureed with the sauce.

- 2 tablespoons extra-virgin olive oil
- ½ pound ground beef or pork, or a combination
- 1 large yellow onion, diced
- 1 medium carrot, diced
- 1 medium celery stalk, diced
- 3 garlic cloves, thinly sliced
- 1 (4-ounce) can tomato paste
- ¼ cup red wine (optional)
- 1 (28-ounce) can crushed tomatoes
- 1 (28-ounce) can tomato puree
- 1 (28-ounce) can tomato sauce
- 1 teaspoon sea salt
- 8 ounces ziti

1. In a large stockpot, warm the oil over medium-high heat. Add the meat and cook, using a wooden spoon to break it up into small pieces, until browned, about 6 minutes. Add the onion, carrot, and celery and sauté, stirring occasionally, until the vegetables are softened, about 6 minutes. Add the garlic and sauté for 1 minute.

2. Add the tomato paste and cook, stirring, until the raw taste of the tomato paste cooks off and it begins to brown, about 3 minutes. Add the red wine and bring to a simmer, stirring to scrape up any tomato paste and browned meat from the bottom of the pot.

3. Add the crushed tomatoes, tomato puree, and tomato sauce and stir to combine. Simmer on low heat with the lid slightly ajar until the sauce is reduced and very flavorful, about 3 hours. Season with salt. Remove from the heat and allow to cool. Reserve 1 cup sauce for serving with your pasta. Transfer the rest of the sauce to storage containers. This sauce will keep in the refrigerator for up to 48 hours and in the freezer for up to 3 months.

4. Meanwhile, bring a large pot of water to a boil. Season the water generously with salt, add the ziti, and cook for 1 minute longer than the package instructions indicate. Drain and set aside any family servings before pureeing.

5. For the puree, add the ziti to a food processor or blender, along with ½ cup sauce per serving. Pulse to break down the pasta and process until you achieve the desired texture. Add more sauce if needed to prevent stickiness. Ziti with meat sauce may be piped into pasta shapes.

6. Test as you go and at time of serving to see if a thickening agent, thickened sauce, or thickened stock is needed; use IDDSI Testing Methods (*iddsi.org*) to help achieve the desired IDDSI level. See pages 42-47.

7. Serve immediately or divide into servings for storage or freezing, following the directions for Serving, page 77.

NUTRITIONAL ANALYSIS PER SERVING | 1 cup
Meat sauce only
235 calories, 6 g fat, 2 g saturated fat, 265 mg sodium, 6 g sugar, 28 g carbohydrates, 3 g fiber, 25.6 g protein

(Ziti nutritional analysis will be on ziti package; different for every brand.)

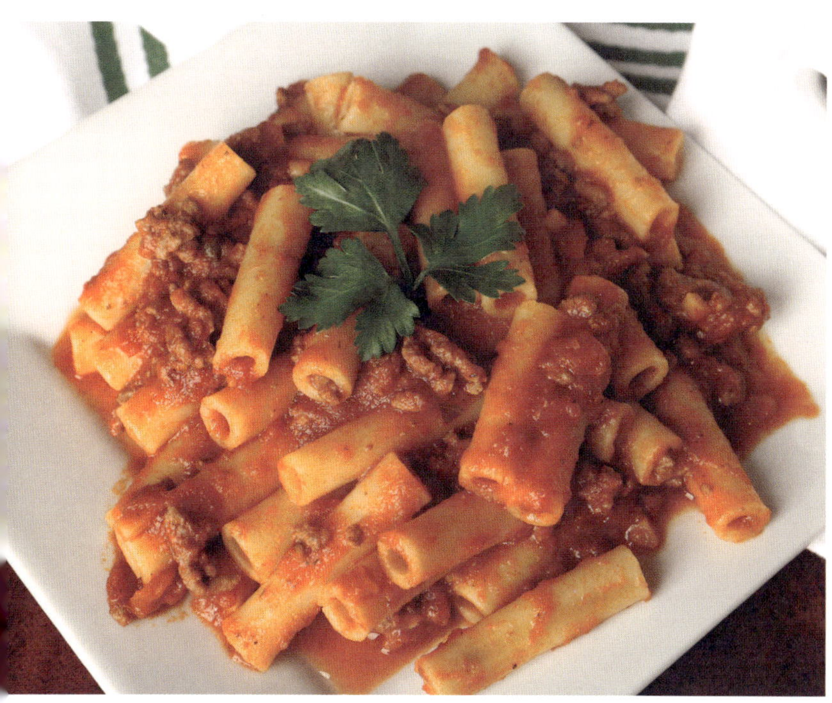

Lasagna

SERVINGS: 6 | IDDSI LEVELS 

This lasagna purees and freezes beautifully. Aside from the convenience, no-boil lasagna noodles are thinner, which makes for a better proportion of carbohydrate to protein and vegetable. The oven-ready noodles also make for a better puree because they are less starchy. This recipe eliminates the traditional mozzarella cheese, which can cause swallowing difficulties.

3 cups ricotta cheese
½ cup grated parmesan, plus more for topping
2 tablespoons finely chopped flat-leaf parsley or parsley paste
2 large eggs, lightly beaten
Sea salt and white pepper
1 quart tomato sauce (from Spaghetti with Tomato Sauce, see page 156), or 1 (32-ounce) jar marinara sauce
1 (9-ounce) package oven-ready lasagna noodles

1. Place a rack in the center of the oven and preheat to 350°F (175°C). In a bowl, mix the ricotta, parmesan, parsley, eggs, and a pinch of salt and white pepper until smooth.

2. Spread 1¼ cups sauce in the bottom of a 9 x 13-inch baking dish. Add a layer of four noodles, overlapping by ¼ inch to create a solid base. Spread ½ cup sauce over the bottom layer of noodles to make sure the noodles have enough sauce to cook properly.

3. Spread 1 cup of the ricotta filling over the sauce, then add a second layer of noodles and cover with ½ cup sauce. Spread another cup of the ricotta filling over the sauce, followed by a third layer of noodles and ½ cup sauce.

4. Finally, spread the last cup of the ricotta filling followed by the final layer of noodles. This uses twelve noodles in all. Spread the remaining 1¼ cups sauce over the top layer of noodles and sprinkle the top with parmesan cheese.

5. Bake until browned and bubbly, 50 minutes. Remove from the oven, setting aside any servings for family meals, and let cool before pureeing.

6. For the puree, transfer the desired number of servings to a food processor and pulse to break up the elements.

Process until you achieve the desired texture. Add sauce if needed to prevent stickiness.

7. Test as you go and at time of serving to see if a thickening agent, thickened sauce, or thickened stock is needed; use IDDSI Testing Methods (*iddsi.org*) to help achieve the desired IDDSI level. See pages 42-47.

8. Serve immediately or divide into servings for storage or freezing, following the directions for Serving, page 77.

NUTRITIONAL ANALYSIS PER SERVING | 4 oz
484 calories, 14 g fat, 8 g saturated fat, 329 mg sodium, 10 g sugar, 61 g carbohydrates, 4 g fiber, 27 g protein

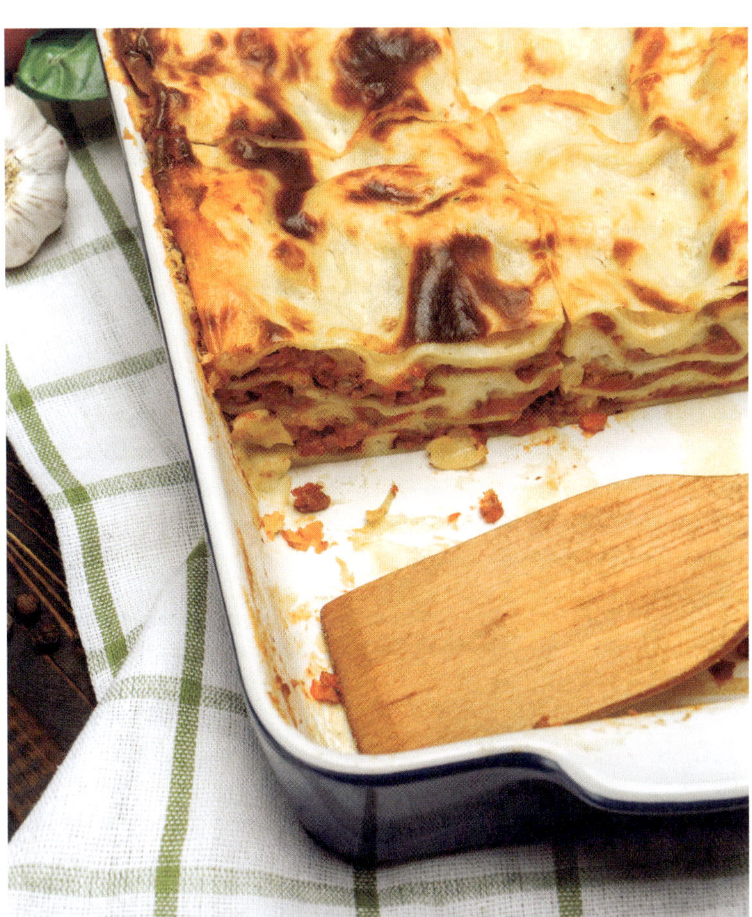

VARIATIONS

For variations on this classic lasagna, add any or a combination of the following to the sauce or in between the filling and the pasta sheets:

- 1 pound **mushrooms**, wiped with a damp cloth, sliced and sautéed
- 1 large **zucchini**, cut into ¼-inch half moons and sautéed, then drained
- 1 can quartered **artichoke hearts**, drained and patted dry, or 1 package frozen artichoke hearts, thawed, drained, and quartered
- 1 pound **spinach**, wilted in a sauté pan and drained
- ½ pound **ground beef**, **ground turkey**, **ground chicken**, or **Italian sausage**, casings removed, browned in 1 tablespoon olive oil

Turkey Meatballs and Spaghetti

SERVINGS: 4 | IDDSI LEVELS 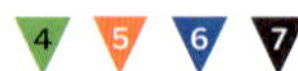

This recipe employs the technique of oven-roasting the meatballs. This eliminates the step of browning meatballs in a pan of oil, which allows you to use less oil and makes for easier cleanup. Meatballs and spaghetti are a delicious classic for the family as well as for a puree. For freezer storage, make a double batch.

2 tablespoons extra-virgin olive oil, divided
1 pound ground turkey
1 large egg
2 tablespoons grated parmesan cheese
2 tablespoons finely chopped flat-leaf parsley or parsley paste
1 garlic clove, grated, or 1 teaspoon garlic paste
¼ cup Italian-style seasoned breadcrumbs, plus more as needed
Sea salt and white pepper
1 quart tomato sauce (from Spaghetti with Tomato Sauce, see page 156), or 1 (32-ounce) jar marinara sauce
8 ounces spaghetti

1. Place a rack in the center of the oven and preheat to 425°F (220°C). Lightly oil a half baking sheet, or use a silicone cupcake sheet placed on a baking sheet.

2. Add the ground turkey to a large mixing bowl along with the egg, parmesan, parsley, garlic, breadcrumbs, 1 teaspoon oil, and a pinch of sea salt and white pepper. Using clean wet hands, mix gently to thoroughly incorporate the mixture.

3. If the mixture is too wet to form meatballs, add additional breadcrumbs, 2 teaspoons at a time. Mix thoroughly, taking care not to overwork the mixture so that the meatballs will not be tough. Cover the bowl and refrigerate for 30 minutes.

4. Using a small cookie scoop, or a tablespoon and your hands (taking care not to pack the mixture tightly), form 1-inch meatballs and transfer them to the baking sheet or to the silicone cupcake sheet.

5. Add the remaining olive oil to a small bowl and, using a pastry brush, paint each meatball with the olive oil. Roast for 15 minutes, turning the meatballs halfway through roasting, until they are light golden brown.
   › **Tip:** You can freeze extra meatballs with sauce in freezer- and oven-safe glass storage containers.

6. Meanwhile, place the sauce in a large saucepan and bring to a simmer over medium-low heat. Transfer the roasted meatballs to the simmering sauce and cook for 20 minutes.

7. Bring a large pot of water to a boil. Season the water generously with salt, add the spaghetti, and cook for 1 minute longer than the package instructions indicate. Drain the spaghetti and set aside any family servings before pureeing, and serve topped with meatballs and sauce.

8. For the puree, break up 3 meatballs per serving into a food processor or high-speed blender. Add ½ cup sauce and about 1 cup cooked spaghetti per serving. Pulse to break down the meatballs and pasta and process until you achieve the desired texture.

9. Test as you go and at time of serving to see if a thickening agent, thickened sauce, or thickened stock is needed; use IDDSI Testing Methods (*iddsi.org*) to help achieve the desired IDDSI level. See pages 42-47.

10. Serve immediately or divide into servings for storage or freezing, following the directions for Serving, page 77.

NUTRITIONAL ANALYSIS PER SERVING | 3 meatballs and ½ cup sauce
120 calories, 5 g fat, 2 g saturated fat, 203 mg sodium, 0 g sugar, 5 g carbohydrates, 0 g fiber, 12 g protein

(Spaghetti nutritional analysis will be on spaghetti package; different for every brand.)

PRO TIP

Instead of turkey, you can use ground beef or a combination of beef with pork or veal. For vegetarian meatballs, use the Vegetarian Almond Lentil Loaf recipe (see page 116) and form the mixture into 1-inch balls.

Linguine with Clam Sauce

SERVINGS: 2 | IDDSI LEVELS 4 5 6 7

A delicious dish, both for anyone with swallowing difficulties and for family and friends. This recipe may be doubled for a group or to stock the freezer. For service, the pureed and thickened pasta may be piped onto a plate to resemble spaghetti. The clam sauce is made separately, pureed and thickened, and added over the top of the dish of piped spaghetti.

- Sea salt
- 4 ounces linguine
- 4 tablespoons extra-virgin olive oil, divided
- 2 garlic cloves, thinly sliced
- 1 (6.5-ounce) can minced clams, with juice
- 1 (8-ounce) bottle clam juice
- 3 tablespoons finely chopped flat-leaf parsley or parsley paste
- ⅛ teaspoon white pepper
- 2 teaspoons fresh lemon juice

1. Bring a large pot of water to a boil. Season the water generously with salt. Add the linguine, stir, and cook for 1 minute longer than the package instructions indicate. Reserve about 1 cup pasta cooking water when you drain the pasta in a colander. Toss the pasta with 1 tablespoon olive oil to prevent it from sticking together and allow the pasta to cool for 5 minutes.

2. Prepare the clam sauce. Add the remaining olive oil to a large sauté pan and set over medium-low heat. Add the garlic and sauté for 1 to 2 minutes. Add the clams, clam juice, parsley, and pepper and simmer for 3 minutes. Add the lemon juice and stir to combine.

3. Remove the clam sauce from the heat and allow to cool. Reserve a portion of the sauce and pasta for family meals.

4. For the puree, transfer the sauce to a food processor or blender. If serving over the piped linguine (see Tip in step 5 below), process until you achieve the desired texture.

5. If pureeing the pasta and the sauce together, add both to a food processor along with 6 tablespoons reserved pasta cooking water per serving, and process until you achieve the desired texture.
   - › **Tip:** For a more exciting presentation, instead of pureeing the pasta with the sauce, transfer 1 serving of the pasta to a food processor or blender. Add 6

tablespoons pasta cooking water and process until you achieve the desired texture. Add more cooking water if necessary to achieve the smooth puree. Transfer the pasta puree to a disposable piping bag and cut off the tip of the bag to form a very narrow opening. Pipe onto a plate, making thin strips in a circular motion, until you have created a plate that resembles a mound of linguine. Cover with plastic wrap until the clam sauce is ready.

6. Test as you go and at time of serving to see if a thickening agent, thickened sauce, or thickened stock is needed; use IDDSI Testing Methods (*iddsi.org*) to help achieve the desired IDDSI level. See pages 42-47.

7. Serve immediately or divide into servings for storage or freezing, following the directions for Serving, page 77.

NUTRITIONAL ANALYSIS PER SERVING | 4 oz
Clam sauce only
243 calories, 14 g fat, 4.7 g saturated fat, 670 mg sodium, 0.6 g sugar, 7.7 g carbohydrates, 0.5 g fiber, 22 g protein

(Linguine nutritional analysis will be on linguine package; different for every brand.)

Zucchini Noodles with Lemon, Spinach, and Asparagus

SERVINGS: 2 | IDDSI LEVELS 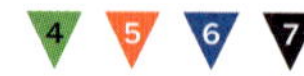

This dish is vegetarian and gluten free. A vegan version may be made by replacing the parmesan cheese with vegan cheese. Veggie noodles have 90 percent fewer calories than pasta. I recommend fresh zucchini spirals made with a home spiral machine, as frozen spirals get mushy when cooked. For a topping, Roasted Mushrooms (see page 182) are a great pairing.

1½ cups zucchini spirals
3 tablespoons extra-virgin olive oil
4 garlic cloves, thinly sliced
1 small bunch asparagus, woody ends trimmed, peeled if skins are tough, and cut into 1-inch pieces
1 cup low-sodium vegetable broth
1 tablespoon fresh lemon juice
¼ teaspoon sea salt
⅛ teaspoon white pepper
1 cup baby spinach leaves
1 teaspoon finely chopped fresh parsley or parsley paste
4 ounces silken tofu, cut into ½-inch dice
¼ cup grated parmesan or vegan parmesan

1. Place the zucchini spirals in a large skillet over medium heat. Cover the pan and steam for 5 minutes, stirring occasionally, until the zucchini is cooked through but not mushy. Transfer the zucchini noodles to a colander and drain. Reserve.

2. Wipe out the skillet, add the olive oil, and warm over medium heat. Add the garlic and cook, stirring frequently, 1 to 2 minutes. Add the asparagus and cook 1 more minute. Add ½ cup vegetable broth and the lemon juice, season with salt and pepper, and bring to a simmer.

3. Simmer until the asparagus is very tender, about 8 minutes. Add the remaining ½ cup vegetable broth and the spinach, parsley, and tofu. Simmer, stirring, until the spinach wilts, about 2 minutes. Add the parmesan and stir until it melts. Remove from the heat and allow to cool for 10 minutes.

4. Add the drained zucchini back to the pan and stir to combine. Set aside any family servings before pureeing.

5. For the puree, add the desired number of ¾-cup portions to a food processor or blender. Pulse to break up the ingredients and process until you achieve the desired texture.

6. Test as you go and at time of serving to see if a thickening agent, thickened sauce, or thickened stock is needed; use IDDSI Testing Methods (*iddsi.org*) to help achieve the desired IDDSI level. See pages 42-47.
   - **Tip:** For serving, if you want, transfer the puree into a disposable piping bag. Cut off the tip of the bag to form a very narrow opening. Pipe onto a plate in a circular motion to create a mound of spaghetti-like spirals. Alternatively, serve the dish by spooning it into a colorful bowl.

7. Serve immediately or divide into servings for storage or freezing, following the directions for Serving, page 77. (If you pipe the whole recipe, any extra piped plates of puree can be placed in a zip-top plastic bag and stored in the fridge for up to 48 hours or in the freezer for up to 3 months.)

NUTRITIONAL ANALYSIS PER SERVING | 1 cup
280 calories, 19.5 g fat, 7.3 g saturated fat, 648 mg sodium, 2.8 g sugar, 11.7 g carbohydrates, 3.5 g fiber, 18.3 g protein

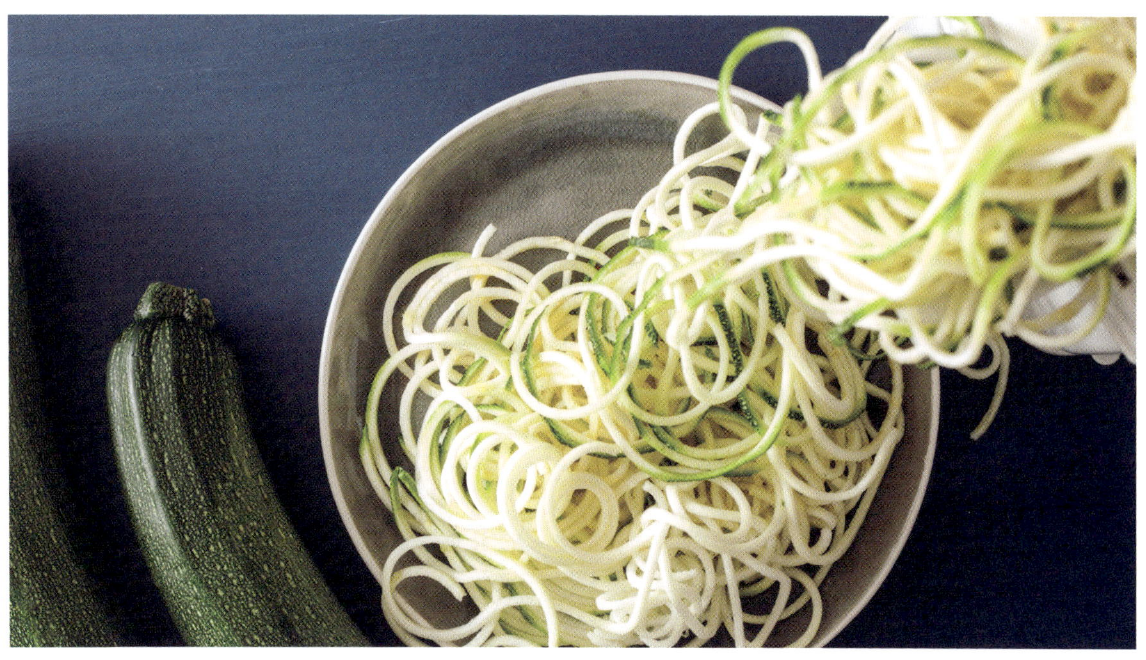

Penne with Pesto

SERVINGS: 2 (PLUS ½ CUP EXTRA PESTO) | IDDSI LEVELS 4  

This is very easy to make, and in addition to pasta, this pesto will flavor a soup, a vegetable, or a protein. Add a teaspoon of pesto to Minestrone (see page 85) or Tomato Sauce (from Spaghetti with Tomato Sauce, see page 156) for added depth of flavor. If you prefer less garlic, reduce the amount of garlic in the recipe. Basil is the important ingredient in making pesto, because of its fragrance and flavor. I have used whole-grain pasta in this recipe, a healthy choice with good flavor. Make sure to cook it until it is tender so it will puree.

8 ounces whole wheat penne
Sea salt
2 garlic cloves
2 cups fresh basil leaves
½ cup extra-virgin olive oil, plus more as needed
¼ cup grated parmesan
¼ cup raw pine nuts

1. Bring a large pot of water to a boil. Season the water generously with salt, add the penne, and cook for 1 minute longer than the package instructions indicate. Reserve ½ cup pasta cooking water. Drain the pasta and set aside.

2. Place the garlic and ¼ teaspoon salt in a food processor. Pulse to mince the garlic. Add the basil and pulse until finely chopped. Use a spatula to scrape down the sides of the food processor. Add half of the olive oil and pulse to puree.

3. Add the parmesan and pine nuts and the rest of the olive oil and puree until you have the consistency of a smooth sauce. Scrape the sides once more and give the pesto an extra buzz to puree the pine nuts well rather than leave them crunchy, as in traditional pesto.
   - **Note:** Store any leftover pesto in a container in the refrigerator for up to 2 weeks or in the freezer for up to a month.

4. In a large bowl, toss the cooked pasta with ¼ cup pesto and ¼ cup pasta water. Add another splash of olive oil or pasta water as needed so that the pasta is saucy and nicely coated. If desired, set aside any family servings before pureeing.

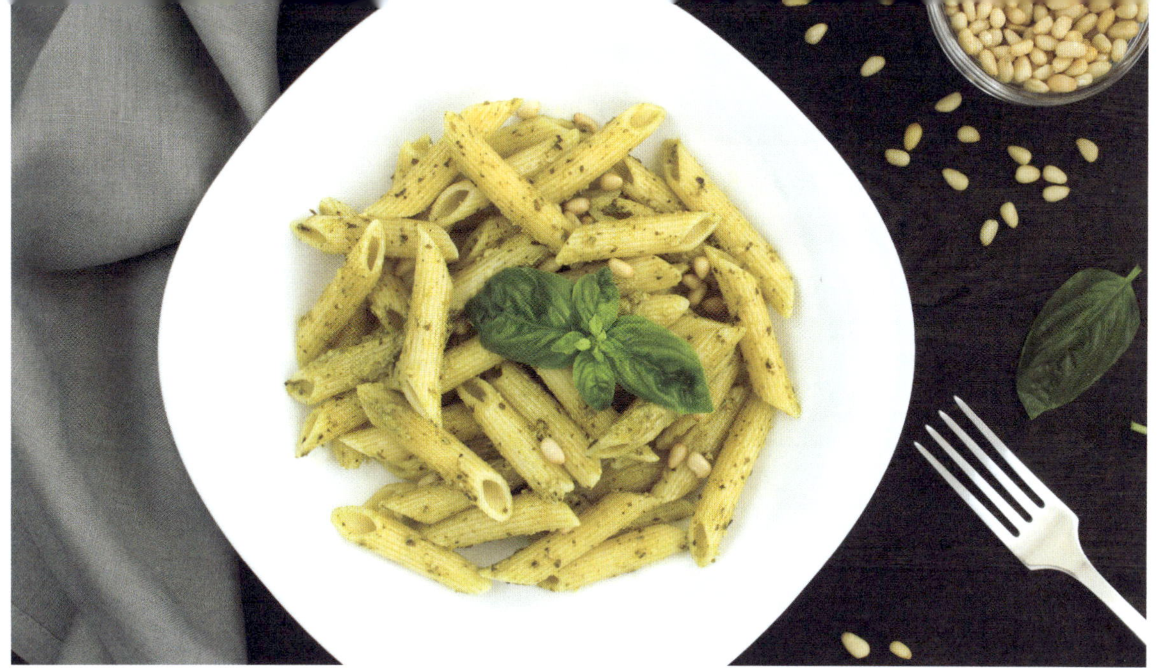

5. For the puree, add the cooked pasta and sauce to a food processor or blender. Pulse to break down the pasta and puree until you achieve the desired texture. Add another splash of pasta water if needed to prevent stickiness.

6. Test as you go and at time of serving to see if a thickening agent, thickened sauce, or thickened stock is needed; use IDDSI Testing Methods (*iddsi.org*) to help achieve the desired IDDSI level. See pages 42-47.

7. Serve immediately or divide into servings for storage or freezing, following the directions for Serving, page 77.

NUTRITIONAL ANALYSIS PER SERVING | 2 tablespoons
Pesto Sauce only
116 calories, 12 g fat, 2 g saturated fat, 83 mg sodium, 0 g sugar, 1 g carbohydrates, 1 g fiber, 1 g protein

(Penne nutritional analysis will be on penne package; different for every brand.)

Vegetable Side Dishes

172 Basic Steamed Vegetables

174 Slow-Baked Sweet Potatoes with Orange

176 Mashed Potatoes

178 Creamed Corn

179 Grilled Summer Vegetables

180 Roasted Winter Vegetables

182 Roasted Mushrooms

183 Roasted Asparagus

184 Ratatouille (Summer Vegetable Ragout)

185 Spinach and Parmesan Sauté

186 Braised Greens

187 Broccoli Parmesan

188 Brussels Sprouts with Shallots

189 Cabbage Sauté

190 Roasted Cauliflower

191 Garlic Green Beans

192 Ginger Carrots

193 Minty Pureed Peas

Steaming is an excellent way to prepare vegetables in the dysphagia kitchen. It is an easy technique for the cook and it preserves flavor and color. Steaming also preserves nutrients that are lost in boiling. It is excellent for batch cooking.

Here is a plan you can follow to stock the freezer with assorted vegetables for quick warming as side dishes for main courses.

I suggest an IDDSI Pureed, Level 4, for vegetable dishes because they make a great accompaniment to a meal. IDDSI Minced & Moist, Level 5, or Soft & Bite-Sized, Level 6, may be used, according to individual assignment by your health-care provider.

Suggested Steaming Times

For best puree results, steam all vegetables until fork tender.

Artichoke hearts	6 minutes
Asparagus	Large: 5 minutes Small: 4 minutes
Brussels sprouts	10 to 12 minutes
Butternut squash or other winter squash, 2-inch pieces	15 minutes
Cabbage, sliced	8 to 12 minutes
Carrot, sliced	7 minutes
Cauliflower and broccoli florets	10 minutes
Corn off the cob	10 to 15 minutes
Green beans	5 to 7 minutes
Kale, chard, collard greens	8 to 10 minutes
Parsnips, sliced	10 minutes
Peas	3 minutes
Spinach	3 to 5 minutes
Turnips, ¼-inch slices	15 minutes
Zucchini, ¼-inch slices	7 minutes

Basic Steamed Vegetables

With steamed vegetables frozen in individual servings, it is easy to add any vegetable to a meal. Just follow the instructions (see Serving, page 77) for thawing and heating in a steamer or on the stovetop. These prepared vegetables can also be added to soups or stews or can be combined to make vegetable soup. They help add variety in the dysphagia kitchen, keeping boredom at bay.

Vegetable purees are also flavorful and suitable additions to family and friend meals. In fact, vegetable purees are often served as the base for a fine-dining meal.

PRO TIP

Keep seasonings simple. Season lightly with salt and white pepper. A little broth helps to make a smooth and flavorful puree. Soy sauce may be used instead of salt. Other options are to season the vegetables with a little olive oil, a squeeze of lemon juice, and a pinch of parmesan cheese. For a quick cream sauce, use a good store-bought Alfredo. I am working on a vegan Alfredo, but it is not yet perfected. Or try a mild, tomato-based curry from Indian cuisine.

1. Choose your favorite vegetables, or experiment to see what appeals to the appetite. Some possibilities include carrots, broccoli, cauliflower, peas, green beans, zucchini, and butternut squash. A favorite of mine is parsnips, a relative of carrots.

2. For one steaming session, prep 1½ pounds of a vegetable, enough for 4 servings of ½ cup to 1 cup each. Peel and cut the vegetables as needed.

3. Vegetables should be cut in same-sized pieces for even cooking. Frozen vegetables work just as well as fresh vegetables and have the same nutrients. They are easy to store and do not go bad. Especially convenient is frozen diced butternut squash because it is already peeled.

4. Steam the vegetables. Fill a steamer basket with vegetables and place it in the steamer of your choice. If using a stovetop method, fill the bottom of a pot large enough to hold the steamer basket with several cups of water (only enough to reach just below the steamer basket), and bring to a boil over high heat. Lower the heat to medium-low, cover the pot with a tight-fitting lid, and steam each vegetable for the amount of time indicated in the list on page 171. (If using another appliance, consult the directions that come with your steamer for cook times.)

5. When steaming time is up, pierce a few of the vegetables with a sharp knife to see if they are tender. Remove the steamer basket. Allow the vegetables to cool. Steaming times for frozen and fresh vegetables are about the same, but I steam frozen vegetables for a minute less, so they do not get mushy. I check for tenderness, for a good puree. If desired, set aside any family servings before pureeing.

6. Puree the vegetables in a food processor or blender with a small amount of the cooking liquid added. To make sure the puree is smooth, rub the puree through a mesh strainer with a silicone spatula. This eliminates any bits of peel, fibrous strings, and seeds. When pureeing vegetables, a blender will break down the vegetables better.

7. Test as you go and at time of serving to see if a thickening agent, thickened sauce, or thickened stock is needed; use IDDSI Testing Methods (*iddsi.org*) to help achieve the desired IDDSI level. See pages 42-47.

8. Serve immediately, or divide into servings for storage or freezing, following the directions for Serving, page 77.

(Dr. Willett's book [see Resources] gives a complete nutritional breakdown for a variety of steamed vegetables.)

PRO TIP

Vegetable puree may be added to store-bought soups and homemade soups and stews, to boost nutrition and enhance flavor. Vegetable puree may also be added to leftover stir-fry, to increase vegetable content and enhance flavor.

Slow-Baked Sweet Potatoes with Orange

SERVINGS: 8 | IDDSI LEVELS 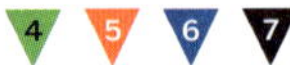

Sweet potatoes are loaded with nutrients, including fiber, antioxidants, vitamins A and C, and manganese. They are delicious with a tart glaze, rather than a more traditional but overly sweet and sugar-laden topping. This recipe was a favorite of my mom's.

- 4 medium sweet potatoes, approximately the same size (about 1½ pounds total)
- 2 tablespoons extra-virgin olive oil
- 2 tablespoons orange marmalade (preferably lower-sugar)
- 1 tablespoon honey or brown sugar (optional)
- 2 tablespoons orange juice
- ⅛ teaspoon ground cinnamon
- Sea salt

1. Place a rack in the center of the oven and preheat to 300°F (150°C). Line a baking sheet with aluminum foil. Wash and dry the potatoes and remove any sharp ends, knots, and blemishes. Puncture each potato three times with a knife to allow steam to escape.

2. Brush the outside of the potatoes with the olive oil and transfer to the prepared baking sheet, leaving room between them for air to circulate. Cover with another sheet of foil. Bake for 90 minutes, until the potatoes are very soft. Remove from the oven, remove the foil, and allow to cool until the sweet potatoes are easy to handle.
   - **Tip:** For family members who do not need puree, simply take the soft-baked potato straight out of the oven and serve, topped with the glaze. Provide an extra bowl of the glaze for additional dipping. If available, tangerine juice is a great substitute for orange juice.

3. For the puree, remove and discard the skins (they should peel away easily) and transfer the sweet potato flesh to a bowl. Use a fork or a potato masher and mash until smooth. Set a mesh strainer or food mill over another large bowl. Working in batches, rub the sweet potatoes through the strainer with a silicone spatula, or through the mill, to remove any remaining fibers.

4. In a small bowl, combine the marmalade and the honey or brown sugar, if needed, with 3 tablespoons warm water. Rub the mixture through a mesh strainer with a silicone spatula—to remove any peel that is not safe for the swallow—into the sweet potato puree. Add the orange juice and cinnamon and season with salt. Stir to combine. If the mashed sweet potato is not smooth enough, transfer to a food processor and puree until smooth.

5. Serve immediately or divide into servings for storage or freezing, following the directions for Serving, page 77.

NUTRITIONAL ANALYSIS PER SERVING | ½ cup
86 calories, 3 g fat, 0 g saturated fat, 30 mg sodium, 1 g sugar, 14 g carbohydrates, 2 g fiber, 1 g protein

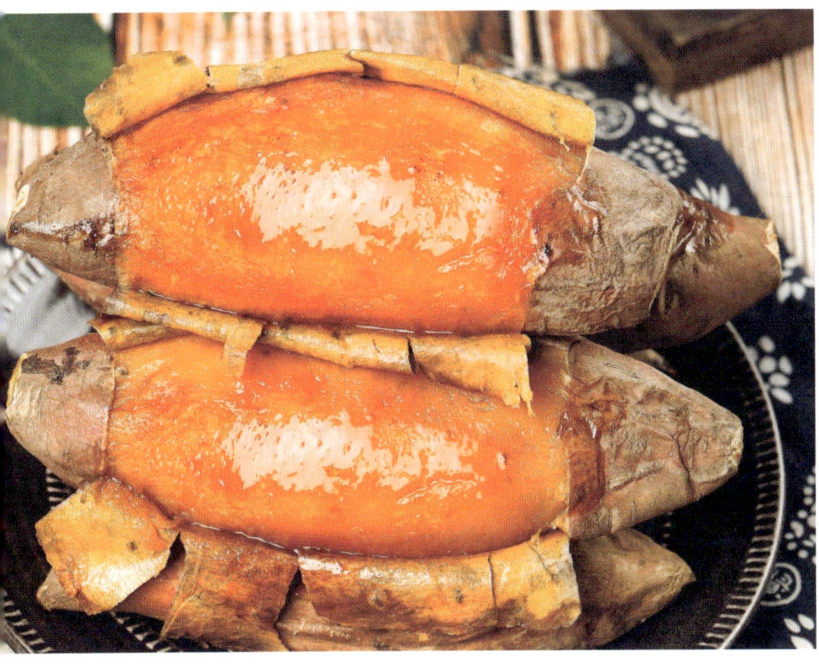

Mashed Potatoes

SERVINGS: 4 | IDDSI LEVELS 

Who would think that making mashed potatoes involves cooking technique? The great French chef Jacques Pépin says that if you have a talent for cooking, technique is the way to showcase your talent. It also saves you time and labor. Technique is everything when it comes to the humble but delicious comfort food of mashed potatoes. My favorite way to make mashed potatoes is to use an Instant Pot or an electric pressure cooker—this takes only 6 minutes. This recipe also includes my mom's secret ingredient for delicious mashed potatoes: a teaspoon of mayonnaise. And don't forget the recipe for Mushroom Gravy (see page 141), homemade and quick. The sauce is the medium of flavor.

2 pounds Yukon Gold potatoes, peeled, cut into 2-inch dice
1 teaspoon sea salt, plus more to taste
1 tablespoon butter or non-trans-fat margarine
½ cup warm milk
1 teaspoon mayonnaise
White pepper

PRO TIP

Mashed potatoes freeze better when mixed with a gravy or a protein and a gravy. When I make dishes such as Roast Turkey Breast with Lemon and Herbs (see page 106), I puree the protein in a food processor with gravy and then gently pulse in the mashed potatoes, just to combine.

1. Add the potatoes, 1 cup water, and 1 teaspoon salt to an electric pressure cooker. Seal the lid and cook on high for 6 minutes. Allow to come down from pressure or use the quick release method to allow steam to escape. The potatoes will be dry, not soggy.

2. If you do not have a pressure cooker, add the potatoes to a large pot, cover with cold water by 2 inches, and season the water with salt. Bring to a boil, lower to a simmer, and cook until the potatoes are tender, about 20 minutes. Drain in a colander and allow them to cool.

3. Once the potatoes have cooled slightly, run them through a potato ricer or food mill, 1 cup at a time, into a bowl. If you do not have a ricer or mill, transfer the potatoes to a large bowl and mash them with a potato masher. Caution: Do not try to mash the potatoes in a food processor or blender, as this will result in what seems like an appliance full of library glue.

4. Add the butter, milk, and mayonnaise, season generously with salt and a pinch of white pepper, and stir until well combined and fluffy.

5. Serve immediately or divide into servings for storage or freezing, following the directions for Serving, page 77.

NUTRITIONAL ANALYSIS PER SERVING | ½ cup
65 calories, 0 g fat, 0 g saturated fat, 11 mg sodium, 0 g sugar, 14 g carbohydrates, 1 g fiber, 3 g protein

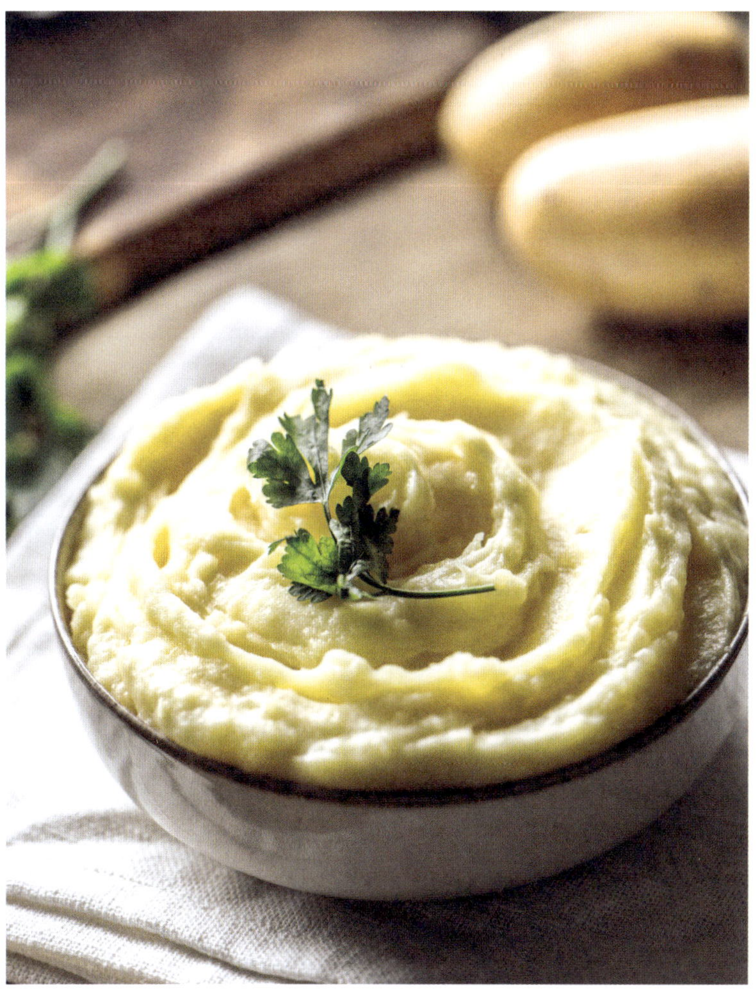

Instant Mashed Potatoes

When you don't have time to make mashed potatoes from scratch, try organic potato flakes from Bob's Red Mill. Prepare according to package directions but add a teaspoon of mayo for richness. These are quite tasty and can also be made using gravy or the reserved pan juices from cooking a chicken or a turkey. Do not over-whip potatoes made from flakes, as they will get gummy.

Creamed Corn

SERVINGS: 4 | IDDSI LEVELS   

Corn makes an excellent side carbohydrate. In summer, I use fresh corn on the cob. In winter, I buy frozen corn. To remove the corn kernels from the cob, I like to use a trick from Ina Garten. Spread a tea towel on your cutting board. Stand an ear of corn on the towel on one end and run a sharp knife down the length of the cob to remove the kernels. The towel keeps the kernels from flying all over the kitchen. It also keeps the counter clean. Transfer the kernels to a bowl.

4 ears fresh corn on the cob, or 1 (10-ounce) package frozen corn kernels
¼ cup sour cream
2 tablespoons whole milk
1 tablespoon butter, non-trans-fat margarine, or extra-virgin olive oil
½ teaspoon sea salt
White pepper

1. Place the corncobs or kernels and 1 cup water into an electric pressure cooker. Seal the lid and cook on high for 6 minutes. Allow to come down from pressure or use the quick release method to allow steam to escape. Alternatively, add the corncobs or kernels to a pot of boiling water. Cook for 6 minutes, drain, and set aside to cool slightly.

2. Once cool enough to handle, remove the kernels from the corncobs and transfer to a bowl. Add the sour cream, milk, butter, salt, and a pinch of white pepper. Stir to coat evenly. If desired, set aside any family servings before pureeing.

3. Add the corn to a food processor or high-speed blender. Process until you achieve the desired texture. Set a mesh strainer over a bowl. Using a silicone spatula, rub the creamed corn through the strainer to remove any tough bits.

4. Test as you go and at time of serving to see if a thickening agent, thickened sauce, or thickened stock is needed; use IDDSI Testing Methods (*iddsi.org*) to help achieve the desired IDDSI level. See pages 42-47.

5. Serve immediately or divide into servings for storage or freezing, following the directions for Serving, page 77.

PRO TIP

Once you've removed the kernels, keep the corncobs in a zip-top bag in the freezer. They are great for flavoring stocks and soups.

NUTRITIONAL ANALYSIS PER SERVING | ¼ cup
134 calories, 6 g fat, 2 g saturated fat, 2.3 mg sodium, 3 g sugar, 18 g carbohydrates, 2 g fiber, 3.2 g protein

Grilled Summer Vegetables

SERVINGS: 4 | IDDSI LEVELS 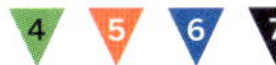

Grilled veggies puree beautifully. The different method of cooking changes the flavor of the vegetables for the summer season. The indoor grill has the benefit of adjustable temperature so that the food does not char, **making it unsafe for the swallow**. The food remains moist and juicy, the most important quality in the dysphagia kitchen. The appliance also allows for an easy cleanup.

1 pound mushrooms, wiped with a damp cloth, stems removed, and sliced
2 medium zucchini (about 1 pound), cut in half vertically and sliced into ¼-inch half moons
2 onions, sliced into ¼-inch rounds, or 1 bunch scallions, cut into 2-inch pieces
2 red bell peppers, seeds and ribs removed, sliced into ½-inch wedges
1 tablespoon extra-virgin olive oil
Sea salt and white pepper
Fresh lemon juice (optional)

1. Heat an indoor electric grill to 375°F (190°C), or set a grill pan over medium-high heat. Place the sliced vegetables in a large bowl, add the olive oil, season with salt and pepper, and toss to coat.

2. Working in batches, spread the vegetables in an even layer on the grill and cook until tender and lightly browned, 3 to 4 minutes per side. Transfer the grilled vegetables to a plate to cool. If desired, set aside any family servings before pureeing.

3. Transfer the vegetables to a food processor or high-speed blender (do this in batches if needed). Add ½ cup water and a squeeze of fresh lemon juice, if desired. Pulse to break up vegetables. Then blend, adding additional water as needed, until smooth.

4. Test as you go and at time of serving to see if a thickening agent, thickened sauce, or thickened stock is needed; use IDDSI Testing Methods (*iddsi.org*) to help achieve the desired IDDSI level. See pages 42-47.

5. Serve immediately or divide into servings for storage or freezing, following the directions for Serving, page 77.

NUTRITIONAL ANALYSIS PER SERVING | 1 cup
156 calories, 1 g fat, 0 g saturated fat, 20 mg sodium, 16 g sugar, 35 g carbohydrates, 9 g fiber, 7 g protein

Roasted Winter Vegetables

SERVINGS: 4 | IDDSI LEVELS 

Prepping the vegetables takes the longest with this dish, but it is well worth it. If you do not have leeks, use a yellow onion or shallots—both roast beautifully. Use whatever is on hand in the fridge. If roasting an entire butternut squash, you will also have enough to create a quick soup or a savory snack. Save the green parts of the leeks in a bag in the freezer and use them when making soup or stock. A good cook wastes nothing.

- 1 butternut squash (about 1½ pounds), halved vertically, seeds removed
- 1 sweet potato, peeled and cut into 2-inch cubes
- 2 leeks, white parts only, cleaned and sliced into 2-inch pieces
- 3 carrots, cut into 2-inch pieces
- 1 parsnip, cut into 2-inch pieces
- 3 small white turnips, peeled and cut into ¼-inch slices
- 3 small beets, peeled and cut into ¼-inch slices
- 3 garlic cloves, peeled
- 2 tablespoons extra-virgin olive oil
- Sea salt and white pepper

1. Preheat oven to 400°F (205°C). Line a baking sheet with parchment paper or aluminum foil. Peel one half of the butternut squash and cut it into 2-inch cubes. (If you have a smaller squash or if you purchased ¾ pound peeled and cut squash, use all of it here. If you have a larger squash, see Roasted Butternut Squash (page 181) for what to do with the other half.)
   - **Tip:** I use a small Chinese cleaver to cut the butternut squash in half vertically, as it requires muscle power. Insert the tip of the cleaver at the top of the squash and lean firmly as you lower the cleaver down the neck and into the body of the vegetable. Simply leveraging your weight ought to do it. If the peel is difficult to remove when the squash is raw, then remove the skin after roasting, when it is soft.
2. On the baking sheet, combine the butternut squash cubes with the other vegetables. Drizzle with the olive oil, season with salt and pepper, and toss to coat. Roast on the center rack for 20 minutes. After 20 minutes, toss the chopped vegetables and drizzle with a few tablespoons of water if they begin to look dry.
3. Continue roasting until the vegetables are very tender and lightly caramelized, another 10 to 20 minutes. Remove the vegetables from the oven and allow to cool. If desired, set aside any family servings before pureeing.

4. Transfer the vegetables to a food processor or high-speed blender (do this in batches if needed). Add ¼ cup water, pulse a few times to break up the vegetables, and puree until smooth. Add more water as needed to achieve the desired texture.

5. Test as you go and at time of serving to see if a thickening agent, thickened sauce, or thickened stock is needed; use IDDSI Testing Methods (*iddsi.org*) to help achieve the desired IDDSI level. See pages 42-47.

6. Serve immediately or divide into servings for storage or freezing, following the directions for Serving, page 77.

NUTRITIONAL ANALYSIS PER SERVING | 1 cup
63 calories, 0.1 g fat, 0 g saturated fat, 6 mg sodium, 3.1 g sugar, 16 g carbohydrates, 2.8 g fiber, 1.4 g protein

Roasted Butternut Squash

Since butternut squash can be large, you might be left with an extra half. If so, place the half, skin on, cut side down, on another prepared baking sheet and roast it in the oven along with the mixed vegetables. This half can be used for another purpose. First remove the seeds. Use a spoon to remove the flesh from the skin and discard the skin. The squash can then be pureed on its own as a vegetable side dish. It can also be pureed with added water or broth (or even a splash of milk or cream) for a quick soup, or used as a base for Butternut Squash Quiche (see page 210).

Roasted Mushrooms

SERVINGS: 4 | IDDSI LEVELS   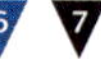

Use any combination of mushrooms that are available at your grocery store or farmer's market. One exception: shiitakes are probably too woody for this dish. If you would like to make a topping or gravy for another dish, double the recipe. Roasted mushroom puree makes a great accompaniment to a burger or a steak with mashed potatoes. The soy sauce brings out the flavor of the mushrooms.

2 tablespoons extra-virgin olive oil
Sea salt and white pepper
1 teaspoon low-sodium soy sauce
1 pound mushrooms, such as baby Bella or cremini, trimmed
½ teaspoon thyme paste (optional)

1. Place a rack in the center of the oven and preheat to 400°F (205°C). Brush a baking sheet with 1 tablespoon olive oil. In a large bowl, mix the remaining olive oil, a pinch of salt and white pepper, and the soy sauce. Add the mushrooms and toss to coat evenly.

2. Transfer the mushrooms to the baking sheet in a single layer, cap-side up if using whole mushrooms.

3. Roast for 12 minutes, or until the mushrooms give up their liquid and become tender. Set aside any family servings before pureeing.

4. For the puree, transfer the mushrooms (and any liquid they have released) to a food processor or high-speed blender. Pulse to break up the mushrooms and process until almost smooth. For an herbal flavor, add the thyme and blend. Add water as needed, 1 tablespoon at a time, and process until you achieve the desired texture.

5. Test as you go and at time of serving to see if thickening is needed; use IDDSI Testing Methods (*iddsi.org*) to help achieve the desired IDDSI level. See pages 42-47.

6. Serve immediately or divide into servings for storage or freezing, following the directions for Serving, page 77.

PRO TIP

For a quickie mushroom gravy, add 1 tablespoon sour cream and 1 tablespoon water or broth to the mushrooms before thickening.

NUTRITIONAL ANALYSIS PER SERVING | ½ cup
68 calories, 7 g fat, 1 g saturated fat, 167 mg sodium, 1 g sugar, 1 g carbohydrates, 0 g fiber, 1 g protein

Roasted Asparagus

SERVINGS: 4 | IDDSI LEVELS 

Most people are familiar with steaming asparagus, but roasting this vegetable gives it intensity of flavor. Pick a bunch where all the stalks are roughly the same size so that they will cook evenly. Thick stalks are better than pencil asparagus for flavor. For a gourmet touch, use white asparagus when in season.

1 pound asparagus, woody ends trimmed, peeled if skins are tough
1 tablespoon extra-virgin olive oil
Sea salt and white pepper
1 teaspoon fresh lemon juice

1. Place a rack in the center of the oven and preheat to 400°F (205°C). Line a baking sheet with parchment paper. In a large bowl, combine the asparagus, oil, and a pinch of salt and white pepper. Toss thoroughly with your hands.

2. Line up the stalks on the baking sheet. Sprinkle lemon juice over the asparagus. Roast until tender, about 12 minutes. Remove from the oven and allow to cool. Set aside any family servings before pureeing.

3. For the puree, transfer the roasted asparagus to a food processor or high-speed blender. Process until you achieve the desired texture. Set a mesh strainer over a bowl. Using a silicone spatula, rub the asparagus through the strainer to remove any fibers.

4. Test as you go and at time of serving to see if a thickening agent, thickened sauce, or thickened stock is needed; use IDDSI Testing Methods (*iddsi.org*) to help achieve the desired IDDSI level. See pages 42-47.

5. Serve immediately or divide into servings for storage or freezing, following the directions for Serving, page 77.

PRO TIP

Roast 2 pounds at once, so you have a delicious ingredient to add to a stir-fry. You can also make a quick asparagus soup by pureeing the asparagus with broth and a splash of coconut milk or heavy cream.

NUTRITIONAL ANALYSIS PER SERVING | 4 oz
52 calories, 4 g fat, 1 g saturated fat, 2 mg sodium, 2 g sugar, 4 g carbohydrates, 2 g fiber, 2 g protein

Ratatouille (Summer Vegetable Ragout)

SERVINGS: 6 | IDDSI LEVELS 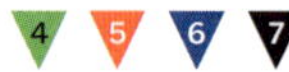

The essence of summer vegetables, this classic Mediterranean dish can be served as a light lunch, a side with a protein such as fish, or paired with grits or polenta. Serve warm or cold. Ratatouille purees and freezes beautifully due to its sauce. The effort of chopping the veggies is well worth it.

4 tablespoons extra-virgin olive oil
1 yellow onion, cut into large dice or thin slices
1 or 2 garlic cloves, thinly sliced
1 red bell pepper, cut into large dice
1 Japanese eggplant, sliced into ⅜-inch-thick rounds
1 zucchini, sliced into ⅜-inch-thick rounds
2 large tomatoes, diced, or 1 (15-ounce) can tomato sauce or diced tomatoes
2 tablespoons chopped fresh flat-leaf parsley or parsley paste
2 tablespoons chopped fresh basil or basil paste
Sea salt and white pepper

1. Preheat the oven to 350°F (175°C) with a rack in the center. In a large skillet, warm 1 tablespoon oil over medium heat. Add the onion and sauté until softened, 3 minutes. Add the garlic and sauté 1 more minute. Transfer to a 9 x 9-inch baking dish.

2. Add the bell pepper to the skillet and sauté until softened, 3 minutes. Transfer to the baking dish. Warm 2 tablespoons oil. Sauté the eggplant until softened, about 5 minutes, and transfer to the baking dish. Warm the remaining 1 tablespoon oil, add the zucchini, and sauté until softened, 3 minutes. Transfer to the baking dish.

3. Add the tomatoes or sauce and the herbs to the vegetables. Season with salt and pepper, stir, cover with foil, and bake for 1 hour until the vegetables are very tender. Remove from oven and allow to cool. Set aside family servings.

4. For the puree, transfer the baked vegetables to a food processor or high-speed blender in batches and process until you achieve the desired texture. Run through a sieve.

5. Test as you go and at time of serving to see if thickening is needed; use IDDSI Testing Methods (*iddsi.org*) to help achieve the desired IDDSI level. See pages 42-47.

6. Serve immediately or divide into servings for storage or freezing, following the directions for Serving, page 77.

NUTRITIONAL ANALYSIS PER SERVING | 1 cup
67 calories, 3 g fat, 0 g saturated fat, 9 mg sodium, 5 g sugar, 11 g carbohydrates, 5 g fiber, 2 g protein

Spinach and Parmesan Sauté

SERVINGS: 2 | IDDSI LEVELS 

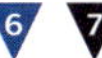

7

Leafy greens are nutrient dense. You can use bagged fresh spinach or a bunch of fresh spinach; make sure to wash thoroughly. You can also use frozen chopped spinach. Spinach will give off water when sautéed, and the liquid may be used for the puree. The spinach can be served with scrambled eggs to make a spinach omelet. Spinach puree freezes beautifully. Make a double recipe if you wish to freeze individual portions for quick meals.

- 1 tablespoon extra-virgin olive oil
- 1 small shallot, thinly sliced (optional)
- 1 garlic clove, thinly sliced (optional)
- 1 bunch spinach, or 1 (10-ounce) package baby spinach
- 1 teaspoon lemon juice
- 2 tablespoons grated parmesan cheese

1. In a large skillet, heat oil over medium-high heat. Sauté the shallot until translucent, about 1 minute. Add the garlic and sauté for 1 more minute. Add the spinach and stir to coat in the flavored oil. Cook for 2 minutes, until all the spinach is wilted. Add the lemon juice and the parmesan and stir until the parmesan melts. Remove from the heat and allow to cool. If desired, set aside any family servings before pureeing.

2. For the puree, add the spinach (along with any liquid in the skillet) to a food processor or high-speed blender and puree until smooth, adding a bit of water as needed to achieve the prescribed texture. Include the garlic in the puree if you like garlic.

3. Test as you go and at time of serving to see if a thickening agent, thickened sauce, or thickened stock is needed; use IDDSI Testing Methods (*iddsi.org*) to help achieve the desired IDDSI level. See pages 42-47.

4. Serve immediately or divide into servings for storage or freezing, following the directions for Serving, page 77.

NUTRITIONAL ANALYSIS PER SERVING | ½ cup
34 calories, 2 g fat, 5 g saturated fat, 53 mg sodium, 0 g sugar, 2.5 g carbohydrates, 1 g fiber, 2 g protein

Braised Greens

SERVINGS: 4 | IDDSI LEVELS 

One cannot overstate the importance of greens. This is a terrific way of incorporating them into the diet. Greens freeze well and may be added to soups and stews. Greens may also be cooked in an Instant Pot or electric pressure cooker, following the manufacturer's instructions for cooking time. The Instant Pot or electric pressure cooker is ideal for the quick cooking of collard greens, since collards normally take a long time and can be tough, but pressure-cooking shortens the process.

1 bunch greens (chard, kale, beet greens, mustard greens, or a combination)
2 tablespoons vegetable oil
1 small onion, diced
1½ cups low-sodium chicken or vegetable broth, plus more as needed
Sea salt and white pepper

1. Remove the stalks from the greens. Roll up the leaves and slice them into ribbons. In a 3-quart pot over medium heat, warm the oil. Add the onion and sauté until translucent, 3 minutes. Add the greens and sauté for 2 minutes. Add broth, plus more as needed to just cover the greens.

2. Season with a pinch of salt and pepper. Bring the broth to a boil, lower the heat to a simmer, and cover with the lid slightly ajar. Cook until the greens are very tender, about 20 minutes. Allow to cool. If desired, set aside any family servings before pureeing.

3. For the puree, add the greens and some of the broth to a food processor or high-speed blender and process until you achieve the desired texture, adding additional broth as needed. (Save leftover broth for using in soups or another puree—it is full of flavor and precious phytochemicals.)

4. Test as you go and at time of serving to see if thickening is needed; use IDDSI Testing Methods (*iddsi.org*) to help achieve the desired IDDSI level. See pages 42-47.

5. Serve immediately or divide into servings for storage or freezing, following the directions for Serving, page 77.

VARIATION

A delicious and nutritious riff on these braised greens is inspired by the classic Italian soup made with **escarole**. Use the Braised Greens method above, swapping the onion for a clove of thinly sliced **garlic**, and the bunch of greens for a head of **escarole**.

NUTRITIONAL ANALYSIS PER SERVING | 4 oz
84 calories, 7 g fat, 1 g saturated fat, 157 mg sodium, 2 g sugar, 5 g carbohydrates, 2 g fiber, 2 g protein

Broccoli Parmesan

SERVINGS: 4 | IDDSI LEVELS 

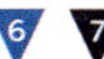

7

This is the classic Italian way of preparing vegetables. It is simple, quick, and tasty. It works for asparagus and spinach as well as broccoli. I find it is a favorite when I do lecture-demonstrations. I often make a double batch because people love it.

1 head broccoli, cut into florets
3 tablespoons extra-virgin olive oil
1 garlic clove, thinly sliced or minced
2 tablespoons fresh lemon juice
2 tablespoons parmesan cheese, grated
Sea salt and white pepper

1. Steam the broccoli until tender (see page 171).

2. In a 12-inch skillet, warm the olive oil over medium-high heat. Add the garlic and sauté for 1 minute. Add the broccoli and stir to coat the broccoli with the oil. Add the lemon juice and the parmesan, and stir in the pan until the cheese melts. Add salt and pepper. Remove from the heat and allow to cool. If desired, set aside any family servings before pureeing.

3. For the puree, add the broccoli to a food processor or high-speed blender and process until you achieve the desired texture, adding a few tablespoons of water as needed to achieve the prescribed texture. Leave in the garlic if you like garlic.

4. Test as you go and at time of serving to see if a thickening agent, thickened sauce, or thickened stock is needed; use IDDSI Testing Methods (*iddsi.org*) to help achieve the desired IDDSI level. See pages 42-47.

5. Serve immediately or divide into servings for storage or freezing, following the directions for Serving, page 77.

NUTRITIONAL ANALYSIS PER SERVING | 4 oz
119 calories, 11 g fat, 2 g saturated fat, 54 mg sodium, 0 g sugar, 4 g carbohydrates, 0 g fiber, 3 g protein

Brussels Sprouts with Shallots

SERVINGS: 4 | IDDSI LEVELS  

My mother adored Brussels sprouts, and this recipe was developed for her. I suggest an IDDSI Pureed, Level 4, for vegetable dishes because they make a great accompaniment to a meal. IDDSI, Minced & Moist, Level 5, or Soft & Bite-Sized, Level 6, may be used.

- 2 tablespoons extra-virgin olive oil
- 1 pound Brussels sprouts, trimmed and halved
- 2 shallots, peeled and thinly sliced
- 1 garlic clove, sliced (optional)
- Sea salt and white pepper
- Dash of maple syrup (optional)

1. Place a rack in the center of the oven and preheat to 375°F (190°C). Brush a baking sheet with 1 tablespoon oil. In a large bowl, combine the Brussels sprouts with the shallots, garlic (if using), the remaining oil, a pinch of salt and white pepper, and maple syrup (if using). Toss to coat thoroughly.

2. Spread the Brussels sprouts on the sheet pan in an even single layer. Roast until tender and lightly caramelized, about 40 minutes. Remove from the oven and allow to cool. If desired, set aside any family servings before pureeing.

3. For the puree, transfer the Brussels sprouts and ¼ cup water to a food processor or high-speed blender. Pulse a few times to break down the vegetables. Puree until smooth, adding more water as needed to achieve a smooth puree. Set a mesh strainer over a bowl. Using a silicone spatula, rub the puree through the strainer to remove any charred particles or dry bits.

4. Test as you go and at time of serving to see if a thickening agent, thickened sauce, or thickened stock is needed; use IDDSI Testing Methods (*iddsi.org*) to help achieve the desired IDDSI level. See pages 42-47.

5. Serve immediately or divide into servings for storage or freezing, following the directions for Serving, page 77.

NUTRITIONAL ANALYSIS PER SERVING | 4 oz
Without maple syrup
99 calories, 7 g fat, 1 g saturated fat, 9 mg sodium, 0 g sugar, 8 g carbohydrates, 3 g fiber, 3 g protein

Cabbage Sauté

SERVINGS: 4 | IDDSI LEVELS 

This is a great side dish to accompany beef or pork. It is also a great vegetarian or vegan dish to combine with a whole grain, such as Rice Congee (see page 196) or Buckwheat (see page 200). The apple adds sweetness to the savory vegetable.

2 tablespoons extra-virgin olive oil
½ yellow onion, thinly sliced
1 garlic clove, minced
½ head of cabbage (1 pound), cored and thinly sliced
1 Golden Delicious apple, peeled, cored, and thinly sliced into half moons (optional)

1. In a large sauté pan, warm the olive oil over medium-low heat. Add the onion and garlic and sauté, stirring frequently, until lightly golden, about 8 minutes. Stir in the cabbage and cook until the cabbage wilts, about 5 minutes.

2. Add the apple and stir to combine. Add ¼ cup water and simmer until the apple is tender, about 5 minutes. Allow the dish to cool. If desired, set aside any family servings before pureeing.

3. For the puree, add the cabbage and 2 tablespoons water to a food processor or high-speed blender. Pulse to break down the cabbage and puree until smooth, adding more water as needed.

4. Test as you go and at time of serving to see if a thickening agent, thickened sauce, or thickened stock is needed; use IDDSI Testing Methods (*iddsi.org*) to help achieve the desired IDDSI level. See pages 42-47.

5. Serve immediately or divide into servings for storage or freezing, following the directions for Serving, page 77.

NUTRITIONAL ANALYSIS PER SERVING | 4 oz
143 calories, 7.3 g fat, 1 g saturated fat, 10 mg sodium, 7.9 g sugar, 19.8 g carbohydrates, 3.1 g fiber, 2.3 g protein

Roasted Cauliflower

SERVINGS: 6 | IDDSI LEVELS  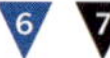

If you do not know cauliflower, here's your chance to get to know this amazing superfood. When pureed, this vegetable has a distinctive nutty flavor gained from roasting.

1 head cauliflower, cored and cut into florets
2 tablespoons extra-virgin olive oil
Salt and white pepper

1. Place a rack in the center of the oven and preheat to 400°F (205°C). Line a baking sheet with parchment paper. In a large bowl, toss the cauliflower florets with the olive oil and a pinch each of salt and white pepper until thoroughly coated. Transfer to the baking sheet and spread into an even, single layer.

2. Roast for about 40 minutes, flipping once halfway through roasting, until very tender and lightly golden. If desired, set aside any family servings before pureeing.

3. For the puree, transfer the cauliflower to a food processor or high-speed blender. Pulse to break up the cauliflower. Add water, as needed, a few tablespoons at a time, and process until you achieve the desired texture.

4. Test as you go and at time of serving to see if a thickening agent, thickened sauce, or thickened stock is needed; use IDDSI Testing Methods (*iddsi.org*) to help achieve the desired IDDSI level. See pages 42-47.

5. Serve immediately or divide into servings for storage or freezing, following the directions for Serving, page 77.

NUTRITIONAL ANALYSIS PER SERVING | 4 oz
66 calories, 4 g fat, 0 g saturated fat, 43 mg sodium, 3 g sugar, 8 g carbohydrates, 4 g fiber, 3 g protein

VARIATIONS

- For **creamed cauliflower**, add 1 heaping tablespoon sour cream to the puree before thickening.
- For the classic flavor profile of **lemon and butter**, add 2 tablespoons melted butter and 2 tablespoons lemon juice to the puree before thickening.
- For a **mild curry**, add several tablespoons of Ethnic Gourmet Calcutta Masala Simmer Sauce.

Garlic Green Beans

SERVINGS: 4 | IDDSI LEVELS   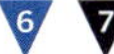

Green beans contain fiber and anti-inflammatory phytochemicals. They may help counteract obesity, diabetes, and heart disease. If using canned green beans, rinse them first, as they are usually higher in sodium.

1 pound green beans, trimmed
3 tablespoons extra-virgin olive oil
2 garlic cloves, thinly sliced
2 tablespoons Italian-style seasoned breadcrumbs
1 tablespoon lemon juice
1 tablespoon parmesan cheese, plus additional if desired

1. Steam the green beans (see page 171).
2. In a large sauté pan, warm the olive oil over medium heat. Add the garlic and cook for 1 minute until soft but not browned. Add the beans to the pan and swirl in the garlic oil.
3. Add the breadcrumbs, lemon juice, and parmesan cheese and stir to make a sauce. Remove from the heat. If desired, set aside any family servings before pureeing.
4. For the puree, transfer the green beans to a food processor or high-speed blender and add ¼ cup water. Pulse to break up the beans and process until you achieve the desired texture, adding more water as needed.
5. Test as you go and at time of serving to see if a thickening agent, thickened sauce, or thickened stock is needed; use IDDSI Testing Methods (*iddsi.org*) to help achieve the desired IDDSI level. See pages 42-47.
6. Serve immediately or divide into servings for storage or freezing, following the directions for Serving, page 77.

VARIATION

This recipe makes a good ingredient for a three-bean salad, which is made with **chickpeas**, **red kidney beans**, and **green beans** in **vinaigrette**. Use the recipe for Vinaigrette Dressing (see page 91) and season to taste; garlic is a common addition. This may be pureed and served as a side dish.

NUTRITIONAL ANALYSIS PER SERVING | 4 oz
154 calories, 11 g fat, 2 g saturated fat, 130 mg sodium, 2 g sugar, 14 g carbohydrates, 4 g fiber, 3 g protein

Ginger Carrots

SERVINGS: 4 | IDDSI LEVELS 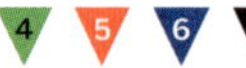

Carrots are a good source of fiber, beta-carotene, and antioxidants. This recipe may be pureed with broth and thickened to make a quick soup. Ginger is excellent for the digestion and as an anti-inflammatory.

4 carrots, peeled, halved lengthwise, and sliced into ¼-inch half moons, or 1 cup baby carrots, sliced into rounds
2 tablespoons extra-virgin olive oil or unsalted butter
1-inch piece fresh ginger, sliced into 1-inch matchsticks, or 2 teaspoons store-bought ginger paste
1 tablespoon honey

1. Steam the carrots (see page 171).

2. In a large skillet over medium-high heat, heat the olive oil or melt the butter. Add the ginger and sauté until fragrant, 1 minute. Stir in the honey to form a ginger glaze. Add the carrots and stir to coat in the glaze. Remove from the heat and allow to cool. If desired, set aside any family servings before pureeing.

3. For the puree, transfer the carrots to a food processor or high-speed blender and add ¼ cup water. Pulse to break up the carrots and process until you achieve the desired texture, adding additional water as needed.

4. Test as you go and at time of serving to see if a thickening agent, thickened sauce, or thickened stock is needed; use IDDSI Testing Methods (*iddsi.org*) to help achieve the desired IDDSI level. See pages 42-47.

5. Serve immediately or divide into servings for storage or freezing, following the directions for Serving, page 77.

NUTRITIONAL ANALYSIS PER SERVING | 4 oz
102 calories, 7 g fat, 1 g saturated fat, 43 mg sodium, 7 g sugar, 10 g carbohydrates, 2 g fiber, 1 g protein

Minty Pureed Peas

SERVINGS: 2 | IDDSI LEVELS 

A great accompaniment for Garlic and Rosemary Lamb Chops (see page 145), these are a tasty and super-simple side dish.

1 cup frozen peas
Sea salt and white pepper
¼ teaspoon mint extract (optional)

1. In a small saucepan over medium-high heat, bring 1 cup water to a simmer. Add the peas and simmer until warmed through, 3 minutes. Drain and allow to cool. If desired, set aside any family servings before pureeing.

2. For the puree, transfer the peas to a mini food processor or small blender, season with a pinch each of salt and pepper, and add the mint extract, if using. Process until you achieve the desired texture, adding a few tablespoons of water as needed. Set a mesh strainer over a bowl. Using a silicone spatula, rub the puree through the strainer to remove any particles of skin.

3. Test as you go and at time of serving to see if a thickening agent, thickened sauce, or thickened stock is needed; use IDDSI Testing Methods (*iddsi.org*) to help achieve the desired IDDSI level. See pages 42-47.

4. Serve immediately or divide into servings for storage or freezing, following the directions for Serving, page 77.

NUTRITIONAL ANALYSIS PER SERVING | 4 oz
31 calories, 0 g fat, 0 g saturated fat, 9 mg sodium, 1.4 g sugar, 5.7 g carbohydrates, 3 g fiber, 2.2 g protein

Whole Grains

196 Rice Congee (Soft Rice Porridge)

198 Quinoa

199 Farro

200 Buckwheat

201 Barley

202 Grits

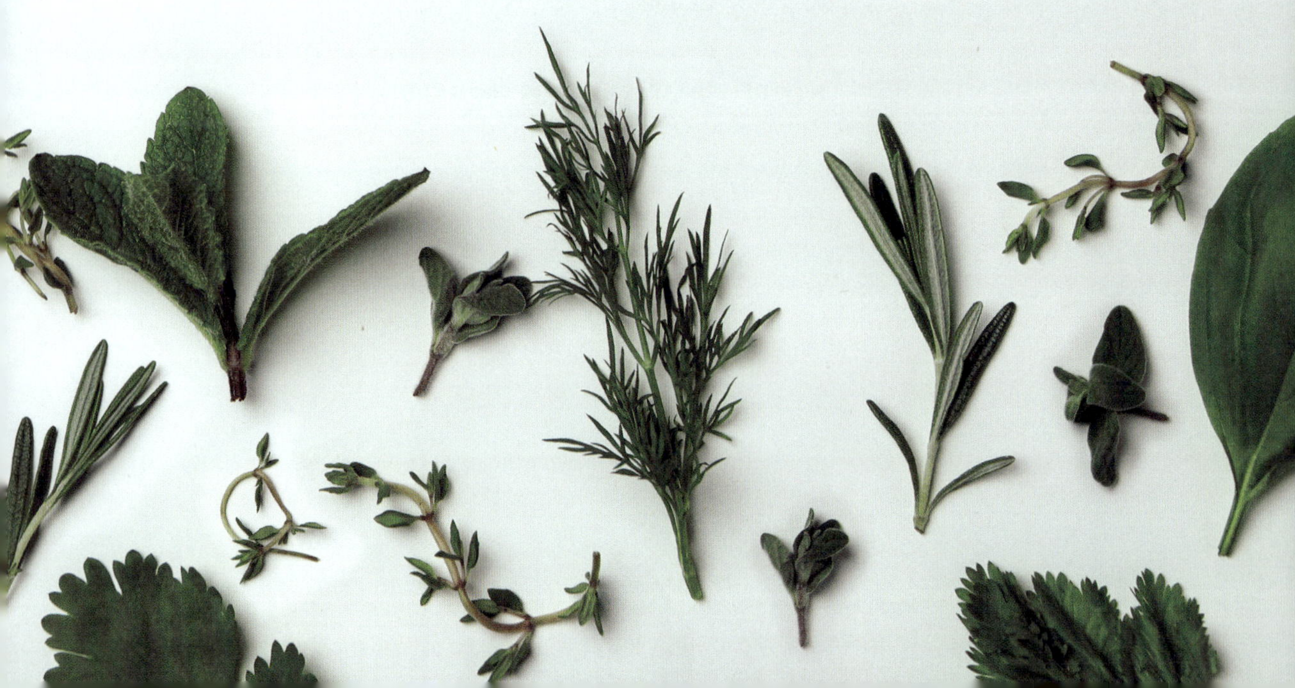

Cooking Whole Grains

The importance of whole grains in the diet cannot be overstated. They are recommended as heart-healthy by the Harvard T.H. Chan School of Public Health Healthy Eating Plate, the American Heart Association, and the American Diabetic Association. They metabolize slowly and do not spike blood sugar, therefore they do not produce a spike in insulin. Whole grains are also a tasty and excellent side dish for a meal.

Cooking grains in batches (also see page 60) means that you can cook once and eat multiple times. Having cooked grains in the refrigerator or freezer also means that you have more choice and variety in the composition of a meal. You can use any sauce with the grain, or use the grain to create other dishes.

Make rice and you have the basis of stir-fried rice and rice pudding. With pressure cooking, the grains may be made in multiple servings and do not require watching—simply set the timer and open it when the pressure comes down naturally.

The basic procedure is the same for all of the grains. The best cooking method is an Instant Pot (or another electric pressure cooker) or a stovetop pressure cooker. Pressure cooking uses steam under pressure to force steam through food, keeping the moisture. The outer coat of the grain softens enough for a smooth puree. You get the benefits of superior nutrients and also get the fiber.

For the patient with swallowing difficulties, the investment in an electric pressure cooker is worth it. Follow the directions for your appliance. After the steam has been released, allow the batch to cool, then puree and add thickener as needed. (Grains can also be cooked on the stovetop. Follow the directions in the individual recipes that follow.)

To store, portion out individual servings into storage containers or zip-top bags and freeze. Stacking the bags flat in the freezer keeps them organized and saves space. One shelf of your freezer could contain frozen individual servings of whole grains, proteins, and vegetables. This allows you to quickly customize a meal anytime—just choose a grain, a portion of protein, and a veggie, and voilà!

Rice Congee (Soft Rice Porridge)

SERVINGS: 8 | IDDSI LEVELS  

Rice congee, or soft rice porridge, has been used in Asia for feeding infants and the elderly for thousands of years. I use brown basmati rice for its flavor, fragrance, and texture. There are several methods of cooking, including pressure cooker or stovetop.

2 cups brown basmati rice
¼ teaspoon sea salt

1. Add the rice to a large mixing bowl and wash it several times with cool tap water, rinsing and draining until the water runs clear. Look for any green kernels or any little stones and remove them.

2. **Pressure cooker method:** Add the rice, 5 cups water, and the salt to a pressure cooker or Instant Pot. Cook on high pressure for 30 minutes. Allow the pot to come down from pressure by natural release. Remove the lid and allow the rice to cool. No matter which cooking method one uses, the rice expands and gives a greater yield.
   - **Tip:** This is a congee. You want it loose, an easily swallowed porridge rather than a firmly textured grain. You want to break down the cell wall and get a creamy texture.

   Stovetop method: Bring the rice, 4 cups water, and the salt to a boil in a large saucepan over medium-high heat. Stir and turn the heat down to low. Cover and simmer for 45 minutes, until the liquid has been absorbed.

3. Watch to make sure the bottom does not burn. If necessary, add another ¼ cup of water. Remove from the heat and allow to rest for 5 minutes; add more water if the rice is dry. Allow to cool.

4. If desired, set aside any family servings before pureeing. For the puree, add the cooked rice to a food processor or blender and process until you achieve the desired texture.

5. Test as you go and at time of serving to see if a thickening agent, thickened sauce, or thickened stock is needed; use IDDSI Testing Methods (*iddsi.org*) to help achieve the desired IDDSI level. See pages 42-47.

6. Serve immediately or divide into servings for storage or freezing, following the directions for Serving, page 77. (Freeze for up to 1 month, not 3 months.)

PRO TIP

Extra portions of Rice Congee from the freezer may be used for making second dishes such as fried rice or rice pudding.

NUTRITIONAL ANALYSIS PER SERVING | 1 cup

Congee with brown basmati rice

160 calories, 1.5 g fat, 0 g saturated fat, 5 mg sodium, 1 g sugar, 34 g carbohydrates, 2 g fiber, 4 g protein

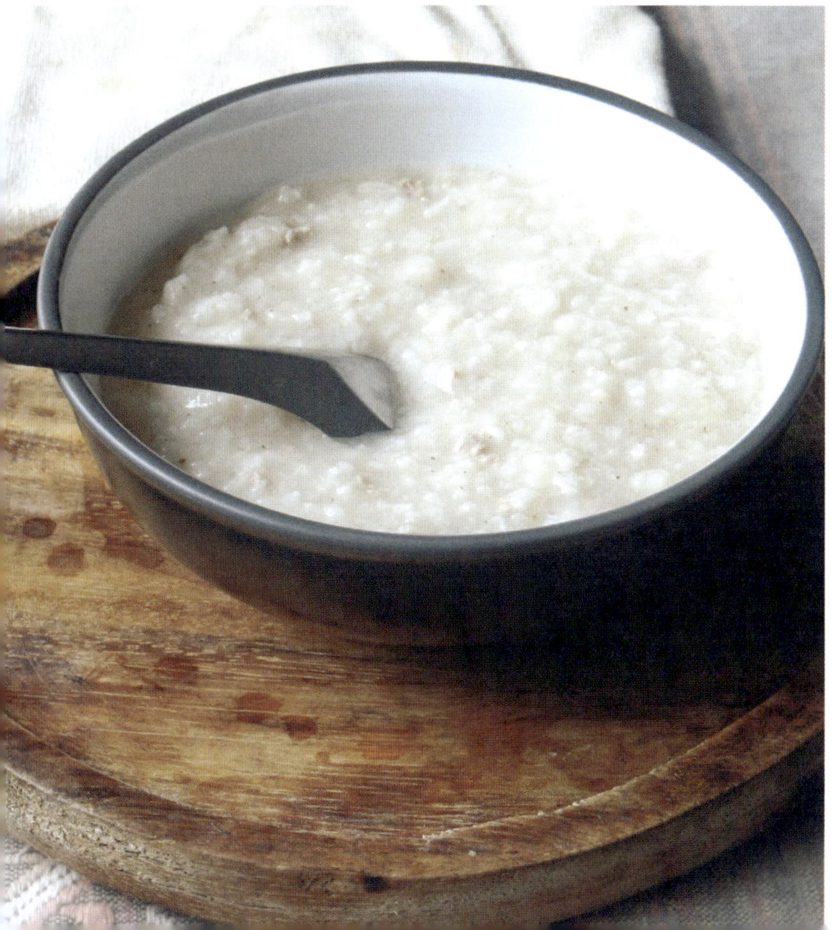

Quinoa

SERVINGS: 4 | IDDSI LEVELS 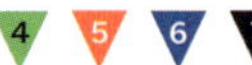

Quinoa is a high-protein grain originally from South America. It makes a great side dish and may be added to soups or stews. This method purees the quinoa with water, but cooked quinoa can also be pureed with broth, soup, or gravy. Cooked quinoa is delicious added to a winter salad of braised greens with roasted mushrooms.

2 cups quinoa
¼ teaspoon sea salt

1. Rinse the quinoa in a mesh strainer to eliminate bitterness.

2. **Pressure cooking method:** Add the quinoa, 2 cups water, and the salt to a pressure cooker or Instant Pot. Cook on high pressure for 1 minute. Allow the pot to come down from pressure by natural release. Remove the lid, fluff the quinoa with a fork, and allow to cool.

   Stovetop method: Bring 3 cups water to a boil in a saucepan over medium-high heat. Add the quinoa and salt, stir, and turn the heat down to low. Cover and simmer for 10 to 15 minutes, until the liquid has been absorbed. Remove from the heat, fluff with a fork, and allow to cool.

3. If desired, set aside any family servings before pureeing. For the puree, add the cooled quinoa and 1½ cups water or broth to a food processor or blender (you may need to do this in two batches). Pulse to break down the grain. Process until you achieve the desired texture.

4. Test as you go and at time of serving to see if thickening is needed; use IDDSI Testing Methods (*iddsi.org*) to help achieve the desired IDDSI level. See pages 42-47.

5. Serve immediately or divide into servings for storage or freezing, following the directions for Serving, page 77. (Freeze for up to 1 month, not 3 months.)

NUTRITIONAL ANALYSIS PER SERVING | 8 oz
156 calories, 3 g fat, 0 g saturated fat, 2 mg sodium, 0 g sugar, 27 g carbohydrates, 3 g fiber, 6 g protein

Farro

SERVINGS: 4-6 | IDDSI LEVELS 

I prefer to use Bob's Red Mill Organic Whole Grain Farro, as I think it has the best flavor. The pressure cooker is the shortest method, or you can soak the grains overnight in water to cut down on cooking time if cooking on a stovetop.

1 cup farro
½ teaspoon salt

1. Rinse the farro in a mesh strainer.
2. **Pressure cooker method:** Add the farro, 3 cups water, and the salt to a pressure cooker or Instant Pot. Cook on high pressure for 20 minutes. Allow the pot to come down from pressure by natural release. Remove the lid, fluff the farro with a fork, and allow to cool.

   Stovetop method: Bring 2 quarts of water or broth to a boil in a pot with salt. Add the farro, then return the heat to medium-high and boil, uncovered, until soft and tender, approximately 30 minutes. Drain off excess liquid, fluff with a fork, and allow to cool. Test for tenderness. If more tenderness is desired, cover and allow to stand for several minutes.
3. If desired, set aside any family servings before pureeing. For the puree, add the cooked farro to a food processor or high-speed blender and process until you achieve the desired texture.
4. Test as you go and at time of serving to see if thickening is needed; use IDDSI Testing Methods (*iddsi.org*) to help achieve the desired IDDSI level. See pages 42-47.
5. Serve immediately or divide into servings for storage or freezing, following the directions for Serving, page 77. (Freeze for up to 1 month, not 3 months.)

NUTRITIONAL ANALYSIS PER SERVING | ½ cup
140 calories, 0 g fat, 0 g saturated fat, 170.5 mg sodium, 0 g sugar, 30 g carbohydrates, 3 g fiber, 6 g protein

Buckwheat

SERVINGS: 4 | IDDSI LEVELS 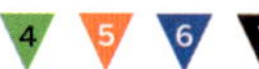

Buckwheat has a nutty, delicious flavor and makes an excellent side dish. Buckwheat is gluten-free and is not a member of the wheat family. It is good for diabetics because it slows the absorption of glucose. I prefer to use Bob's Red Mill Organic Whole Grain Buckwheat Groats.

1 cup whole-grain buckwheat groats, lightly toasted in a dry cast-iron or stainless steel skillet
¼ teaspoon salt

1. **Pressure cooker method:** Add the toasted buckwheat, 1¾ cups water or broth, and the salt to a pressure cooker. Secure the lid. Cook on high pressure for 12 minutes. Allow the pot to come down from pressure by natural release. Unlock and remove the lid. Fluff the buckwheat with a fork, and allow to cool.

   Stovetop method: Bring 2½ cups water or broth to a boil in a pot on the stove. Add the toasted buckwheat and salt. Return to a boil, then reduce the heat to a simmer, cover, and cook until tender, about 15 minutes. Drain off excess liquid, fluff with a fork, and allow to cool.

2. If desired, set aside any family servings before pureeing. For the puree, add the cooked buckwheat to a food processor or blender and process until you achieve the desired texture.

3. Test as you go and at time of serving to see if a thickening agent, thickened sauce, or thickened stock is needed; use IDDSI Testing Methods (*iddsi.org*) to help achieve the desired IDDSI level. See pages 42-47.

4. Serve immediately or divide into servings for storage or freezing, following the directions for Serving, page 77. (Freeze for up to 1 month, not 3 months.)

NUTRITIONAL ANALYSIS PER SERVING | 8 oz
92 calories, 0.6 g fat, 0.1 g saturated fat, 4 mg sodium, 0.9 g sugar, 19.9 g carbohydrates, 2.7 g fiber, 3.4 g protein

Barley

SERVINGS: 4 | IDDSI LEVELS 

Barley has a nutty, delicious flavor and may be added to soups or bowls, or served as a side dish. I recommend Bob's Red Mill Pearl Barley.

1 cup pearled barley
1 teaspoon salt

1. Rinse the barley in a mesh strainer.
2. **Pressure cooker method:** Combine barley, 4 cups water, and the salt in a pressure cooker or Instant Pot. Cook on high pressure for 20 minutes. Allow the pot to come down from pressure by natural release. Remove the lid, fluff the barley with a fork, and allow to cool.

   Stovetop method: Bring 2 quarts water to a boil in a pot and add the barley and salt. Return to medium-high heat and boil, uncovered, until soft, 25 to 30 minutes. Drain off excess liquid, fluff with a fork, and allow to cool.
3. If desired, set aside any family servings before pureeing. For the puree, add the cooked barley to a food processor or high-speed blender and process until you achieve the desired texture.
4. Test as you go and at time of serving to see if a thickening agent, thickened sauce, or thickened stock is needed; use IDDSI Testing Methods (*iddsi.org*) to help achieve the desired IDDSI level. See pages 42-47.
5. Serve immediately or divide into servings for storage or freezing, following the directions for Serving, page 77. (Freeze for up to 1 month, not 3 months.)

NUTRITIONAL ANALYSIS PER SERVING | 1 cup
89 calories, 0.6 g fat, 0 g saturated fat, 101 mg sodium, 0.2 g sugar, 18.4 g carbohydrates, 4.3 g fiber, 3.1 g protein

Grits

SERVINGS: 8-10 | IDDSI LEVELS 

Grits are made from cornmeal and are a close cousin to polenta. The recommended kinds are stone-ground, unenriched, and coarse. They may be flavored to suit your palate. I prefer Bob's Red Mill Creamy White Corn Grits.

1 cup white corn grits
Milk, as needed (see method)
½ teaspoon salt
1 tablespoon unsalted butter
4 tablespoons grated parmesan cheese
¼ teaspoon garlic powder
¼ teaspoon onion powder

1. **Pressure cooker method:** Add the grits, 3½ cups water, ½ cup milk, and salt to a pressure cooker or Instant Pot. Cook on high pressure for 10 minutes. Allow the pot to come down from pressure by natural release.

   Stovetop method: Bring 2 cups water and 2 cups milk to a boil in a pot and add the salt and grits. Reduce the heat to low. Cook for about 30 minutes, stirring occasionally, until the liquid is absorbed and the grits are creamy. Remove from heat.

2. Season with the butter, parmesan cheese, garlic powder, and onion powder. Stir to combine thoroughly. Cover and let stand for 1 to 2 minutes.

3. If desired, set aside any family servings before pureeing. For the puree, add the cooked grits to a food processor or blender and process until you achieve the desired texture.

4. Test as you go and at time of serving to see if a thickening agent, thickened sauce, or thickened stock is needed; use IDDSI Testing Methods (*iddsi.org*) to help achieve the desired IDDSI level. See pages 42-47.

5. Serve immediately or divide into servings for storage or freezing, following the directions for Serving, page 77. (Freeze for up to 1 month, not 3 months.)

NUTRITIONAL ANALYSIS PER SERVING | ¼ cup
182 calories, 1 g fat, 0 g saturated fat, 479 mg sodium, 0.4 g sugar, 38 g carbohydrates, 2 g fiber, 4 g protein

Legumes and Pulses

204 Beans

206 Brown Lentils

Legumes are defined as members of the bean family: kidney beans, cannellini beans, and black beans are all legumes. Pulses include lentils and garbanzo beans (chickpeas).

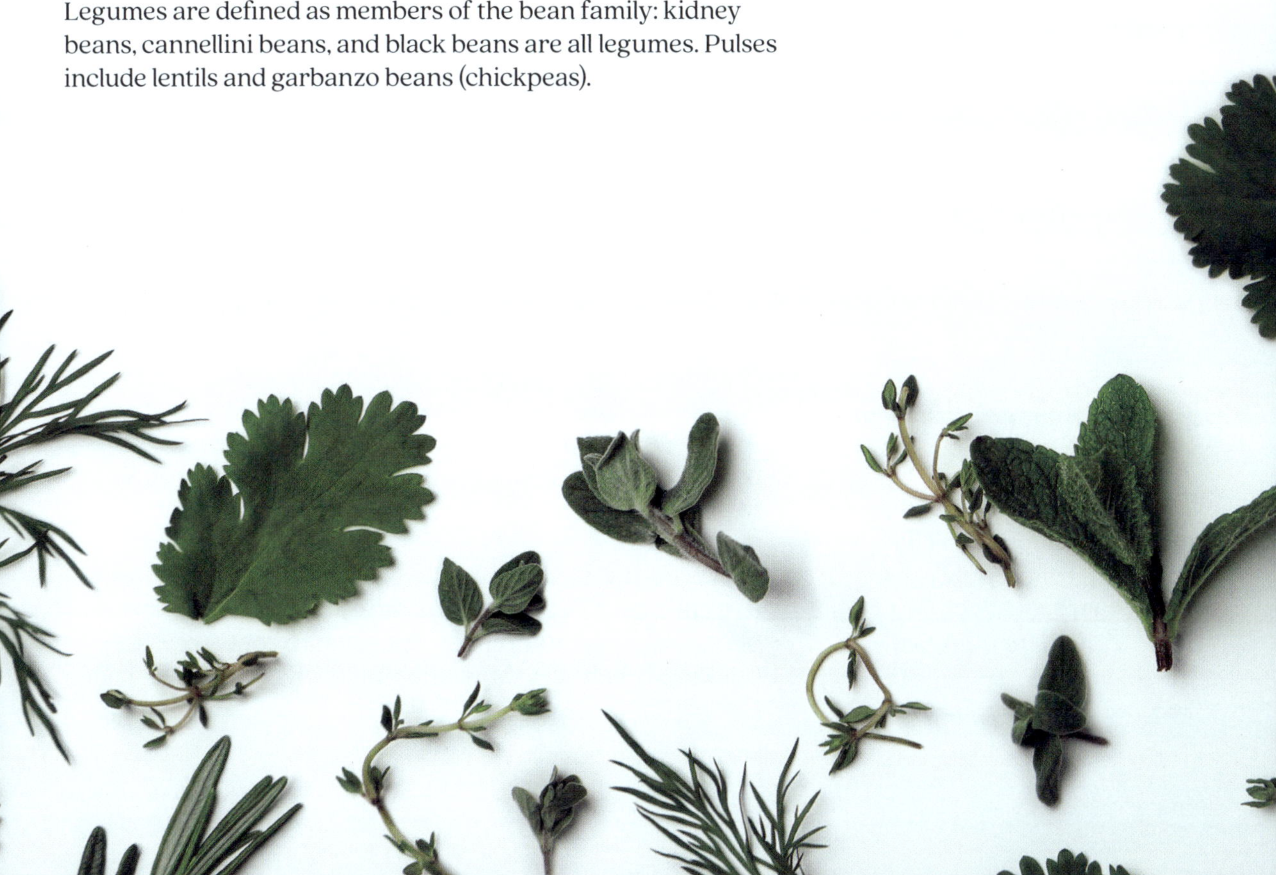

Beans

SERVINGS: 6-12 | IDDSI LEVELS   

Beans are an important source of protein, especially for vegetarians and vegans. One can make beans in a pressure cooker without presoaking. This stress-free method of cooking is a big labor and time-saver. The cooking methods are the same for all beans, but each type of bean has a different cooking time. A great way to serve beans is with Rice Congee (see page 196) for the classic dish of rice and beans. This is a favorite in the Cuban kitchen. Red beans and rice is a staple in New Orleans.

2 cups dry beans, rinsed and sorted
1 onion, sliced
1½ teaspoons salt

1. **Pressure cooker method:** Add the beans and onion to a pressure cooker or Instant Pot. Cover with about 1½ inches of water over the level of the beans. (Do not fill the inner pot of your Instant Pot more than half full.) Add herbs and spices: a bay leaf or oregano and parsley for cannellini or chickpeas; cumin for pinto beans.
   - **Note:** Soaking is not necessary for pressure-cooked beans. If not pressure cooking, beans will cook faster if they are soaked. If they are not soaked, the cooking time will be longer.

   Stovetop method: If you have time, soak the beans overnight in water to rehydrate. Then drain and cook as follows. Add the beans and onion to a pot. Cover with about 1 inch of water over the level of the beans. Add herbs and spices: a bay leaf or oregano and parsley for cannellini or chickpeas; cumin for pinto beans.

2. **Pressure cooker method:** Cook on high for the amount of time specified in the following chart. Allow the pressure to come down by natural release. Remove the lid, remove bay leaf, and stir to combine. Allow the beans to cool.

   Stovetop method: Bring the beans to a boil, then lower to a simmer. Check the beans after 1 hour for tenderness. If they are not tender, continue to cook and check. Cooking times vary depending upon the type and age of the beans.

PRO TIP

2 cups of dry beans weighs roughly 1 pound; two cups uncooked beans yield 6 cups when cooked, or 6 to 12 servings depending on the dish.

3. If desired, set aside any family servings before pureeing. For the puree, add the cooked beans to a food processor or blender and process until you achieve the desired texture.

4. Test as you go and at time of serving to see if a thickening agent, thickened sauce, or thickened stock is needed; use IDDSI Testing Methods (*iddsi.org*) to help achieve the desired IDDSI level. See pages 42-47.

5. Serve immediately or divide into servings for storage or freezing, following the directions for Serving, page 77. (Freeze for up to 1 month, not 3 months.)

NUTRITIONAL ANALYSIS PER SERVING* | ½ cup
115 calories, 0.5 g fat, 0 g saturated fat, 1 mg sodium, 0.3 g sugar, 20 g carbohydrates, 8 g fiber, 8 g protein

(Dr. Willett's book (see Resources) gives a complete nutritional breakdown for a variety of beans.)

Cooking times on high pressure	
Black beans	30 minutes
Chickpeas	40 minutes
Kidney beans	35 minutes
Pinto beans	25 minutes
Navy beans	25 minutes
Great northern beans	35 minutes

Brown Lentils

YIELD: 2 CUPS | IDDSI LEVELS 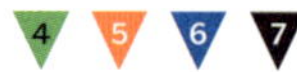

Lentils are a powerhouse of nutrition, providing protein for those on vegetarian and vegan diets. They may be used to make delicious soups and stews and used as a side dish. A variety of lentils may be found in your local market, including green lentils, French green lentils, brown lentils, and black lentils. Check packages for cooking times. There is no need to soak lentils in advance of cooking. Red lentils do not do well in an Instant Pot or pressure cooker.

1 cup brown lentils
2 cups water or vegetable broth
¼ teaspoon Italian seasoning
¼ teaspoon garlic powder
1 bay leaf
½ teaspoon salt

1. **Pressure cooker method:** Rinse and pick over the lentils, discarding any broken lentils or stones. Add the lentils, water or broth, and seasonings to a pressure cooker or Instant Pot. Cook on high pressure for 10 minutes. Allow the pot to come down from pressure by natural release. Remove the lid. If you added a bay leaf earlier, remove it. Allow the lentils to cool. Add the salt and stir to mix.

   Stovetop method: Rinse and pick over the lentils, discarding any broken lentils or stones. Add the lentils, water or broth, and seasonings to a saucepan. Bring to a rapid simmer over medium-high heat. Lower the heat to a gentle simmer and cook uncovered, for twenty to thirty minutes. Add water as needed to make sure the lentils are just covered. Lentils are done when tender. If you added a bay leaf earlier, remove it. Allow the lentils to cool. Add the salt and stir to mix.

2. If desired, set aside any family servings before pureeing. For the puree, add the cooked lentils to a food processor or blender and process until you achieve the desired texture.

3. Test as you go and at time of serving to see if a thickening agent, thickened sauce, or thickened stock is needed; use IDDSI Testing Methods (*iddsi.org*) to help achieve the desired IDDSI level. See pages 42-47.

4. Serve immediately or divide into servings for storage or freezing, following the directions for Serving, page 77. (Freeze for up to 1 month, not 3 months.)

NUTRITIONAL ANALYSIS PER SERVING | ¼ cup
169 calories, 0.1 g fat, 0 g saturated fat, 298 mg sodium, 1 g sugar, 30.4 g carbohydrates, 5.1 g fiber, 11.8 g protein

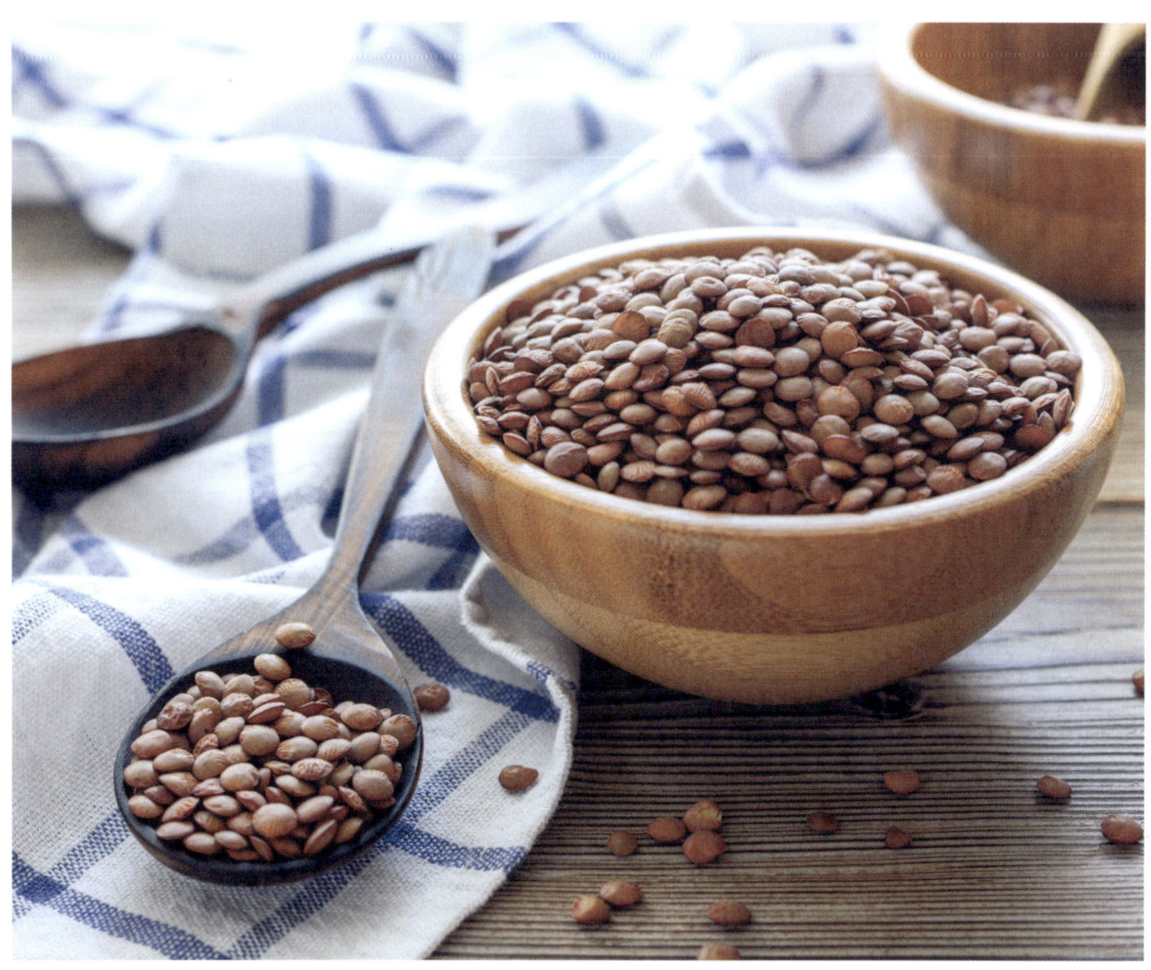

Breakfasts

209 Steel-Cut Oatmeal with Yogurt and Honey

210 Butternut Squash Quiche

212 Blintzes with Blueberry Sauce and Sour Cream *(Blueberry Sauce)*

214 Scrambled Eggs and Mashed Potatoes

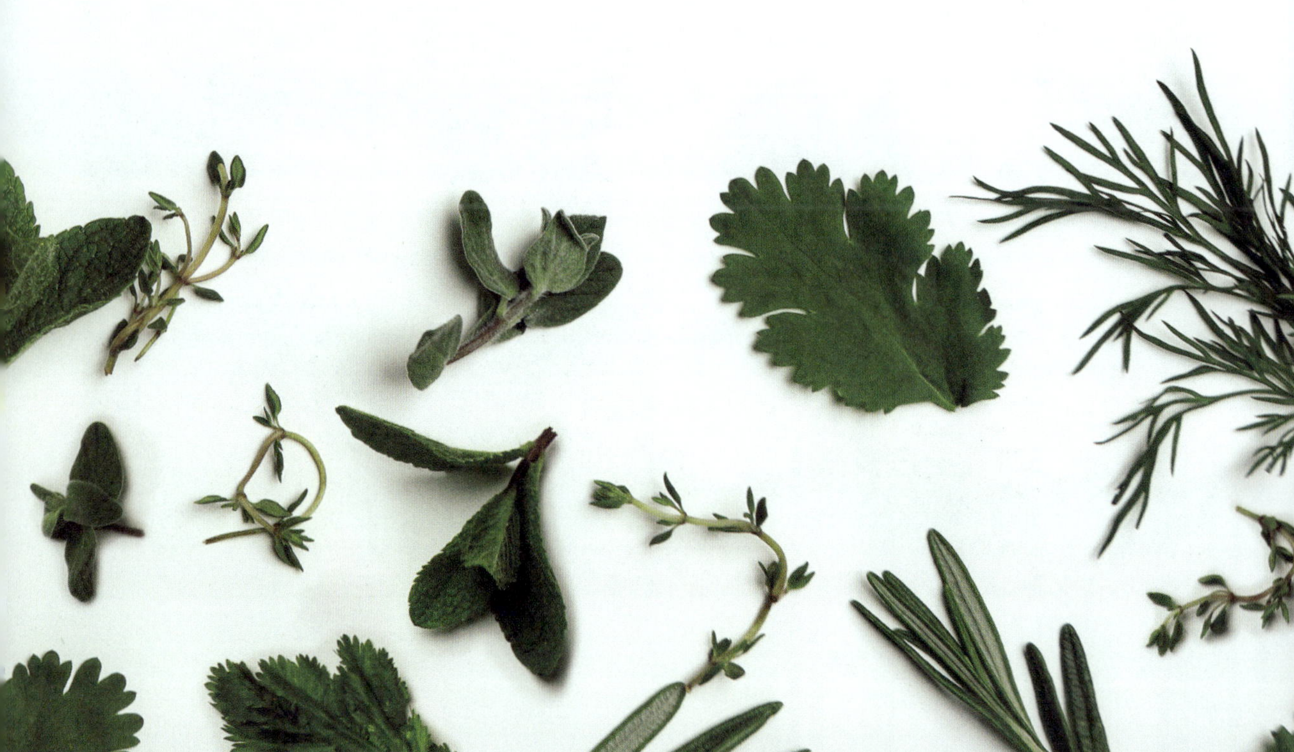

Steel-Cut Oatmeal with Yogurt and Honey

SERVINGS: 1 | IDDSI LEVELS 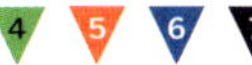

Steel-cut oats are less processed and have more fiber and less sugar than the packaged instant oatmeal varieties. For a labor-saving device, I use a mini rice cooker. It makes smooth oatmeal, and you don't have to stand over the stove and stir.

1 cup water
¼ cup steel-cut oats, 5-minute variety
Sea salt
Ground cinnamon (optional)
⅓ medium banana*, sliced into ¼-inch slices (optional)
½ cup whole milk
¼ cup whole Greek yogurt
1 teaspoon honey

** Check with your healthcare provider to see if you can include pureed banana. This will boost the nutrient level.*

1. **Rice cooker method:** In a rice cooker, combine the water, oats, a pinch of salt, and a dash of cinnamon, if using. Cook according to the rice cooker instructions, or until the oatmeal is soft. If it needs more time, continue cooking until the grains are very tender. Add extra water, several tablespoons at a time, if the oatmeal dries out.

   Stovetop method: Bring the water to a boil in a small saucepan set over high heat. Stir in the oats, a pinch of salt, and a dash of cinnamon, if using. Lower the heat to medium-low and simmer, stirring occasionally and adding liquid as needed, until the oats are tender, about 20 minutes.

2. If desired, set aside any family servings before pureeing. For the puree, once the oatmeal cools, transfer it to a food processor or high-speed blender. Add the banana, if using, and pulse to break it up. Add the milk, yogurt, and honey. Process until you achieve the desired texture.

3. Test as you go and at time of serving to see if thickening is needed; use IDDSI Testing Methods (*iddsi.org*) to help achieve the desired IDDSI level. See pages 42-47.

4. Serve immediately or divide into servings for storage or freezing, following the directions for Serving, page 77.

NUTRITIONAL ANALYSIS PER SERVING | 8 oz
351 calories, 4 g fat, 1 g saturated fat, 68 mg sodium, 50 g sugar, 76 g carbohydrates, 6 g fiber, 8 g protein

Butternut Squash Quiche

SERVINGS: 8 | IDDSI LEVELS 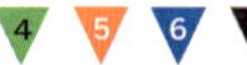

For the person with a swallowing disorder, the quiche filling is a custard, Level 4 IDDSI. For family and friends, the crust may be served with the dish.

- 1 store-bought or homemade pie crust (see page 101)
- 2 tablespoons extra-virgin olive oil
- ½ cup sliced mushrooms
- 1½ teaspoons low-sodium soy sauce
- ½ cup yellow onion, thinly sliced
- 2 cups cooked, pureed butternut squash (see page 181)
- ¼ cup milk (could substitute water for depth of veggie flavor)
- 4 extra-large eggs, lightly beaten
- 4 ounces goat cheese, room temperature
- 1 tablespoon chopped fresh thyme leaves or thyme paste

1. Place a rack in the center of the oven and preheat to 375°F (190°C).

2. Press the pie crust into an even layer in a 9-inch tart pan with a removable bottom. Place the pan on a baking sheet. Prick the crust with a fork several times. Bake for 10 minutes, until the surface of the crust is dry to the touch. Remove from the oven and allow to cool.

3. Meanwhile, in a skillet or sauté pan, add 1 tablespoon olive oil over medium-low heat. Add the mushrooms and cook, stirring occasionally, until they are soft and give up their liquid, about 10 minutes. Add the soy sauce. Remove the mushrooms from the pan and set aside on a plate.

4. Add 1 tablespoon olive oil, raise the heat to medium-high, and sauté the onion until it is lightly golden, about 3 minutes. Remove from the heat and allow to cool.

5. Place the onion and mushrooms in a food processor or high-speed blender. Pulse a few times to break up the vegetables, then puree to a smooth consistency, adding warm water, a tablespoon at a time if necessary, to get a smooth puree. Add the butternut squash, milk, beaten eggs, goat cheese, and thyme. Blend until smooth.

6. Add the quiche filling to the cooled crust. Bake for 15 minutes. Lower the oven temperature to 350°F (175°C) and bake for an additional 35 minutes, or until a toothpick or knife inserted into the filling comes out clean. Transfer the quiche to a cooling rack to cool.

7. Slice and serve portions for family meals. The quiche filling, scooped out of the crust, is IDDSI Level 4 and can be enjoyed by the person with swallowing difficulties without pureeing.

8. If you wish to serve the crust, place the desired number of slices in a food processor or high-speed blender. Add 1 to 2 tablespoons warm water or broth per slice. Process until you achieve the desired texture. Test as you go and at time of serving to see if a thickening agent, thickened sauce, or thickened stock is needed; use IDDSI Testing Methods (*iddsi.org*) to help achieve the desired IDDSI level. See pages 42-47.

9. Serve immediately or divide into servings for storage or freezing, following the directions for Serving, page 77.

NUTRITIONAL ANALYSIS PER SERVING | 1 cup (1 slice)
1 slice quiche with crust
221 calories, 13 g fat, 5 g saturated fat, 155 mg sodium, 1 g sugar, 19 g carbohydrates, 1 g fiber, 6 g protein

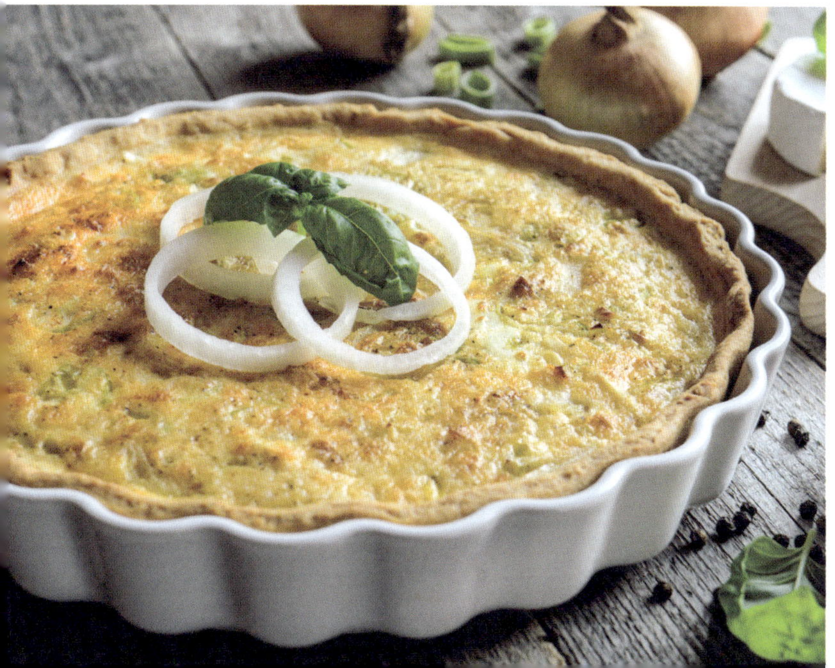

PRO TIP

If I do not have time to roast butternut squash to make the quiche, I use Birds Eye Southland frozen pureed butternut squash from the freezer section of the grocery store as the base for the quiche. I thaw it in the fridge before adding it to the recipe. You can also use 21 ounces of fresh cubed butternut squash. Cook in the microwave for about 8 minutes. Remove the skin if it is not peeled off. According to a recipe tester, this is perfect for puree. Once the squash is pureed, run it through a mesh sieve to eliminate fibers, skin, and seeds, **which are not safe for the swallow**.

Blintzes with Blueberry Sauce and Sour Cream

SERVINGS: 3 | IDDSI LEVELS  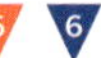

Blintzes are crepe-like pancakes filled with a ricotta and cream cheese mixture and were a favorite of the gangster Meyer Lansky. Blintzes are generally available at supermarkets, but if you want to make your own, recipes can be found online.

1 batch of homemade cheese blintzes (see link above) or frozen purchased blintzes
2 teaspoons unsalted butter or non-trans-fat margarine
Blueberry Sauce (see page 213) (may be made with frozen blueberries)
Low-fat sour cream

1. Make the homemade blintzes according to the recipe and freeze any extras in a zip-top bag. Use freshly made blintzes or defrost frozen blintzes in the refrigerator for 2 hours. In a small nonstick pan, melt the butter or margarine. Add the cooked blintzes and warm. Or add the frozen blintzes and cook following the package directions.

2. For family meal servings, top each blintz with a generous amount, several tablespoons, of Blueberry Sauce and a dollop of sour cream.

3. For the puree, cool the blintzes. Break up 2 blintzes per serving into a food processor or blender. Add 2 tablespoons Blueberry Sauce and 1 tablespoon sour cream for each blintz. Process until you achieve the desired texture.

4. Test as you go and at time of serving to see if a thickening agent, thickened sauce, or thickened stock is needed; use IDDSI Testing Methods (*iddsi.org*) to help achieve the desired IDDSI level. See pages 42-47.

5. Serve immediately or divide into servings for storage or freezing, following the directions for Serving, page 77.

NUTRITIONAL ANALYSIS PER SERVING | 2 blintzes
358 calories, 21 g fat, 8 g saturated fat, 176 mg sodium, 17 g sugar, 30 g carbohydrates, 0 g fiber, 11 g protein

PRO TIP

When you puree any dish with ricotta cheese, the volume increases because of the incorporated air; one serving will look much larger after pureeing than before. The blintzes are light in taste and texture because of the air, but the nutritional content is the same. The added volume does not change the nutrients.

Blueberry Sauce

YIELD: 1 CUP | IDDSI LEVELS 

Any homemade fruit sauce is more delicious and nutritious than the flavored syrups for pancakes you can buy bottled. This sauce has the added virtue of flexibility—add it to oatmeal or any other hot cereal or to ice cream for a nutrition boost, and it can be made from blackberries, raspberries, strawberries, cherries, mango, or kiwi.

- 1 pint blueberries, washed, or 8 ounces frozen blueberries
- 2 tablespoons fresh lemon juice
- ¼ cup maple syrup, honey, or agave syrup
- 2 tablespoons cornstarch

1. Place the blueberries and 1 cup water in a high-speed blender. Blend on high until the fruit is liquefied. Run the liquefied fruit through a mesh strainer lined with cheesecloth.

2. Place the strained blueberry puree in a saucepan and set over medium-high heat. Bring to a boil, then reduce the heat to medium-low. Add the lemon juice and sweetener and simmer gently for 5 minutes.

3. In a small bowl, whisk the cornstarch with 2 tablespoons water to make a slurry. Add the slurry to the sauce, return the heat to medium-high, and bring the sauce back to a boil. Cook, stirring occasionally, until the sauce is thickened and the raw taste of cornstarch disappears.

4. Remove from the heat and allow the sauce to cool for 10 minutes; set aside any desired family servings.

5. Test as you go and at time of serving to see if a thickening agent, thickened sauce, or thickened stock is needed; use IDDSI Testing Methods (*iddsi.org*) to help achieve the desired IDDSI level. See pages 42-47.

6. Serve immediately, refrigerate for up to 48 hours, or freeze for up to 3 months. Store in ½-cup individual servings (for pureeing two blintzes).

NUTRITIONAL ANALYSIS PER SERVING | ½ cup
123 calories, 0 g fat, 0 g saturated fat, 2 mg sodium, 25 g sugar, 29 g carbohydrates, 2 g fiber, 1 g protein

Scrambled Eggs and Mashed Potatoes

SERVINGS: 1 | IDDSI LEVELS 

I found that it was difficult to puree home fries for a classic American accompaniment to breakfast, because there were hard particles in the puree. The mashed potatoes deliver flavor and are a good substitute for home fries.

3 large eggs, lightly beaten
1½ tablespoons milk
1 tablespoon unsalted butter or non-trans-fat margarine
½ cup Mashed Potatoes (see page 176)

1. In a small bowl, beat the eggs and milk. Melt the butter in a nonstick skillet over medium-low heat. Add the eggs to the pan, reduce the heat to low, and cook, stirring with a silicone spatula, until the desired consistency is reached.

2. Remove the pan from the heat. The eggs should be the consistency of custard, IDDSI Level 4 (see page 44).

3. Warm the mashed potatoes for 30 seconds in the microwave. The mashed potatoes should be the consistency of custard, IDDSI Level 4, when prepared according to the recipe.

4. For serving, place the eggs in one dish and potatoes in a second dish and alternate bites.

5. Make this on the day it is to be consumed. Do not store in the freezer. May be held overnight in the fridge.

PRO TIP

To round out this classic American breakfast, try pureeing two chicken-and-apple sausages (I like Applegate Naturals). Heat the frozen sausages in a pan over medium-low heat until warmed through, 4 to 5 minutes per side. Place the sausages in a food processor and add a little water or broth to process until you achieve the desired texture. Test as you go and at time of serving to see if a thickening agent, thickened sauce, or thickened stock is needed; use IDDSI Testing Methods (*iddsi.org*) to help achieve the desired IDDSI level. See pages 42-47.

NUTRITIONAL ANALYSIS
221 calories, 10 g fat, 3 g saturated fat, 147 mg sodium, 2 g sugar, 19 g carbohydrates, 2 g fiber, 15 g protein

Smoothies

216 The Motor City Shake *(Toasted Cashew Cream)*

218 The Memphis Shake

219 The Manhattan Shake

220 Mango Lassi

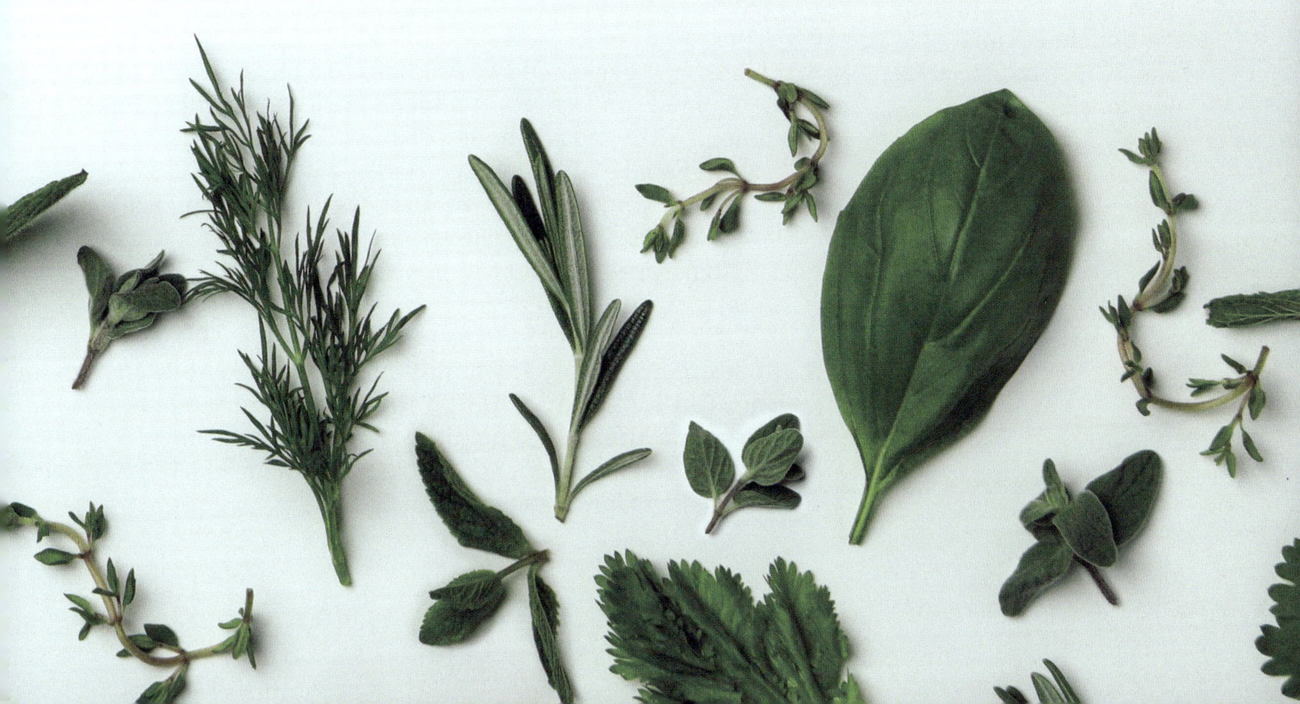

The Motor City Shake

SERVINGS: 3 | IDDSI LEVEL 

This is a warm sweet potato pie shake with an optional whipped topping and optional caramel sauce. The orange juice balances the sweetness of the sweet potato. Coconut milk provides fat for proper absorption of vitamin A. Use more or less of the soft-baked sweet potato to get the correct thickness. You can substitute canned sweet potato with no added sugar, if time is too short to slow-bake the sweet potato.

4 medium sweet potatoes, or 1 (15-ounce) can sweet potato puree
1 tablespoon vegetable oil
1 cup coconut milk or whole milk
2 tablespoons orange juice
⅛ teaspoon ground cinnamon
⅛ teaspoon ground allspice
1⁄16 teaspoon ground cloves
Honey or stevia to taste
CocoWhip topping or Toasted Cashew Cream (see page 217) (optional)
Store-bought caramel sauce, such as St. Dalfour (optional)

1. Place a rack in the center of the oven and preheat to 300°F (150°C). Wash and dry the potatoes and cut off any sharp ends or blemishes. Puncture each potato three times with a knife to allow steam to escape.

2. Place the potatoes in a baking dish, leaving room between them for air to circulate. Brush the skins with the oil and cover tightly with aluminum foil. Bake for 90 minutes, until very soft. Remove from oven and allow to cool.

3. Once cool, remove and discard the potato skins, scraping out the potato flesh and transferring it to a large mixing bowl. Mash with a fork until soft and smooth. Using a silicone spatula, rub the mash through a mesh strainer to remove any fibers.

4. Transfer the mashed sweet potato to a blender with the milk, juice, and spices, and blend until thoroughly combined. Taste and add honey or stevia if you would like a sweeter shake.
   - **Tip:** If you would like to serve the shake warm, transfer to a pot and warm over medium-low heat. I use a high-speed blender for making this, set on warming setting for 2 minutes.

5. If desired, set aside any family servings before thickening. Test for Level 3 IDDSI. If the shake is thick enough without adding thickener, it is all right to consume. If it is not thick enough, add thickener to achieve Level 3 IDDSI. See *iddsi.org* and pages 45-47.

6. Serve immediately, topped with Toasted Cashew Cream and caramel sauce, if using, or divide into servings for storage or freezing, following the directions for Serving, page 77.

NUTRITIONAL ANALYSIS PER SERVING | 1 cup
Without Cashew Cream
372 calories, 10.1 g fat, 2.5 g saturated fat, 140 mg sodium, 28.7 g sugar, 63.3 g carbohydrates, 7.8 g fiber, 9.3 g protein

Toasted Cashew Cream

YIELD: 1 CUP | IDDSI LEVEL 

If you do not wish to prepare your own Toasted Cashew Cream, you can substitute 1 cup frozen coconut milk whipped dessert topping, available in supermarkets—I like So Delicious CocoWhip. For either topping, add one half pump of gel thickener or half scoop of powder to bind the whipped topping.

Recipe courtesy of Dr. Denise Pickett-Bernard, PhD, RDN, LDN.

1 cup raw cashews
¾ cup water, plus extra for blending
2 tablespoons maple syrup

1. Place the cashews in a dry skillet over medium-low heat and toast, stirring frequently, until lightly golden, 2 to 4 minutes. Transfer the cashews to a high-speed blender.

2. Add ¾ cup water and the maple syrup and blend until completely smooth. Add more water, if necessary, to get a pureed thickness. Best to always make this fresh.

NUTRITIONAL ANALYSIS PER SERVING | 2 tablespoons
137 calories, 5.8 g fat, 1.2 g saturated fat, 4 mg sodium, 15.5 g sugar, 20.9 g carbohydrates, 0.4 g fiber, 1.9 g protein

The Memphis Shake

SERVINGS: 2 | IDDSI LEVEL 

It is said that the peanut butter and banana sandwich was Elvis Presley's favorite. This recipe uses peanut butter powder, because it is low in fat and blends easily. You can substitute 1 tablespoon smooth peanut butter. I know the King liked bacon. Since you cannot puree bacon, I like to use bacon dust on top of the shake to get the flavor. It can be purchased online—I like Bacon Lovers Seasoning by Flavor God.

2 bananas*, cut into 1-inch chunks, frozen
2 tablespoons organic peanut butter powder, whisked with 2 tablespoons water until smooth
½ cup whole milk or nondairy milk, chilled
Honey or stevia, to taste
Bacon Lovers Seasoning by Flavor God (optional)

** Check with your healthcare provider to see if you can include pureed banana. This will boost the nutrient level.*

1. Add the bananas, hydrated peanut butter powder, milk, and sweetener to a blender. Blend until smooth, adding more milk if needed.

2. If desired, set aside any family servings before thickening. Test for Level 3 IDDSI. If the shake is thick enough without adding thickener, it is all right to consume. If it is not thick enough, add thickener to Level 3 IDDSI. See *iddsi.org* and pages 45-47.

3. Sprinkle bacon dust on top of the shake, if using, and serve immediately (this is best consumed fresh). The extra serving may be refrigerated and served within 24 hours. Before serving, simply blend it up to mix the thickener well.

NUTRITIONAL ANALYSIS PER SERVING | 4 oz
279 calories, 1.6 g fat, 0.4 g saturated fat, 64 mg sodium, 55.4 g sugar, 62.3 g carbohydrates, 3.2 g fiber, 1.6 g protein

The Manhattan Shake

SERVINGS: 2 | IDDSI LEVEL 

The flavor of this shake is nostalgic for me; it was a favorite when I was in school. This orange and vanilla shake makes an excellent midmorning or midafternoon snack.

2 navel oranges
1 banana*, cut into 1-inch chunks, frozen
1 cup vanilla almond milk
1 teaspoon vanilla extract
1 scoop whey vanilla protein powder or plant-based protein powder
1 cup ice

** Check with your healthcare provider to see if you can include pureed banana. This will boost the nutrient level.*

1. Juice the oranges into the pitcher of a blender. Add the banana, almond milk, vanilla extract, protein powder, and ice. Pulse to break up the ingredients and blend until smooth.

2. If desired, set aside any family servings before thickening. Test for Level 3 IDDSI. If the shake is thick enough without adding thickener, it is all right to consume. If it is not thick enough, add thickener to achieve Level 3 IDDSI . See *iddsi.org* and pages 45-47.

3. Serve immediately (this is best consumed fresh). The extra serving may be refrigerated and served within 24 hours. Before serving, simply blend it up to mix the thickener well.

NUTRITIONAL ANALYSIS PER SERVING | 8 oz
297 calories, 4.5 g fat, 1.6 g saturated fat, 160 mg sodium, 15.1 g sugar, 26.8 g carbohydrates, 1.4 g fiber, 37.1 g protein

Mango Lassi

SERVINGS: 2 | IDDSI LEVEL 

Lassi is a refreshing Indian yogurt shake made with fruit, fruit juice, and yogurt. A probiotic-rich fermented food, yogurt supports digestion, while fresh fruit adds fiber. Store in the fridge overnight and drink within 24 hours; it is best served fresh. Lassi does not have the high sugar content of a classic American milkshake made with ice cream. This recipe can be doubled or tripled for several people.

2 tablespoons honey, optional, whisked
1 cup frozen mango chunks
1 cup buttermilk, or ¾ cup Greek yogurt plus ¼ cup buttermilk
½ tablespoon fresh lime juice (from ½ lime)
1 scoop whey protein powder or plant-based protein powder, optional
½ teaspoon ginger juice or ½ teaspoon dried ginger, optional

1. Dissolve the honey in 2 tablespoons hot water. Add the mango to a high-speed blender and pulse to break up the fruit.

2. Add the dissolved honey, buttermilk, lime juice, protein powder, and ginger juice, or dried ginger, if using. Blend until smooth.

3. If desired, set aside any family servings before thickening. Test for Level 3 IDDSI. If the shake is thick enough without adding thickener, it is all right to consume. If it is not thick enough, add thickener to achieve Level 3 IDDSI. See *iddsi.org* and pages 45-47.

4. Serve immediately (this is best consumed fresh). The extra serving may be refrigerated and served within 24 hours. Before serving, simply blend it up to mix the thickener well.

VARIATION

Try making lassi with **fresh melon** or **ripe bananas**.

NUTRITIONAL ANALYSIS PER SERVING | 8 oz
346 calories, 4.2 g fat, 2.2 g saturated fat, 117 mg sodium, 32.5 g sugar, 39.8 g carbohydrates, 1.5 g fiber, 40.7 g protein

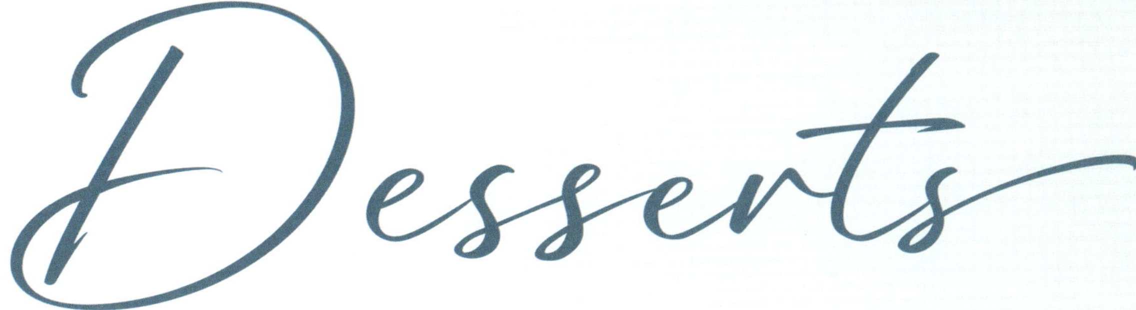

Desserts

222 Cathie G.'s Banana Cream Pie

224 Texas Sheet Cake with Oh-So-Delicious Chocolate Frosting

226 Pumpkin Flan

228 Thickened Ice Cream

229 The Ice Cream Sandwich

230 Raspberry "Ice Cream"

232 Homemade Vanilla Pudding

233 Homemade Chocolate Pudding

234 Cheesecake Puree

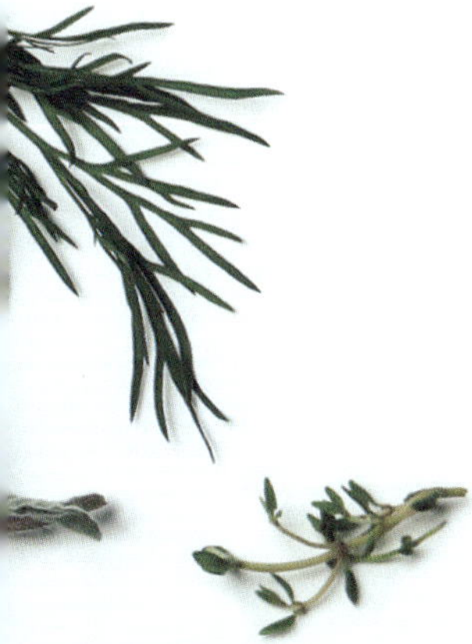

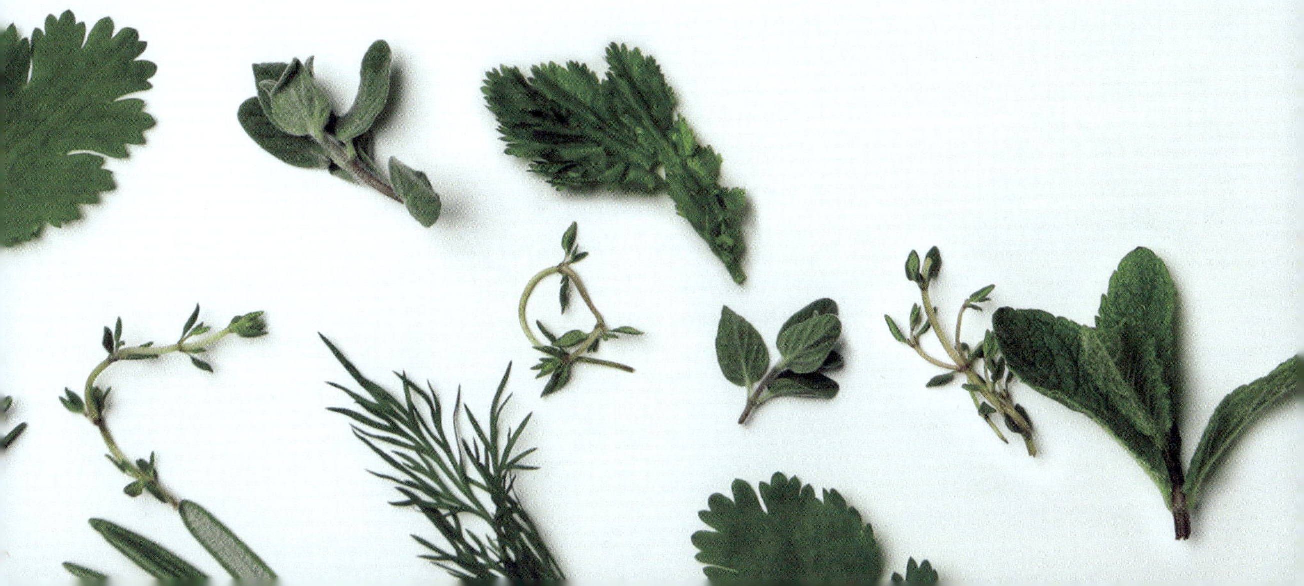

Cathie G.'s Banana Cream Pie

SERVINGS: 4 | IDDSI LEVELS   

I experimented for a long time to create this recipe. Banana Cream Pie was my mom's favorite dessert. The trick to making this pie for the puree kitchen is a flavorful banana puree—don't try to make this with bright yellow, firm bananas. Choose fruit with well-browned skins, but avoid black and squishy bananas. You may substitute almond or oat milk for the dairy milk. The ingredients are layered in a clear glass for a pretty parfait effect. If you wish, put the whipped topping in a pastry bag fitted with a star tip for a professional look.

FOR THE CRUST

3 cups graham cracker crumbs (about 12 graham crackers processed in a food processor)
2 tablespoons raw cane sugar or Truvia Sweet Complete Granulated stevia
½ teaspoon ground cinnamon, more if desired

FOR THE PUDDING

4 very ripe bananas, coarsely mashed
2½ cups whole milk or milk of choice, divided
2 tablespoons pure maple syrup
2 tablespoons coconut oil or unsalted butter, melted
Pinch of sea salt
Pinch of ground turmeric, for color
3 tablespoons cornstarch
1 cup thawed frozen coconut milk whipped dessert topping (see Tip)

To make the crust:

1. Pulse the graham cracker crumbs, sugar or stevia, and cinnamon in a food processor or blender until finely ground into a sand-like texture. Add about 6 tablespoons very hot water, pulse, and let soften, adding more water if needed.

2. Test as you go and at time of serving to see if a thickening agent, thickened sauce, or thickened stock is needed; use IDDSI Testing Methods (*iddsi.org*) to help achieve the desired IDDSI level. See pages 42-47. This is your crust. It is the base of the dessert. Spread the crust mixture evenly into 4 serving bowls. Refrigerate to chill and set while you make the pudding.

To make the pudding:

1. Process the bananas in a food processor or blender until very smooth and lump-free. Add 2 cups milk, maple syrup, coconut oil, salt, and turmeric and pulse to combine.

2. Put the cornstarch in a medium saucepan. Add the remaining ½ cup milk and whisk until smooth. Add the banana mixture and whisk until combined. Cook over medium heat, whisking constantly, until simmering.

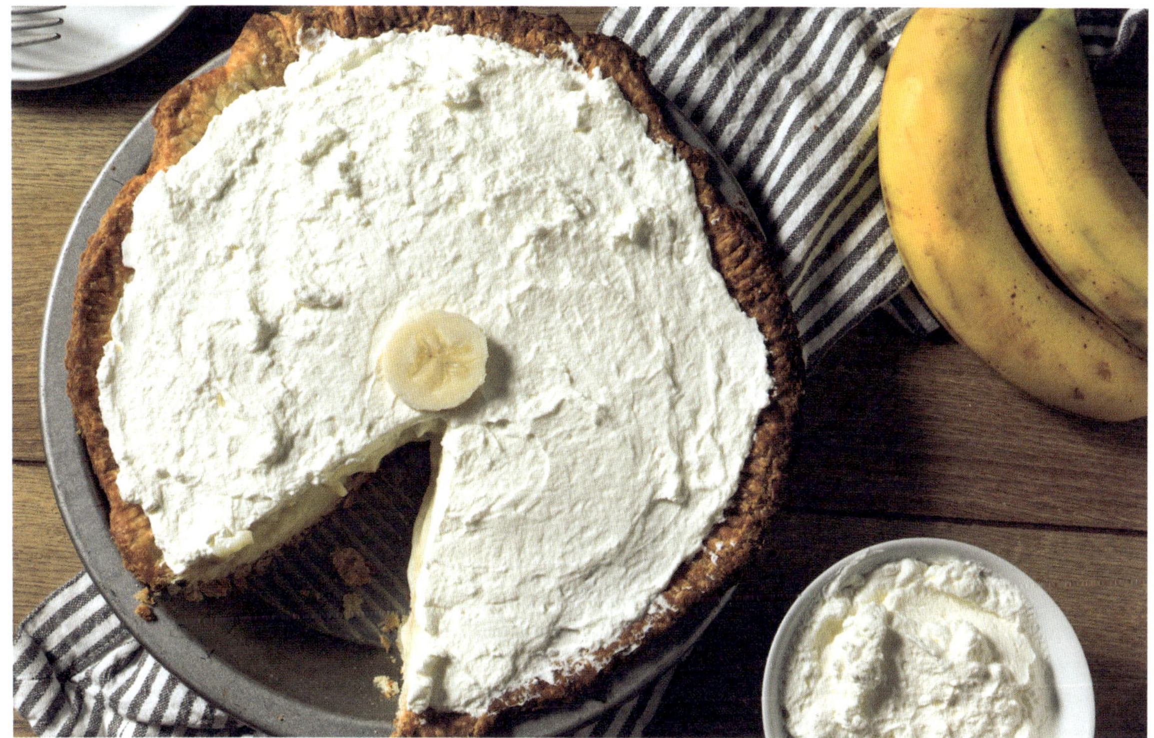

3. Reduce the heat to low and simmer, still whisking to avoid scorching on the bottom, for 1 minute. Divide the pudding evenly among 4 serving bowls over the crust.

4. Let stand until cooled, about 30 minutes. Cover with plastic wrap and refrigerate until chilled, at least 4 hours. Serve chilled, topped with the whipped topping. This may be stored covered in the refrigerator for up to 2 days (I do not recommend freezing this).
   - **Tip:** I prefer whipped coconut milk topping (my favorite is So Delicious CocoWhip), because freshly whipped dairy cream tends to separate as it stands. Add one half pump of gel thickener or half scoop of powder to bind the whipped topping.

NUTRITIONAL ANALYSIS PER SERVING | ½ cup
285 calories, 12 g fat, 6 g saturated fat, 145 mg sodium, 20 g sugar, 43 g carbohydrates, 3 g fiber, 3 g protein

Texas Sheet Cake with Oh-So-Delicious Chocolate Frosting

SERVINGS: 12 | IDDSI LEVELS 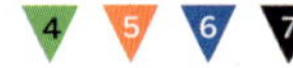

This flat chocolate cake is naturally moist and blends into a smooth, crumb-free puree. The frosting is made with Nocciolata, a hazelnut-cocoa spread that will remind you of another Italian nut spread. But I prefer Nocciolata because it doesn't have trans fats, is generally more nutritious, and has a smoother texture for the swallow. For an extra treat, serve with whipped coconut milk topping (see Tip, page 225, step 8).

FOR THE CAKE

Nonstick cooking spray for the pan
2 cups whole-wheat pastry flour
1¾ cups sugar
1 teaspoon baking soda
½ teaspoon sea salt
½ cup (1 stick) unsalted butter, cut into pieces
⅓ cup natural cocoa powder, such as Hershey's
1 cup sour cream
2 large eggs
1 teaspoon vanilla extract

FOR THE FROSTING

1 cup organic chocolate hazelnut spread, preferably Nocciolata
¾ cup full-fat sour cream, plus more as needed for the puree
2 tablespoons whole milk, plus more as needed

1. To make the cake, position a rack in the center of the oven and preheat to 350°F. Spray the inside of an 18 x 13-inch half-sheet pan with nonstick spray.
2. Whisk the flour, sugar, baking soda, and salt together in a medium bowl. Bring 1 cup water, the butter, and the cocoa powder to a boil in a medium saucepan over high heat, stirring until the butter is melted. Add to the flour mixture and whisk until combined. Add the sour cream, the eggs, and vanilla and whisk again to combine.
3. Spread evenly in the prepared pan. Bake until the cake springs back when lightly pressed on top and pulls away slightly from the sides, 20 to 22 minutes. Let cool completely.
4. To make the frosting, mash the hazelnut spread and ¾ cup sour cream together with a sturdy spoon or silicone spatula to a pudding-like consistency, adding milk by the tablespoon, as needed. Transfer to a pastry bag fitted with a ½-inch star tip.
5. If desired, set aside any family servings before pureeing, and serve with frosting piped onto the cake.

6. To puree the cake, break up the desired number of servings into a food processor or blender. Pulse the cake into crumbs. Add 2 tablespoons sour cream per serving and 3 tablespoons very hot water and process into a puree, adding more water, 1 tablespoon at a time, as needed. Transfer to a bowl.

7. Test as you go and at time of serving to see if a thickening agent, thickened sauce, or thickened stock is needed; use IDDSI Testing Methods (*iddsi.org*) to help achieve the desired IDDSI level. See pages 42-47. Divide the pureed cake portions evenly among serving or storage bowls with 1 or 2 tablespoons of frosting piped over top.

8. Serve with thickened whipped topping (see Tip, page 223), if desired, or cover with plastic wrap and refrigerate for up to 48 hours or freeze for up to 1 month.
   - **Tip:** I prefer whipped coconut milk topping (my favorite is So Delicious CocoWhip), because freshly whipped dairy cream tends to separate as it stands. Add one half pump of gel thickener or half scoop of powder to bind the whipped topping.

NUTRITIONAL ANALYSIS PER SERVING | 4 oz
Chocolate cake only
220 calories, 8.9 g fat, 5.6 g saturated fat, 29.3 mg sodium, 321 g sugar, 35.1 g carbohydrates, 1.2 g fiber, 2.6 g protein

---

NUTRITIONAL ANALYSIS PER SERVING | 1 tablespoon
Frosting only
33 calories, 2 g fat, 1 g saturated fat, 5 mg sodium, 2 g sugar, 3 g carbohydrates, 0 g fiber, 0 g protein

Pumpkin Flan

SERVINGS: 4 | IDDSI LEVEL 

A perfect dessert for a holiday meal. I use St. Dalfour Organic Caramel Sauce for its convenience. It contains natural sugars as opposed to refined sugar. This caramel sauce is a go-to quickie ingredient. It has the consistency of honey. As I have been told by three speech-language pathologists, **if the caramel is of the same thickness as the custard, the dish is safe for the swallow.** Dipping sauce may be Level 3 IDDSI, Moderately Thick. Caramel sauce is optional. **As always, clear this dish with your healthcare provider.**

4 teaspoons store-bought caramel sauce, such as St. Dalfour
4 large eggs, room temperature, lightly beaten
1½ cups whole milk or coconut milk
½ cup maple syrup
¾ cup pumpkin puree, unseasoned
1 teaspoon ground cinnamon
¼ teaspoon ground allspice
1½ teaspoons ground ginger
⅛ teaspoon ground cloves
¼ teaspoon salt

EQUIPMENT
Aluminum foil
4 (6-ounce) porcelain ramekins, oven and dishwasher safe, available online and in stores

1. Make an aluminum foil sling for four 6-ounce (¾ cup) porcelain custard ramekins. For each sling, fold a 12-inch-long piece of aluminum foil into thirds lengthwise. Place under the ramekin and fold the tops together to secure the sling.

2. This is your device for removing the ramekins from the pressure cooker. Using a ramekin as a stencil, cut four disks from another sheet of foil to cover the top of the custard in each ramekin. Place 1 teaspoon caramel sauce into the bottom of each ramekin. Swirl the ramekin so the caramel covers the bottom.

3. In a medium bowl, whisk the eggs, milk, and maple syrup until smooth. Add the pumpkin puree and spices and whisk until blended thoroughly. Divide the mixture among the ramekins.

4. Cover the top of each ramekin with a foil disk and place each in its foil sling.

5. **Pressure cooker method:** Lower the ramekins into the steamer rack of the pressure cooker. Fill the bottom of the pressure cooker with water, just below the steamer rack. Cook on high pressure for 20 minutes; allow pressure to release naturally.

Stovetop method: Alternatively, place a steamer basket in a large pot on the stove, add water to fill just below the base of the basket, and bring the water to a boil. Carefully lower the ramekins into the steaming basket. Lower the heat, cover, and steam until the custard is just set, 30 to 45 minutes.

6. Once done, remove the lid and transfer the ramekins to a cooling rack to cool completely. Refrigerate for 4 hours before serving.

7. To serve, gently remove the aluminum foil cover from the custard. Run a knife under warm water and loosen the custard by running the knife around the edge of the ramekin. Using a saucer or a shallow bowl, cover the top of the ramekin and flip it to turn the custard out. The caramel will be on top. Serve immediately, or store, covered, in the refrigerator for up to 2 days. (I do not recommend freezing.)

NUTRITIONAL ANALYSIS PER SERVING | 4 oz
205 calories, 11.2 g fat, 3.8 g saturated fat, 157 mg sodium, 10.8 g sugar, 12.4 g carbohydrates, 0.5 g fiber, 14 g protein

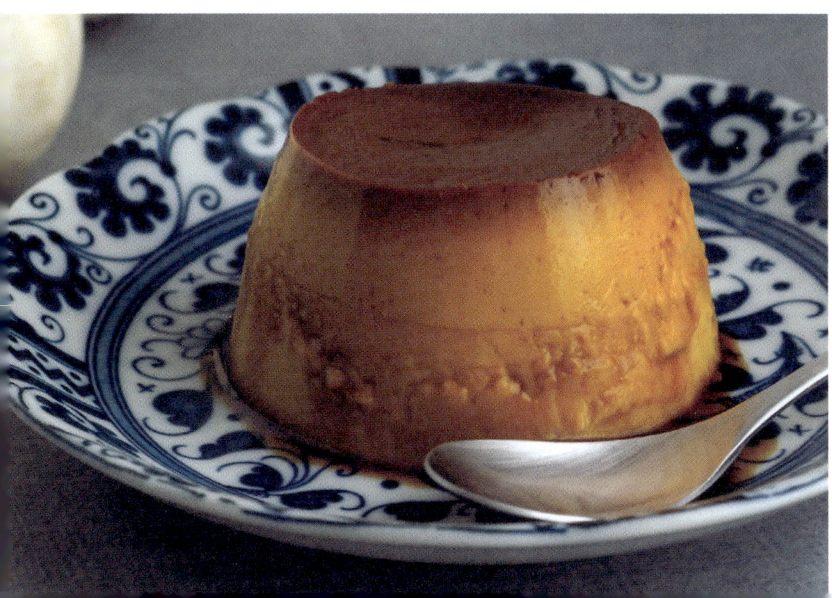

Thickened Ice Cream

SERVINGS: 1 | IDDSI LEVEL 

Why would a person with dysphagia want homemade frozen dessert? The answer is simple: variety.

Ice cream is the most popular and most beloved dessert in America. Commercially available thickened desserts only come in basic flavors. When you want your favorite ice cream and your favorite ice cream is not available, here is the answer. Using this recipe, you can thicken your favorite ice cream. It is important to thicken the ice cream so that it will not melt down to a liquid but remain safe for the swallow. **Get clearance from your healthcare provider to thicken your favorite ice cream if it contains fruit (such as cherries) or nuts.** Do not attempt to thicken ice cream that contains marshmallows, sprinkles, hard candy, toffee, or cookie bits, **as these are not safe for the swallow.**

1 cup ice cream

1. Let the ice cream soften for 15 minutes at room temperature or in the refrigerator. Put the softened ice cream in a blender. Puree on high for 10 seconds, until completely smooth. If any particles remain in the blended ice cream, use a silicone spatula to rub it through a mesh strainer set over a medium bowl.

2. Test for Level 4 IDDSI. If the ice cream is thick enough without adding a thickener, it is all right to consume; if needed, add a thickening agent. See *iddsi.org* and pages 45-47. Serve immediately, or refreeze. Can be stored in the freezer for up to 1 week.

NUTRITIONAL ANALYSIS PER SERVING

For a nutritional analysis of your favorite flavors, see the package of ice cream.

The Ice Cream Sandwich

SERVINGS: 1 | IDDSI LEVEL 

This is a deconstructed dessert recipe for the classic ice cream sandwich, using chocolate cake and thickened vanilla ice cream. It is festive. Designed to delight. A treat for the eyes and the palate. Since this is a quickie recipe, I am recommending a store-bought cake, preferably without icing (or with the icing removed); alternatively, you can make your favorite cake with no icing. To make a diabetic version of this dessert, buy no-sugar-added ice cream and a no-sugar-added cake, as your healthcare provider recommends.

2 servings store-bought chocolate cake, without icing
2 tablespoons sour cream
¼ cup Thickened Ice Cream (see page 228)

1. Break up the cake into a food processor or blender. Pulse several times to break down the cake into granules. Add 2 tablespoons warm water and the sour cream and puree to combine. Add 2 more tablespoons warm water, as needed, and process until you achieve the desired texture.

2. Test for Level 4 IDDSI. If the cake puree is thick enough without adding a thickener, it is all right to consume; if needed, add a thickening agent. See *iddsi.org* and pages 45-47.

3. To serve an ice cream sandwich, spread 2 tablespoons of the cake puree in the base of a small bowl. Spread the thickened ice cream over the top. Top with 2 more tablespoons cake puree. Place in the freezer for 10 minutes to firm up before serving. Can be stored in the freezer for up to 1 week.

NUTRITIONAL ANALYSIS PER SERVING

See the packages of the cake, sour cream, and ice cream; brands and flavors will vary.

Raspberry "Ice Cream"

YIELD: 3 CUPS | IDDSI LEVEL 

These instructions are for a raspberry "ice cream" that remains in a pudding consistency when it melts. It uses food thickener to achieve this result. This recipe uses whole dairy milk, but it may be made dairy-free by substituting nondairy milk, such as coconut milk, soy milk, cashew milk, or almond milk. The best choices are whole milk or coconut milk. The texture will be thinner with nondairy milks. I used a stevia-based sweetener, Truvia Sweet Complete Granulated, a powder that has no aftertaste, rather than refined white sugar.

1 pound frozen raspberries
1 cup whole milk or nondairy milk
1½ to 2 tablespoons Truvia Sweet Complete Granulated stevia or sugar, plus more if desired

1. Add the frozen fruit to a food processor or high-speed blender. Pulse just until the fruit is liquefied. With a silicone spatula, scrape down the sides of the container and rub the puree through a mesh strainer to eliminate any skin, fiber, or seeds.

2. Add the milk and sweetener and process until smooth. Use a spatula to scrape down the sides of the container. This will ensure that the texture is consistent throughout the puree. For each cup fruit, use the same amount of thickener you would use to thicken 4 ounces of liquid to IDDSI Level 4.

3. For gel thickener, this is double the amount of IDDSI Level 3 thickener. For powder thickeners, follow the manufacturer's directions. Test for Level 4 IDDSI (see *iddsi.org* and pages 45-47). If the "ice cream" is thick enough without adding additional thickener, it is all right to consume. If needed, add more thickening agent.

4. Transfer the puree to glass storage containers, cover, and store in the freezer. Soften in the refrigerator for 1 to 2 hours before serving. Don't store in the freezer for more than 1 week for the best texture.

VARIATIONS

Use other frozen fruits instead of raspberries: **peaches**, **pineapple**, **mangoes**, **blueberries**, or **cherries**. Pineapple is best used with a nutrition extractor like a Nutribullet, which will pulverize the cell walls, because pineapple is fibrous. The recipe calls for frozen fruit, but you can substitute fresh fruit by freezing it in a plastic zip bag in the freezer for two hours before using.

NUTRITIONAL ANALYSIS PER SERVING | ½ cup
43 calories, 0.5 g fat, 0.3 g saturated fat, 12 mg sodium, 4.1 g sugar, 9.7 g carbohydrates, 3 g fiber, 1.3 g protein

Cook-and-Serve Pudding

The instant pudding mix that you buy in boxes in the grocery store contains sugar, preservatives, and additives. The pudding recipes on pages 232 and 233 use stevia powder. Each recipe makes five batches of pudding mix; each batch contains four servings. There is enough, in other words, for family and friends. Stored on a shelf in a cool dry place, the pudding mixes last for a month. Freeze the mix and it will last three months. For a vegan version, substitute coconut milk powder and coconut milk or cream.

Making the pudding takes less than 10 minutes on the stove. And the cleanup is easy, too, if you get the pudding pot rinsed in hot water right away. If you would like to top your pudding with whipped cream, I recommend a whipped coconut topping (I like So Delicious CocoWhip) because, unlike dairy whipped cream, it will not separate. Use whipped cream only if you are thickening a small amount for immediate consumption.

PRO TIP

Make a chocolate topping as follows: Test your favorite chocolate syrup for Pureed, IDDSI Level 4. If the topping is the same thickness as the frozen dessert, it will be safe for the swallow. Add a thickener if needed. Transfer topping to a chef's squirt bottle for ease in adding to desserts.

Homemade Vanilla Pudding

SERVINGS: 20 (YIELD: 5 ½-CUP BATCHES DRY MIX; 1 BATCH SERVES 4) | IDDSI LEVEL 

This instant pudding mix contains no added sugar, additives, or preservatives. It is made with vanilla powder, which is easier to use than vanilla extract. Make the pudding mix, and store it in a cool dry container. Make a batch using 1/2 cup of the mix to serve as a dessert. Serve with fruit sauce or whipped topping, or use to make rice pudding.

FOR MIX

1 cup Truvia Sweet Complete Granulated stevia
1 cup cornstarch
¾ cup nonfat dry milk powder
½ teaspoon sea salt
2 teaspoons vanilla powder

FOR VANILLA PUDDING

2 cups whole milk

Rice Pudding

To make rice pudding, add 1 cup pureed Rice Congee (see page 196) to a serving of vanilla pudding and stir. Serve warm or chilled. The rice is pureed and the pudding is custard, so this dish is ready to serve just after being mixed.

1. In a medium bowl, whisk together the stevia, cornstarch, milk powder, salt, and vanilla powder. Transfer to an airtight container with a lid. Store in a cool, dry place for up to 1 month, or in the freezer for up to 3 months.

2. Add 2 cups whole milk to a saucepan and whisk in ½ cup pudding mix until thoroughly dissolved. Bring the milk mixture to a boil over medium-high heat.

3. Use an instant-read or candy thermometer to check the temperature. Once it reaches 203°F, reduce the heat and simmer, stirring constantly, until the pudding thickens, about 5 minutes. The pudding should coat the back of a spoon. If it is not thickening enough, add more mix as needed.

4. Transfer the pudding to a large glass bowl and allow to cool for 10 minutes. Cover with plastic wrap pressed directly on the surface to keep it from forming a skin. Refrigerate for at least 2 hours before serving. Top with whipped coconut topping (see Tip, page 225), if desired. Store in the fridge for up to 48 hours (I do not recommend freezing this.)

NUTRITIONAL ANALYSIS PER SERVING | ½ cup
30 calories, 1 g fat, 0.7 g saturated fat, 153 mg sodium, 10.8 g sugar, 29.2 g carbohydrates, 0 g fiber, 7 g protein

Homemade Chocolate Pudding

SERVINGS: 20 (YIELD: 5 ½-CUP BATCHES DRY MIX; 1 BATCH SERVES 4) | IDDSI LEVEL 

This homemade chocolate pudding mix is better than anything off the shelf. It is made with a flavorful top-quality cocoa powder and vanilla powder. Good cocoa powder means non–Dutch process when making puddings. Natural food stores carry organic brands. Ghirardelli is a good brand available in supermarkets. This is easier than melting chocolate to make pudding.

FOR MIX

1¼ cups Truvia Sweet Complete Confectioners stevia
1¼ cup cornstarch
1 cup nonfat milk powder
½ cup good cocoa powder, non–Dutch process
½ teaspoon sea salt
1 teaspoon vanilla powder
½ teaspoon espresso powder (optional*)

FOR CHOCOLATE PUDDING

2 cups whole milk
2 tablespoons sugar-free chocolate syrup

** Adding espresso powder brings out the chocolate flavor. Another method: While bringing the milk to a boil, add 1 teaspoon freshly brewed coffee.*

1. In a medium bowl, whisk together the stevia, cornstarch, milk powder, cocoa powder, salt, vanilla powder, and espresso powder (if using). Transfer the pudding mix to an airtight container with a lid. Store in a cool, dry place for up to 1 month, or in the freezer for up to 3 months.

2. Add 2 cups whole milk to a saucepan and whisk in ½ cup pudding mix until thoroughly dissolved. Add the sugar-free chocolate syrup. Bring the milk mixture to a boil over medium-high heat.

3. Use an instant-read or candy thermometer to check the temperature. Once it reaches 203°F, reduce the heat and simmer, stirring constantly, until the pudding thickens, about 5 minutes. The pudding should coat the back of a spoon. If it is not thickening enough, add more mix as needed.

4. Transfer the pudding to a large glass bowl and allow to cool for 10 minutes. Cover with plastic wrap pressed directly on the surface to keep it from forming a skin. Refrigerate for at least 2 hours before serving. Top with whipped coconut topping (see Tip, page 225), if desired. Store in the fridge for up to 48 hours (I do not recommend freezing this.)

NUTRITIONAL ANALYSIS PER SERVING | ½ cup
205 calories, 3.2 g fat, 2.2 g saturated fat, 132 mg sodium, 8.3 g sugar, 41.7 g carbohydrates, 6.2 g fiber, 8.8 g protein

Cheesecake Puree

SERVINGS: 1 | IDDSI LEVELS 

Great desserts are a necessity for the dysphagia patient—they add calories and nutrition to the diet. This is an easy recipe that uses a good store-bought cheesecake. You can cut one serving of cheesecake from a family dessert, or many bakery departments in supermarkets sell single servings of cheesecake. This cheesecake is especially delicious with a cherry fruit sauce (see Blueberry Sauce, page 213, and make it with cherries instead).

1 slice cheesecake
1 tablespoon milk, plus more as needed
1 teaspoon vegetable oil
Fruit sauce (see Blueberry Sauce, page 213), optional

1. Scrape the cheesecake filling off the crust and put the filling in a food processor or blender. Add the milk and blend until smooth, adding more milk, 1 tablespoon at a time, as needed to get a pudding consistency. Scrape the pureed filling into a small bowl and set aside.

2. Add the crust to the food processor or blender. Add 1 tablespoon very hot water. Pulse the crust until it liquefies. Add 1 teaspoon vegetable oil and puree until all cracker grains have disappeared and you have a smooth puree.

3. Test as you go and at time of serving to see if a thickening agent, thickened sauce, or thickened stock is needed; use IDDSI Testing Methods (*iddsi.org*) to help achieve the desired IDDSI level. See pages 42-47.

4. To serve, spoon the crust into a glass serving bowl. Top with the cheesecake filling and fruit sauce, if using. This is best consumed the day it is made.

NUTRITIONAL ANALYSIS PER SERVING | 1 slice cheesecake, 4 oz
Without fruit sauce
581 calories, 41 g fat, 18 g saturated fat, 793 mg sodium, 39 g sugar, 46 g carbohydrates, 0.7 g fiber, 10 g protein

Acknowledgments

I am grateful to the medical review team at Mayo Clinic, including Tara Schmidt, RDN, LD; Anne Kulinski, M.S., CCC-SLP, BCS-S; Callie Rancourt, RDN, LD; and Janelle Hatlevig, O.T., BCPR; and to the Mayo Clinic Press team, including Daniela Rapp, Alan Bradshaw, Amanda Knapp, Dana Noble, Jenny Krueger, Kelly Hahn, and Larry Dorfman, who have helped shape this book and bring it to as many readers as possible.

I greatly benefited from the support of my mother's primary care physician, Dr. Manuel Martinez; David Fagen, SLP; Kathleen Oliver, dietitian, and her colleague Rachel Morris; Mary Spremulli, SLP, the founder of Voice Aerobics; and Debra Tarakovsky, SLP. All of them generously shared their knowledge with me.

Thanks to Denise Pickett-Bernard, PhD, RDN, LDN, one of the pioneers of functional medicine, for putting my first guidebook on the reading list for dietitians when she was assistant dean of nutrition at Life University.

Susan Bratton, the founder of Savor Foods, a food company dedicated to the nutrition of cancer patients, has been very supportive.

My old school friend Heidi Pines, head of long-term care at Aetna Insurance for some twenty years, was familiar with the healthcare system in Florida. She offered me expert information and support in this process.

Elizabeth Daley, president of the National Foundation of Swallowing Disorders: thanks for posting my webinar on how to puree the Thanksgiving meal.

Jonathan Waller, founder of the Dysphagia Café website: thanks for informative interviews and posting my blog on the caregiver point of view on the website. Thanks for the idea for the blintz shake.

Thanks to the support I received from God's Love We Deliver's Lisa Zullig. Thanks to the Bayfront

Medical Center and Fawcett Hospital in Florida, who nominated me for an award given by Innovations in Alzheimer's Care. Thanks also to the AARP family caregiving support group on Facebook and the Leeza Gibbons Care Connections group.

Many thanks to Dr. Walter Willett, of the Harvard T.H. Chan School of Public Health, who has been kind enough to be supportive and give me interview time, and to my knowledgeable and expert contributors Karen Sheffler and Theresa Richard, who have made the book immeasurably better and more useful.

And to my tireless agent and editor, BJ Berti, who has worked hard to support my vision and make this book a success: without you it wouldn't have happened! I owe you my heartfelt thanks for all that you have done and your contributions to the book.

I owe thanks to John Holahan, founder of Simply Thick, and Matthew Done, the creator of Slō Drinks.

Thanks to Rick Rogers, who helped with invaluable ideas and suggestions on the recipes, and to Megan Litt, who took over from Rick.

Andrew Cullum, The iddsi Guy, who specializes in dining with dignity for seniors in healthcare facilities in the United Kingdom, offered valuable suggestions in regard to the plating of pureed foods.

Finally, I must acknowledge my mother, the late great Cathie G., for teaching me how to cook. As I said to her, "It's a good thing you were such a good mother and taught me how to cook, because now I am the mother and you are my baby, and I am feeding you your own food."

Resources

Bread

IDDSI YouTube Video, “Preparing a Minced & Moist (IDDSI Level 5) Sandwich” (*www.youtube.com/watch?v=W7bOufqmz18*).

Guide to the IDDSI Framework by Andrew Cullum, the iddsi guy (*www.birchallfoodservice.co.uk/app/uploads/2024/05/IDDSI-Framework-Guide.pdf*). Directions for making bread into a sandwich or a wrap: Scroll down to the page “Bread.”

Dysphagia general resources

American Speech Language Hearing Association (*www.asha.org*).

Dysphagia Outreach Project (*www.dysphagiaoutreach.org*): A nonprofit organization whose mission is to collect and distribute dysphagia supplies to individuals in need.

Liquid Hope, Organic Whole Foods Feeding Tube Formula (*www.functionalformularies.com/product/liquid-hope/*).

Lyons Health Labs (*www.hormelhealthlabs.com/resources/category/recipes/?goal =0_b43d3998f6-7212472834-523917149&mc_cid=7212472834&mc_eid=d19e4ca163/*). Offers a range of products for dysphagia diets, product guides, information about dysphagia, and recipes.

Mayo Clinic Health Newsletter, *https://links.e.response.mayoclinic.org/Newsletter-SignUp*.

National Foundation of Swallowing Disorders (*swallowingdisorderfoundation.com*).

New York University’s Steinhardt School, “What Is Dysphagia?” 2018 (*www.youtube.com/watch?v=MuajiHaA1Zs*). A short video in which faculty members discuss causes of dysphagia and how it’s treated.

FDA sites

US Food and Drug Administration, “HFP Education Resource Library” (*www.fda.gov/food/resources-you-food/hfp-education-resource-library*).

US Food and Drug Administration, "Buy, Store & Serve Safe Food" (*www.fda.gov/food/consumers/buy-store-serve-safe-food*).

IDDSI

All resources and documents published by IDDSI are available on the IDDSI website (*iddsi.org/resources*).

IDDSI, "The IDDSI Framework (the Standard)," 2019 (*iddsi.org/framework/IDDSI-framework*).

IDDSI, "Testing Methods," n.d. (*iddsi.org/framework/testing-methods*).

IDDSI, "Not Enough Cooks in the Kitchen: Sparking Team-and-Evidence-Based Implementation of IDDSI," YouTube, posted May 15, 2024, by IDDSI (*www.youtube.com/watch?v=6NQ8uWrhTZI*).

IDDSI training webinars are available online. Good introductions are "IDDSI 101 for Food Service Workers, Certified Nursing Assistants, and Caregivers," 2022 (*www.youtube.com/watch?v=9tRoJ31Mz30*) and "IDDSI 201 Testing Methods for Food Service Workers," 2002 (*www.youtube.com/watch?v=7C0lZOhMULw*).

IDDSI Food preparation tips

Country Range, "A Guide to the IDDSI Framework: Texture Modified Meal Solutions" (*countryrange.co.uk/wp-content/uploads/2024/05/17041-CRG-IDDSI-Guide-CR-04_LR-compressed.pdf*) offers an excellent summary of IDDSI at a glance (including levels and testing), a useful technique for pureeing bread and making sandwiches and rolls, and great photos of piped food.

CountryRange, "Country Range Makes IDDSI Guidelines Easy to Swallow For Care Caterers" (*countryrange.co.uk/news/country-range-makes-iddsi-guidelines-easy-to-swallow-for-care-caterers/*).

John Holahan's YouTube channel (*www.youtube.com/@SimplyThickJohn*), offers short videos on thickening, with excellent instructions on how to thicken a variety of foods and beverages, including thick stock and thick ice cubes. He also posts on TikTok (*www.tiktok.com/@simplythickjohn?lang=en*).

Modern Dysphagia Cooking: Turn Family Favorites into Dysphagia-Friendly Dishes, by Laurie Berger, John Holahan, Paul Haefner, and Nancy A. Yezzi (Simply Thick, 2023), shows how to take ingredients and recipes through IDDSI solid food levels 4, 5, 6, and 7.

Lyons Health Labs (formerly Hormel Health Labs)

"Caring for Caregivers," 2022 (*www.hormelhealthlabs.com/resources/caring-for-caregivers*).

"Tips for Managing Dysphagia at Home During the Holidays," 2021 (*www.hormelhealthlabs.com/resources/tips-for-managing-dysphagia-at-home-during-the-holidays*).

Pill Swallow Gel

Gloup is a pill swallow gel to help those with difficulty swallowing their pills. Gloup is distributed now in the USA by PatCom Medical. (Gloup was formerly known as Phazix in the USA at *Phazix.com*). Gloup has two versions: "Forte" is an extremely thick consistency and has sugar added. "Zero" is made with Xylitol and is moderately thick. See *www.pillswallowgel.com*.

Piping, and more photos of piped food

See the iddsi guy: *www.theiddsiguy.com/*.

Safe food handling

US Food and Drug Administration, "Safe Food Handling" (*www.fda.gov/food/buy-store-serve-safe-food/safe-food-handling*).

Soups

Vitamix, "Homemade, Made Easy" (*www.vitamix.com/us/en_us/what-you-can-make/hot-soups*).

SwallowStudy by Karen Sheffler

"Caring for Caregivers During COVID-19 Crisis & Beyond," 2020 (*swallowstudy.com/caring-for-caregivers-during-covid-19-crisis-beyond*).

"Dysphagia Resources" (n.d.) (*swallowstudy.com/resources-2*).

"International Dysphagia Diet Standardisation Initiative (IDDSI) Resources" (n.d.) (*swallowstudy.com/iddsi-resources*).

"Pneumonia Alphabet Soup (Part 1)," 2016 (*swallowstudy.com/pneumonia-alphabet-soup-part-1*).

"7 IDDSI Updates," 2022 (*swallowstudy.com/7-iddsi-updates*).

Theresa Richard

Access to tools, resources, and mentors to help SLPs serve their patients with confidence is at Med SLP Collective (*medslpcollective.com*).

Book by Theresa Richard: *So You're Having Trouble Swallowing* (*theresarichard.com*).

Podcast by Theresa Richard: *Swallow Your Pride* (*swallowyourpridepodcast.com*).

YouTube: *theresarichard.com/youtube.*

Thickeners

Lyons/Hormel Health Labs (*www.hormelhealthlabs.com/products*) offers pre-thickened liquids, thickener powder, protein and nutrition shakes, frozen purees, meals, and more. Their clear-gum-based thickener called Thick & Easy® Clear Instant Food & Beverage Thickener can be purchased in powder form or in ready-to-serve containers.

ParapharmaTech (*www.healthierthickening.com/*) makes Purathick for adults and children and Gelmix Infant Thickener. Gelmix is a USDA organic thickener specifically formulated for infant/pediatric use. Developed to thicken breast milk and formula for reflux and swallowing problems.

Simply Thick (*simplythick.com*) offers a range of thickeners, funnels, kits, and dysphagia resources. They have a Best Practices for IDDSI compliant food prep webinar available at *youtu.be/szow6iKO37c?si=l2LJsXFoYABlZTjl.*

Slō Drinks (*slodrinks.com*) offers a thickening syrup that can be used with both hot and cold drinks (including carbonated drinks), milkshake mixes, and a liquid that makes it easier to swallow pills.

Thick-It (*thickit.com*) produces several types of thickeners, Clear Advantage ready-to-drink thickened beverages (including water), and purees. The company's website also offers information on how to use its products and a list of additional resources.

Sources

Introduction

Harvard TH Chan School of Public Health, “Healthy Eating Plate,” *https://nutritionsource.hsph.harvard.edu/healthy-eating-plate/.*

IDDSI (*https://iddsi.org/resources*).

Mayo Clinic Integrative Medicine and Health Program, *https://www.mayoclinic.org/departments-centers/integrative-medicine-health/.*

Mayo Clinic *Aging Forward* (podcast), *https://mcpress.mayoclinic.org/podcasts/aging-forward/.*

National Foundation of Swallowing Disorders, “Deciphering Dysphagia,” September 28, 2016, *https://swallowingdisorderfoundation.com/deciphering-dysphagia.*

Walter Willett, *Eat, Drink and Be Healthy: The Harvard Medical School Guide to Healthy Eating;* Free Press, 2017.

What Is a Swallowing Disorder? Coping with Change

Complications

Attrill S, White S, Murray J, Hammond S, Doeltgen S. Impact of oropharyngeal dysphagia on healthcare cost and length of stay in hospital: A systematic review. *BMC Health Serv Res.* 2018;18(1):594.

Emotional Effects of Dysphagia

Ekberg O, Hamdy S, Woisard V, Wuttge-Hannig A, Ortega P. Social and psychological burden of dysphagia: Its impact on diagnosis and treatment. *Dysphagia*. 2002;17(2):139–146.

Swallowing and Swallowing Issues

Butler SG, Stuart A, Markley L, Feng X, Kritchevsky SB. Aspiration as a function of age, sex, liquid type, bolus volume, and bolus delivery across the healthy adult life span. *Ann Otol Rhinol Laryngol*. 2018;127(1):21–32.

Miller RM, Groher ME. Speech-language pathology and dysphagia: A brief historical perspective. *Dysphagia*. 1993;8(3):180–184.

Robbins J, Butler SG, Daniels SK, et al. Swallowing and dysphagia rehabilitation: Translating principles of neural plasticity into clinically oriented evidence. *J Speech Lang Hear Res*. 2008;51(1):S276–S300.

Swallowing Evaluation

Carnaby-Mann G, Lenius K. The bedside examination in dysphagia. *Phys Med Rehabil Clin N Am*. 2008;19(4):747–768.

Garand KL, McCullough G, Crary M, Arvedson JC, Dodrill P. Assessment across the life span: The clinical swallow evaluation. *Am J Speech Lang Pathol.* 2020;29(2S):919–933.

Kahrilas PJ, Lin S, Rademaker AW, Logemann JA. Impaired deglutitive airway protection: A videofluoroscopic analysis of severity and mechanism. *Gastroenterology.* 1997;113(5):1457–1464.

Langmore SE, Schatz K, Olsen N. Fiberoptic endoscopic examination of swallowing safety: A new procedure. *Dysphagia*. 1988;2(4):216–219.

Martin-Harris B, Canon CL, Bonilha HS, Murray J, Davidson K, Lefton-Greif MA. Best practices in modified barium swallow studies. *Am J Speech Lang Pathol.* 2020;29(2S):1078–1093.

Thickening

Lam P, Stanschus S, Zaman R, Cichero JAY. The International Dysphagia Diet Standardisation Initiative (IDDSI) Framework: The Kempen pilot. *BJNN.* 2017;13(Sup2):S18–S26.

Miles A, McFarlane M, Scott S, Hunting A. Cough response to aspiration in thin and thick fluids during FEES in hospitalized inpatients. *Int J Lang Commun Disord.* 2018;53(5): 909–918.

Nativ-Zeltzer N, Kuhn MA, Imai DM, et al. The effects of aspirated thickened water on survival and pulmonary injury in a rabbit model. *Laryngoscope.* 2018;128(2):327–331.

Treatment

American Geriatrics Society Ethics Committee and Clinical Practice and Models of Care Committee. American Geriatrics Society feeding tubes in advanced dementia position statement. *J Am Geriatr Soc.* 2014;62(8):1590–1593.

Carnaby-Mann GD, Crary MA. McNeill dysphagia therapy program: A case-control study. *Arch Phys Med Rehabil.* 2010;91(5):743–749.

Crary MA, Carnaby GD, LaGorio LA, Carvajal PJ. Functional and physiological outcomes from an exercise-based dysphagia therapy: A pilot investigation of the McNeill Dysphagia Therapy Program. *Arch Phys Med Rehabil.* 2012;93(7):1173–1178.

Kleim JA, Jones TA. Principles of experience-dependent neural plasticity: Implications for rehabilitation after brain damage. *J Speech Lang Hear Res.* 2008;51(1):S225–S239.

Logemann JA. *Evaluation and treatment of swallowing disorders.* 2nd ed. Pro-Ed; 1998.

McKenna VS, Zhang B, Haines MB, Kelchner LN. A systematic review of isometric lingual strength-training programs in adults with and without dysphagia. *Am J Speech Lang Pathol.* 2017;26(2):524–539.

Sapienza C, Troche M, Pitts T, Davenport P. Respiratory strength training: Concept and intervention outcomes. *Semin Speech Lang.* 2011;32(1):21–30.

Sapienza CM. Respiratory muscle strength training applications. *Curr Opin Otolaryngol Head Neck Surg.* 2008;16(3):216–220.

Shaker R, Kern M, Bardan E, et al. Augmentation of deglutitive upper esophageal sphincter opening in the elderly by exercise. *Am J Physiol.* 1997;272(6 Pt 1):G1518–1522.

Steele CM, Bayley MT, Peladeau-Pigeon M, et al. A randomized trial comparing two tongue-pressure resistance training protocols for post-stroke dysphagia. *Dysphagia.* 2016;31(3):452–461.

Sze WP, Yoon WL, Escoffier N, Rickard Liow SJ. Evaluating the training effects of two swallowing rehabilitation therapies using surface electromyography—chin tuck against resistance (CTAR) exercise and the Shaker exercise. *Dysphagia.* 2016;31(2):195–205.

Yoon WL, Khoo JK, Rickard Liow SJ. Chin tuck against resistance (CTAR): New method for enhancing suprahyoid muscle activity using a Shaker-type exercise. *Dysphagia.* 2014;29(2):243–248.

You Have Dysphagia: What's Next?

Aspiration Pneumonia

Langmore SE, et al. Predictors of aspiration pneumonia: How important is dysphagia? *Dysphagia.* 1998;13(2);69–81.

Langmore SE, et al. Predictors of aspiration pneumonia in nursing home residents. *Dysphagia.* 2002;17(4);298–307.

Caregiving

Namasivayam-MacDonald AM, Shune SE. The burden of dysphagia on family caregivers of the elderly: A systematic review. *Geriatrics*. 2018;3(2);30. *https://doi.org/10.3390/geriatrics3020030.*

Namasivayam-MacDonald AM, Shune SE. The influence of swallowing impairments as an independent risk factor for burden among caregivers of aging parents: A cross-sectional study. *Geriatr Nurs*. 2020;41(2);81–88. *https://doi:10.1016/j.gerinurse.2019.06.008.*

Shune SE, Namasivayam-MacDonald AM. Swallowing impairments increase emotional burden in spousal caregivers of older adults. *J Appl Gerontol.* 2020;39(2);172–180. *https://doi:10.1177/0733464818821787.*

Shune SE, Resnick E, Zarit SH, Namasivayam-MacDonald AM. Creation and initial validation of the Caregiver Analysis of Reported Experiences with Swallowing Disorders (CARES) screening tool. *Am J Speech Lang Pathol.* 2020;29(4);2131–2144. *https://doi.org/10.1044/2020_AJSLP-20-00148.*

Texture-Modified Foods

Cichero JAY, Steele C, Duivestein J, et al. The need for international terminology and definitions for texture-modified foods and thickened liquids used in dysphagia management: Foundations of a global initiative. *Curr Phys Med Rehabil Rep.* 2013;1;280–291. *https://doi.org/10.1007/s40141-013-0024-z.*

Cichero JAY, Lam P, Steele CM, et al. Development of international terminology and definitions for texture-modified foods and thickened fluids used in dysphagia management: The IDDSI Framework. *Dysphagia*. 2016;32;293–314. *https://doi.org/10.1007/s00455-016-9758-y.*

Larsen D, Vansant M, Eisenhardt M. Characterizing gelatin-based desserts using international dysphagia diet standardisation initiative testing methods. *Perspectives of the ASHA Special Interest Groups*. 2024;9(1);262–272. *https://doi.org/10.1044/2023_PERSP-23-00159.*

Steele CM, Alsanei WA, Ayanikalath S, et al. The influence of food texture and liquid consistency modification on swallowing physiology and function: A systematic review. *Dysphagia*. 2015;30;2–26. *https://doi.org/10.1007/s00455-014-9578-x.*

About the Author and Contributors

Diane Wolff is the author of the independently published award-winning Essential Puree Library. She is also a speaker for dysphagia caregiver groups and professional groups. When her mother, who had dementia, was diagnosed with dysphagia, she asked Diane to care for her. Diane agreed but did not know where to start. After much experimentation, wide research, consultations with healthcare professionals, and others, through trial and error, she arrived at a series of best practices and delicious recipes with the encouragement of her mother's primary care physician. Born from her strong desire to share what she has learned about cooking for someone with dysphagia, this is the book she wishes she had when caring for her mother.

Dr. Walter Willett is professor of epidemiology and nutrition, and director of the Thich Nhat Hanh Center for Mindfulness in Public Health Nutrition, at the Harvard T.H. Chan School of Public Health, professor of medicine at Harvard Medical School, and author of *Eat, Drink and Be Healthy: The Harvard Medical School Guide to Healthy Eating.*

Theresa Richard, M.A., CCC-SLP, BCS-S, is the author of *So You're Having Trouble Swallowing*, and the founder of the MedSLP Collective. She hosts the *Swallow Your Pride* podcast.

Karen Sheffler, M.S., CCC-SLP, BCS-S, is a medical speech-language pathologist and a board-certified specialist in swallowing and swallowing disorders.

Andrew Cullum is the founder and director of The iddsi Guy. He offers comprehensive training programs tailored specifically to the needs of nursing care homes and equips chefs and caregivers with the expertise to provide IDDSI-compliant meals that are both nutritious and delicious.

Index

See also Recipes and Ingredients Index on page 250.

A

Alzheimer's disease, 32
American Speech-Language-Hearing Association (ASHA), 22
appliances, kitchen, 55–59
  blender, 56–57
  food processor, 56
  indoor grill, 58–59
  pressure cooker, 58
  slow cooker, 58
  steamer, 59
Ashford, John R., 37
aspiration
  coughing and, 9, 13–14
  emotional impact of, 15
  exercise and, 28
  feeding independence and, 31
  IDDSI levels and, 44–49
  liquid medications and, 52
  myths and misconceptions of, 17–19
  silent aspiration, 13–14, 26
  swallowing and, 13–14
  vinegar and, 67, 96
aspiration pneumonia, 20, 26
  feeding independence and, 31
  prevention and risk reduction, 27, 28, 34–36
assessment of dysphagia, 14–15

B

baby food, 9
bacteria, food safety and, 59, 62, 70
bacteria, mouth, 26, 35, 37–38
bacterial lung infection. *See* aspiration pneumonia
baking supplies, 66
batch cooking method (The System), 55, 60–63, 139
  cooking day tips, 62–63
  food storage and labeling, 63
  serving freezer foods, 77
  shopping and cooking schedules, 63
  Steamed Parchment Parcels, 78
  steaming and, 171
  whiteboard meal-tracking, 63
beans and legumes, pantry, 65
bedridden patients, 26, 35, 36
blenders, 56–57
Bob's Red Mill, 133, 177, 199, 200, 201, 202
boil-in-bag method, 77

C

Carewell Home Health Products, 69
cheesecloth, 60
Child, Julia, 63
chin tuck technique, 17, 19, 30, 31
choking, 20
  emotional impact of, 15
  IDDSI levels and, 42–45
  risk reduction, 28–29, 36, 40, 50
  swallowing efficiency and, 26
  as symptom, 13
chronic obstructive pulmonary disease (COPD), 36
compensatory strategies, 28, 30–32
condiments, 66
congestive heart failure (CHF), 36
cornbread, pureeing, 139
cornstarch-based thickeners, 53, 70
coughing, 20, 22, 26
  improving coughing ability, 27, 36–37
  safer swallowing strategies and, 30
  as symptom, 13

Covid-19 pandemic, 10
Cullum, Andrew, 245

D

dehydration, 13, 20, 36, 47
delirium, 36
dementia, 9, 26, 32
desserts, frozen, 67
diet texture modification, 31–32
distractions while eating, 32
dry mouth, 25, 33, 35, 38, 42, 43, 45
dysphagia
  assessment of, 14–15
  causes of, 19
  diagnosis of, 9–10
  diet modifications for, 19
  emotional impact of, 15–16
  FAQs, 19–23
  myths and misconceptions about, 17–18
  oropharyngeal dysphagia, 24
  pharyngoesophageal dysphagia, 24–25
  risks and complications of, 20
  social situations and, 20–21
  statistics, 9
  treatment plans for, 27–28
Dysphagia Research Society (DRS), 22

E

ear, nose, and throat (ENT) doctor, 25, 27, 37
environmental strategies, 32–33
ethnic, family, and regional recipes, 71–72

F

feeding tube. *See* tube feeding and feeding tubes
fiberoptic endoscopic evaluation of swallowing (FEES), 14, 24
flossing, 37
Flow Test, IDDSI, 34, 44–49, 52–53
food aversion, 25
food mill, 59–60
food processor, 56
frailty, 36, 37
freezer checklist, 67. *See also* pantry and freezer
fruit, frozen, 67
Funnel, IDDSI, 34, 48–49, 52

G

Garten, Ina, 11, 114, 178
gastroenterologist, 25, 27
gastrostomy tube, 35. *See also* tube feeding and feeding tubes
Ghirardelli, 233
grains, pantry, 65–66

H

healthcare facilities
  chefs and, 73
  dysphagia management in, 28–29
  IDDSI implementation in, 40
  responsibilities of, 22
  self-advocacy in, 21–22
Healthy Eating Plate (Harvard T.H. Chan School of Public Health), 10, 195
herb paste, pantry, 66, 81
holiday and travel tips, 33–34
hospitals and hospitalization, 10, 21–22, 40
host resistance, 36
humidification, 33
hyposalivation, 35. *See also* dry mouth

I

IDDSI. *See* International Dysphagia Diet Standardisation Initiative
immunosuppression, 36
indoor grill, 58–59
infection control, 34–36
instant mashed potatoes, 177
integrative medicine, 72–73
International Dysphagia Diet Standardisation Initiative (IDDSI), 10
  IDDSI Flow Test, 34, 44–49, 52–53
  IDDSI Fork Drip Test, 44–47, 51–52
  IDDSI Fork Pressure Test, 40, 42–45, 50
  IDDSI Spoon Tilt Test, 44–47, 50–51, 52

International Dysphagia Diet Standardisation Initiative (IDDSI), continued
implementation of, 40
levels and testing summary chart, 42–49
person-centered care, 39–40
standardized diet framework, 31–32, 39, 41
testing methods, 39–40
using testing methods in kitchens, 50–53

L

legumes and pulses, pantry, 65
lentils. *See* legumes and pulses
lighting and visuals while eating, 32–33
LightLife, 111

M

malnutrition, 13, 20, 36
meal delivery services, 65
meat and seafood, frozen, 67
mesh strainer, 60
modified barium swallow study (MBSS), 14, 24
mouth hygiene. *See* oral hygiene and infection control
mouthwash, 37–38

N

nasogastric tube, 35. *See also* tube feeding and feeding tubes
National Foundation of Swallowing Disorders (NFOSD), 22
neurological disorders, 9, 19, 65
neurologist, 25, 27
Ninja blenders, 57–58
Nocciolata, 224
nursing homes, 21–22
nutrition and integrative medicine, 72–73

O

occupational therapist, 27, 36, 37
oils and vinegars, pantry, 66–67
oral hygiene and infection control, 37–38. *See also* dry mouth
oral moisturizer, 38
oropharyngeal dysphagia, 24
otolaryngologist, 25, 27, 37

P

pancake mixes, prepackaged, 66
pantry and freezer, 63–67
freezer checklist, 67
pantry checklist, 64–67
Parkinson's disease, 26
pasta, pantry, 64–65
patient rights, 21
Pépin, Jacques, 66, 112, 127, 133, 176
person-centered care, 21, 22, 23, 29, 40
pharmacies, 9, 69
pharmacist, 25, 31
pharyngoesophageal dysphagia, 24–25
Phazix, 31
physical therapist, 27, 36, 37
pills, swallowing, 31
piping techniques, 74–75
pneumonia. *See* aspiration pneumonia
polypharmacy, 35
potato ricer, 59
Presley, Elvis, 218
pressure cooker, 58
psychiatrist, 25
Puck, Wolfgang, 147
pulmonary clearance, 36

R

ready-made meals, 65
reduced systemic immunologic response, 36
registered dietitian nutritionist (RDN), 19, 25, 27
rehabilitation exercises, 27–28
residue, food, 14, 26, 27, 30
Richard, Theresa, 10, 245

S

sauces with pureed foods, 70
seafood, frozen, 67
self-advocacy, 21–22

Sheffler, Karen, 10, 245
silent aspiration, 13–14, 26
skilled nursing facility, 38, 40
slow cooker, 58
snacks, 70–71
So Delicious CocoWhip, 217, 223, 225, 231
social isolation, 15, 20
spatulas, silicone, 60
speech-language pathologist (SLP), 13–17, 19, 22–25, 27, 30–31
spices, seasonings, herb pastes, and condiments, 66
St. Dalfour Organic Caramel Sauce, 216, 226
steamer, 59, 77
swallowing, 12–14
  coughing during or after, 13
  efficiency and, 26
  interventions and strategies, 17–18
  phases of, 12–13
  safer swallowing treatment plan, 29–32
  safety and, 13, 26
swallowing evaluation, 14–15, 17, 19, 22, 24–26
sweeteners, pantry, 67
syringe, 10 mL, 34, 44–49, 52
System, The. *See* batch cooking method

T

thickener packets, 34
thickeners, 69–70
  choosing to use, 17
  cornstarch-based thickeners, 53, 70
  gum-based thickeners, 53, 70
  IDDSI Flow Test and, 52, 53
  IDDSI levels and, 46–47
  medications and, 31
  mouthwash and, 38
  orange juice and, 53
  powdered thickeners, 53, 70
  storage of, 70
  temperature and, 53
  traveling and, 34
  variability of, 53
Thrive Ice Cream, 71
tomato products, pantry, 64
tools and utensils, kitchen, 59–60
tooth brushing and toothpaste, 37–38
traditional Chinese medicine (TCM), 73
travel tips, 33–34
Truvia Sweet Complete stevia, 222, 230, 232, 233
tube feeding and feeding tubes, 18, 25, 35, 47

U

utensils, kitchen. *See* tools and utensils, kitchen

V

vegetable peeler, 60
vegetables, frozen, 67
videofluoroscopic swallow study (VFSS), 14, 24
vinegars, pantry, 66–67
visual appeal of food, 72, 74–75
Vitamix, 57, 58

W

weight loss, 20, 22, 36
whisks, 60
whole grains, pantry, 65–66
Wondra flour, 66, 102, 104, 141, 153

X

xerostomia, 35. *See also* dry mouth

Z

Zullig, Lisa, 63

Recipes and Ingredients Index

A

artichokes
- steaming times, 171
- variation of Lasagna, 161

asparagus
- Asparagus and Mushroom Pot Pie, 112–113
- Cod and Vegetable Parcels, 122–123
- Roasted Asparagus, 183
- steaming times, 171
- variation of Broccoli Parmesan, 187
- Zucchini Noodles with Lemon, Spinach, and Asparagus, 166–167

Asparagus and Mushroom Pot Pie, 112–113

Avocado Salad, Tuna, 92–93

B

Baked Cod with Lemon and Mashed Potatoes, 121

Banana Cream Pie, Cathie G.'s, 222–223

Barbecue Sauce, 143

Barbecued Pork Loin, 142–143

barley
- cooking methods, 201
- Mushroom Barley Soup, 87
- Sausage and Rice Stuffed-Peppers, 150–151

Basic Steamed Vegetables, 172–173

beans. *See* green beans; legumes and pulses

beef
- Beef Stew, 134–135
- Mild Steak Chili, 138–139
- Pot Roast, 136–137
- Shepherd's Pie, 133
- Stuffed Cabbage, 148–149
- variation of Lasagna, 160–161
- variation of Mom's Turkey Meatloaf, 108–109
- variation of Turkey Meatballs and Spaghetti, 162–163
- Ziti with Meat Sauce, 158–159

Beef Stew, 134–135

beets
- Braised Greens (beet greens), 186
- Red Beet Salad with Ranch Dressing, 96
- Roasted Winter Vegetables, 180–181

bell peppers
- Grilled Summer Vegetables, 179
- Onion and Pepper Smother Gravy, 153
- Ratatouille (Summer Vegetable Ragout), 184
- Sausage and Peppers, 152
- Sausage and Rice Stuffed-Peppers, 150
- Tempeh, Black Bean, and Veggie Chili, 111
- Vegetable Curry, 117–118

Blintzes with Blueberry Sauce and Sour Cream, 212–213

Blueberry Sauce, 213

Braised Greens, 186

Breadcrumbs, Fresh, 127

Broccoli Parmesan, 187

Brown Lentils, 206–207

Brussels Sprouts with Shallots, 188

Buckwheat, 200

Butternut Squash Quiche, 210–211

C

cabbage
Cabbage Sauté, 189
Stuffed Cabbage, 148–149
Summer Slaw, 97
Cabbage Sauté, 189
carrots
Basic Steamed Vegetables, 172
Beef Stew, 134–135
Chawan Mushi (Japanese Teacup Soup), 88
Chicken Pot Pie, 100
Cod and Vegetable Parcels, 122–123
Cornish Game Hens with Pan Gravy, 102–103
Ginger Carrots, 192
Matzo Ball Soup, 82–83
Minestrone, 85
Mushroom Barley Soup, 87
Pork Fried Rice, 144
Pot Roast, 136–137
Roasted Winter Vegetables, 180
Spaghetti with Tomato Sauce, 156–157
Split Pea Soup, 84
Summer Slaw, 97
Vegetable Curry, 118
Vegetarian Almond Lentil Loaf, 116–117
Ziti with Meat Sauce, 158–159
Cathie G.'s Banana Cream Pie, 222–223
cauliflower
Roasted Cauliflower, 190
steaming times, 171
Vegetable Curry, 118–119
Celery Root Remoulade, 94–95
Chawan Mushi (Japanese Teacup Soup), 88
Cheesecake Puree, 234
chicken
Chawan Mushi (Japanese Teacup Soup), 88
Chicken Marsala, 104–105
Chicken Pot Pie, 100–101
Chunk Chicken Salad, 98
Matzo Ball Soup, 82–83
variation of Lasagna, 161
variation of Mom's Turkey Meatloaf, 108–109
variation of Pork Fried Rice, 144
variation of Shrimp and Vegetable Stir-Fry, 130–131
variation of Stuffed Cabbage, 148
Chicken Marsala, 104–105
Chicken Pot Pie, 100–101
chili
Mild Steak Chili, 138–139
Tempeh, Black Bean, and Veggie Chili, 111
chocolate
Homemade Chocolate Pudding, 233
Texas Sheet Cake with Oh-So-Delicious Chocolate Frosting, 224–225
Chunk Chicken Salad, 98
Classic Roast Loin of Pork, 140–141
Cod and Vegetable Parcels, 122–123
Congee, Rice (Soft Rice Porridge), 196–197
corn
Creamed Corn, 178
Grits, 202
steaming times, 171
Cornish Game Hens with Pan Gravy, 102–103
Crab Cake, New England, 126–127
Creamed Corn, 178
Cucumber Salad with Red Onion, Tomato, 90–91
curry
variation of Roasted Cauliflower, 190
Vegetable Curry, 118–119

E

eggplant
Eggplant Parmesan with Ricotta Topping, 114–115
Ratatouille (Summer Vegetable Ragout), 184
Eggplant Parmesan with Ricotta Topping, 114–115
eggs
Butternut Squash Quiche, 210–211
Scrambled Eggs and Mashed Potatoes, 214
ethnic, family, and regional recipes, 71–72

F

Farro, 199
fish and seafood
  Baked Cod with Lemon and Mashed Potatoes, 121
  Chawan Mushi (Japanese Teacup Soup), 88
  Cod and Vegetable Parcels, 122–123
  Linguine with Clam Sauce, 164–165
  New England Crab Cakes, 126–127
  Salmon in Puff Pastry, 124–125
  Shrimp, Cheese, and Spinach-Stuffed Portobellos, 128–129
  Shrimp and Vegetable Stir-Fry, 130–131
  Tuna Avocado Salad, 92–93
  variation of Pork Fried Rice, 144
Fresh Breadcrumbs, 127
fruit
  Blueberry Sauce, 213
  Cabbage Sauté (apple), 189
  Cathie G.'s Banana Cream Pie, 222–223
  Mango Lassi, 220
  Manhattan Shake (banana), 219
  Memphis Shake (banana), 218
  Pineapple Honey Mustard Glaze, 147
  Raspberry "Ice Cream," 230
  Steel-Cut Oatmeal with Yogurt and Honey (banana), 209
  Summer Slaw (apple and pear), 97

G

Garlic and Rosemary Lamb Chops, 145
Garlic Green Beans, 191
Ginger Carrots, 192
gravy
  Cornish Game Hens with Pan Gravy, 102–103
  Herb Gravy, 107
  Mushroom Gravy, 141
  Onion and Pepper Smother Gravy, 153
green beans
  Basic Steamed Vegetables, 172–173
  Garlic Green Beans, 191
  steaming times, 171
greens
  Braised Greens, 186
  steaming times, 171
  variation of Stuffed Cabbage, 148
Grilled Summer Vegetables, 179
  steaming times, 179
Grits, 202

H

herb paste
  Roast Turkey Breast with Lemon and Herbs, 106
  Roasted Tomato Soup, 80–81
  Spaghetti with Tomato Sauce, 156
Holiday Ham, 146–147
Homemade Chocolate Pudding, 233
Homemade Vanilla Pudding, 232

I

Ice Cream, Thickened, 228
Ice Cream Sandwich, 229

J

Japanese Teacup Soup, 88

L

lamb
  Garlic and Rosemary Lamb Chops, 145
  variation of Beef Stew, 135
Lasagna, 160–161
Lassi, Mango, 220
legumes and pulses
  Brown Lentils, 206–207
  cooking methods, 204–205
  Mild Steak Chili, 138–139
  Minestrone, 85
  Split Pea Soup, 94
  Tempeh, Black Bean, and Veggie Chili, 111
  Vegetarian Almond Lentil Loaf, 116–117
Linguine with Clam Sauce, 164–165

M

Mango Lassi, 220
Manhattan Shake, 219

Mashed Potatoes, 176–177
Matzo Ball Soup, 82–83
Memphis Shake, 218
Mild Steak Chili, 138–139
Minestrone, 85
Minty Pureed Peas, 193
Mom's Turkey Meatloaf, 108–109
Motor City Shake, 216–217
Mushroom Barley Soup, 87
Mushroom Gravy, 141
mushrooms
  Asparagus and Mushroom Pot Pie, 112–113
  Butternut Squash Quiche, 210–211
  Chicken Marsala, 104–105
  Grilled Summer Vegetables, 179
  Mushroom Barley Soup, 87
  Mushroom Gravy, 141
  Roasted Mushrooms, 182
  Shrimp, Cheese, and Spinach–Stuffed Portobellos, 128–129
  Tempeh, Black Bean, and Veggie Chili, 111
  variation of Lasagna, 160–161

N

New England Crab Cakes, 126–127

O

Oatmeal with Yogurt and Honey, Steel-Cut, 209
Onion and Pepper Smother Gravy, 153

P

Parchment Parcels, Steamed, 78
parsnips
  Basic Steamed Vegetables, 172–173
  Matzo Ball Soup, 82–83
  Roasted Winter Vegetables, 180–181
  steaming times, 171
pasta
  Lasagna, 160–161
  Linguine with Clam Sauce, 164–165
  Minestrone, 85
  Penne with Pesto, 168–169
  Spaghetti with Tomato Sauce, 156–157
  Stuffed Shells, 155
  Turkey Meatballs and Spaghetti, 162–163
  Ziti with Meat Sauce, 158–159
peas
  Basic Steamed Vegetables, 172
  Beef Stew, 134–135
  Chicken Pot Pie, 100
  Minty Pureed Peas, 193
  Pork Fried Rice, 144
  Vegetable Curry, 118–119
Penne with Pesto, 168–169
peppers. *See* bell peppers
Pineapple Honey Mustard Glaze, 147
Pink Remoulade, 95
pork
  Barbecued Pork Loin, 142
  Classic Roast Loin of Pork, 140
  Holiday Ham, 146–147
  Pork Fried Rice, 144
  variation of Mom's Turkey Meatloaf, 108–109
  variation of Stuffed Cabbage, 148–149
  variation of Turkey Meatballs and Spaghetti, 162–163
  Wonton Soup, 86
  Ziti with Meat Sauce, 158–159
  See also sausage
Pork Fried Rice, 144
Pot Pie Crust, 101
Pot Roast, 136–137
potatoes
  Beef Stew, 134–135
  Mashed Potatoes, 176–177
  Scrambled Eggs and Mashed Potatoes, 214
  Shepherd's Pie, 133
  Vegetable Curry, 118–119
potstickers. *See* Wonton Soup
Pudding, Homemade Chocolate, 233
Pudding, Homemade Vanilla, 232
Pudding, Rice, 232
Puff Pastry, Salmon in, 124–125
pulses. *See* legumes and pulses
Pumpkin Flan, 226–227

Q

Quiche, Butternut Squash, 210–211
Quinoa, 198

R

Ranch Dressing, 93
Raspberry "Ice Cream," 230
Ratatouille, 184
Red Beet Salad with Ranch Dressing, 96
rice
- Pork Fried Rice, 144
- Rice Congee (Soft Rice Porridge), 196–197
- Sausage and Rice–Stuffed Peppers, 150–151

Rice Congee (Soft Rice Porridge), 196–197
Rice Pudding, 232
Roast Turkey Breast with Lemon and Herbs, 106–107
Roasted Asparagus, 183
Roasted Butternut Squash, 181
Roasted Cauliflower, 190
Roasted Mushrooms, 182
Roasted Tomato Soup, 80–81
Roasted Winter Vegetables, 180–181

S

Salmon in Puff Pastry, 124–125
sausage
- Sausage and Peppers, 152–153
- Sausage and Rice–Stuffed Peppers, 150–151

Sausage and Peppers, 152–153
Sausage and Rice–Stuffed Peppers, 150–151
Scrambled Eggs and Mashed Potatoes, 214
Shepherd's Pie, 133
shrimp
- Chawan Mushi (Japanese Teacup Soup), 88
- Shrimp, Cheese, and Spinach–Stuffed Portobellos, 128–129
- Shrimp and Vegetable Stir-Fry, 130–131
- variation of Pork Fried Rice, 144

Shrimp, Cheese, and Spinach–Stuffed Portobellos, 128–129
Shrimp and Vegetable Stir-Fry, 130–131
Slow-Baked Sweet Potatoes with Orange, 174–175
Spaghetti with Tomato Sauce, 156–157
spinach
- Salmon in Puff Pastry, 124–125
- Shrimp, Cheese, and Spinach–Stuffed Portobellos, 128–129
- Spinach and Parmesan Sauté, 185
- steaming times, 171
- variation of Broccoli Parmesan, 187
- variation of Lasagna, 160–161
- Wonton Soup, 86
- Zucchini Noodles with Lemon, Spinach, and Asparagus, 166–167

Spinach and Parmesan Sauté, 185
Split Pea Soup, 94
squash, summer. *See* zucchini
squash, winter
- Basic Steamed Vegetables, 172
- Butternut Squash Quiche, 210–211
- Pumpkin Flan, 226–227
- Roasted Butternut Squash, 181
- Roasted Winter Vegetables (butternut squash), 180–181
- steaming times, 171
- Tempeh, Black Bean, and Veggie Chili, 111

Steamed Parchment Parcels, 78
Steel-Cut Oatmeal with Yogurt and Honey, 209
Stuffed Cabbage, 148–149
Stuffed Shells, 155
Summer Slaw, 97
Summer Vegetable Ragout, 184
sweet potato
- Holiday Ham, 146
- Lamb and Sweet Potato Stew, 135
- Motor City Shake, 216
- Roasted Winter Vegetables, 180–181
- Slow-Baked Sweet Potatoes with Orange, 174–175
- Vegetable Curry, 118–119

T

Tempeh, Black Bean, and Veggie Chili, 111
Texas Sheet Cake with Oh-So-Delicious Chocolate Frosting, 224–225
Thickened Ice Cream, 228
three-bean salad. *See* Garlic Green Beans
Toasted Cashew Cream, 217
tofu
- variation of Chawan Mushi (Japanese Teacup Soup), 88
- variation of Sausage and Rice–Stuffed Peppers, 150–151
- variation of Shrimp and Vegetable Stir-Fry, 130–131
- variation of Stuffed Cabbage, 148–149
- Vegetable Curry, 118–119
- Zucchini Noodles with Lemon, Spinach, and Asparagus, 166–167

Tomato Cucumber Salad with Red Onion, 90–91
tomatoes
- Minestrone, 85
- Pot Roast, 136
- Ratatouille, 184
- Roasted Tomato Soup, 80–81
- Spaghetti with Tomato Sauce, 156–157
- Tempeh, Black Bean, and Veggie Chili, 111
- Tomato Cucumber Salad with Red Onion, 90
- Ziti with Meat Sauce, 158–159

Tuna Avocado Salad, 92–93
turkey
- Mom's Turkey Meatloaf, 108–109
- Roast Turkey Breast with Lemon and Herbs, 106–107
- Turkey Meatballs and Spaghetti, 162–163
- variation of Lasagna, 160–161
- variation of Mild Steak Chili, 138–139
- variation of Stuffed Cabbage, 148–149

Turkey Meatballs and Spaghetti, 162–163
turnips
- Roasted Winter Vegetables, 180–181
- steaming times, 171

V

Veal and Rosemary Stew, 135
vegan recipes
- adaptations for pudding recipes, 231
- Beans, 204–205
- Brown Lentils, 206–207
- Cabbage Sauté, 189
- Minestrone, 85
- Roasted Tomato Soup, 80–81
- Spaghetti with Tomato Sauce, 156–157
- Split Pea Soup, 84–85
- Tomato Cucumber Salad with Red Onion, 90–91
- variation of Shrimp and Vegetable Stir-Fry, 130–131
- variation of Vegetarian Almond Lentil Loaf, 116–117
- variation of Zucchini Noodles with Lemon, Spinach, and Asparagus, 166–167

Vegetable Curry, 118–119
Vegetarian Almond Lentil Loaf, 116–117
Vinaigrette Dressing, 91

W

Wonton Soup, 86

Z

Ziti with Meat Sauce, 158–159
zucchini
- Cod and Vegetable Parcels, 122–123
- Grilled Summer Vegetables, 179
- Ratatouille (Summer Vegetable Ragout), 184
- Shrimp and Vegetable Stir-Fry, 130–131
- steaming times, 171
- variation of Lasagna, 160–161
- Vegetable Curry, 118–119
- Zucchini Noodles with Lemon, Spinach, and Asparagus, 166–167

Zucchini Noodles with Lemon, Spinach, and Asparagus, 166–167

Image Credits COVER, CREDIT: everydayplus / iStock / Getty Images Plus via Getty Images | COVER, CREDIT: Yuliya Taba / E+ via Getty Images | COVER, CREDIT: Larissa Veronesi / Moment via Getty Images | p. 8, CREDIT: izhairguns / iStock / Getty Images Plus via Getty Images | p. 16, CREDIT: Edalin / iStock / Getty Images Plus via Getty Images | p. 54, CREDIT: izhairguns / iStock / Getty Images Plus via Getty Images | p. 57, CREDIT: knape / iStock / Getty Images Plus via Getty Images | p. 64, CREDIT: NataliaAlkema / iStock / Getty Images Plus via Getty Images | p. 68, CREDIT: izhairguns / iStock / Getty Images Plus via Getty Images | p. 76, 79, 89, 99, 110, 120, 132, 154, 170, 194, 203, 208, 215, 221, CREDIT: AtlasStudio / iStock / Getty Images Plus via Getty Images | p. 81, CREDIT: juefraphoto / iStock / Getty Images Plus via Getty Images | p. 91, CREDIT: Ken Cave / iStock / Getty Images Plus via Getty Images | p. 93, CREDIT: VICUSCHKA / Moment via Getty Images | p. 95, CREDIT: zia_shusha / iStock / Getty Images Plus via Getty Images | p. 101, CREDIT: bonchan / iStock / Getty Images Plus via Getty Images | p. 105, CREDIT: margouillatphotos / iStock / Getty Images Plus via Getty Images | p. 109, CREDIT: Brian Hagiwara / The Image Bank via Getty Images | p. 113, CREDIT: fotografiche / iStock / Getty Images Plus via Getty Images | p. 115, CREDIT: Carlo A / Moment via Getty Images | p. 117, CREDIT: cheche22 / iStock / Getty Images Plus via Getty Images | p. 119, CREDIT: bhofack2 / iStock / Getty Images Plus via Getty Images | p. 123, CREDIT: Sarsmis / iStock / Getty Images Plus via Getty Images | p. 127, CREDIT: LauriPatterson / E+ via Getty Images | p. 129, CREDIT: Nikolay_Donetsk / iStock / Getty Images Plus via Getty Images | p. 131, CREDIT: Ravsky / iStock / Getty Images Plus via Getty Images | p. 139, CREDIT: rudisill / E+ via Getty Images | p. 143, CREDIT: HandmadePictures / iStock / Getty Images Plus via Getty Images | p. 147, CREDIT: VeselovaElena / iStock / Getty Images Plus via Getty Images | p. 149, CREDIT: -lvinst- / iStock / Getty Images Plus via Getty Images | p. 151, CREDIT: LauriPatterson / E+ via Getty Images | p. 153, CREDIT: EzumeImages / iStock / Getty Images Plus via Getty Images | p. 157, CREDIT: instamatics / E+ via Getty Images | p. 159, CREDIT: Imagesbybarbara / iStock / Getty Images Plus via Getty Images | p. 161, CREDIT: repinanatoly / iStock / Getty Images Plus via Getty Images | p. 167, CREDIT: OlgaMiltsova / iStock / Getty Images Plus via Getty Images | p. 169, CREDIT: Liudmyla Yaremenko / iStock / Getty Images Plus via Getty Images | p. 175, CREDIT: Hubei territory Network Technology Co., Ltd/ 500px / 500px Asia via Getty Images | p. 177, CREDIT: SimpleImages / Moment via Getty Images | p. 197, CREDIT: aodaodaod / iStock / Getty Images Plus via Getty Images | p. 207, CREDIT: SMarina / iStock / Getty Images Plus via Getty Images | p. 211, CREDIT: NoirChocolate / iStock / Getty Images Plus via Getty Images | p. 223, CREDIT: bhofack2 / iStock / Getty Images Plus via Getty Images | p. 227, CREDIT: c11yg / iStock / Getty Images Plus via Getty Images